DESIGNING PRESCHOOL INTERVENTIONS

The Guilford School Practitioner Series

EDITORS

STEPHEN N. ELLIOTT, PhD
University of Wisconsin–Madison

JOSEPH C. WITT, PhD
Louisiana State University, Baton Rouge

Recent Volumes

Behavior Change in the Classroom: Self-Management Interventions
EDWARD S. SHAPIRO and CHRISTINE L. COLE

ADHD in the Schools: Assessment and Intervention Strategies
GEORGE J. DuPAUL and GARY STONER

School Interventions for Children of Alcoholics
BONNIE K. NASTASI and DENISE M. DeZOLT

Entry Strategies for School Consultation
EDWARD S. MARKS

Instructional Consultation Teams: Collaborating for Change
SYLVIA A. ROSENFIELD and TODD A. GRAVOIS

Social Problem Solving: Interventions in the Schools
MAURICE J. ELIAS and STEVEN E. TOBIAS

Academic Skills Problems: Direct Assessment and Intervention, Second Edition
EDWARD S. SHAPIRO

Brief Intervention for School Problems: Collaborating for Practical Solutions
JOHN J. MURPHY and BARRY L. DUNCAN

Advanced Applications of Curriculum-Based Measurement
MARK R. SHINN, *Editor*

Medications for School-Age Children: Effects on Learning and Behavior
RONALD T. BROWN and MICHAEL G. SAWYER

DSM-IV Diagnosis in the Schools
ALVIN E. HOUSE

Effective School Interventions
NATALIE RATHVON

Designing Preschool Interventions: A Practitioner's Guide
DAVID W. BARNETT, SUSAN H. BELL, and KAREN T. CAREY

Designing Preschool Interventions

A PRACTITIONER'S GUIDE

◆◆◆

David W. Barnett
Susan H. Bell
Karen T. Carey

◆

THE GUILFORD PRESS
New York   London

© 1998 The Guilford Press
A Division of Guilford Publications, Inc.
72 Spring Street, New York, NY 10012
www.guilford.com

Printed in the United States of America

This book is printed on acid-free paper.

Last digit is print number: 9   8   7   6   5   4   3   2

Library of Congress Cataloging-in-Publication Data

Barnett, David W., 1946–
    Designing preschool interventions : a practitioner's guide / David
W. Barnett, Susan H. Bell, Karen T. Carey.
        p.   cm.—(The Guilford school practitioner series)
    Rev. ed. of: Designing interventions for preschool learning and
behavior problems. 1st ed. c1992.
    Includes bibliographical references (p.   ) and index.
    ISBN 1-57230-491-X (hc.)   ISBN 1-57230-823-0 (pbk.)
    I. Problem children—Education (preschool).   2. Behavior disorders
in children.   3. Behavior modification.   4. Socialization.
I. Bell, Susan H.   II. Carey, Karen T., 1952–   . III. Barnett,
David W., 1946–   Designing interventions for preschool learning and
behavior problems.   IV. Title.   V. Series.
LC4801.B36   1999
649'.153—dc21   99-33760
                                                                      CIP

About the Authors

♦

David W. Barnett, PhD, earned his doctorate in school psychology from Indiana State University and is currently Professor of School Psychology at the University of Cincinnati. He has served as a mental health consultant to Head Start for over 20 years and as a principal investigator for the Ohio Early Childhood Intervention Project. Dr. Barnett has published widely on topics pertaining to school psychology practice and early intervention.

Susan H. Bell, PhD, earned her doctorate in school psychology from the University of Cincinnati and is currently Assistant Professor of Developmental Psychology and Child Development at Georgetown College in Georgetown, Kentucky. Dr. Bell has coordinated an interdisciplinary team serving preschool children in Raleigh, North Carolina. More recently, she directed the Ohio Early Childhood Intervention Project and served as behavioral consultant to the Arlitt Child and Family Research and Education Center at the University of Cincinnati. Her research interests include early intervention for children with learning problems and severe behavioral challenges, families of children with developmental disabilities, and intervention-based assessment.

Karen T. Carey, PhD, earned her doctorate in school psychology from the University of Cincinnati. She currently serves on the faculty at California State University, Fresno, where she coordinates the School Psychology Program. For over 20 years, she has worked as a practicing school psychologist. Dr. Carey has been actively involved in the National Association of School Psychologists, the California Association of School Psychologists, and Division 16 of the American Psychological Association. She has published widely on issues in school psychology and in Spring 1998 was given the Provost's award for excellence in graduate teaching and research at California State University, Fresno.

Acknowledgments

♦

We extend our gratitude to Northern Kentucky Head Start in Newport, Kentucky. This center has served as a training site for school psychology students at the University of Cincinnati (UC) since 1978. For many years, Madhavi Parikh, as director of the center, encouraged innovation in practice. Now, for many more years, Joan Menning has served as director in an exemplary way. Both helped create expectations for excellence and gave critical support for research and training. All UC students had opportunities to help design, implement, and evaluate a wide range of interventions for children, teachers, and parents. They conducted many studies that helped alter the ways that services were provided. We also thank Maxine Walker, the Head Start secretary for many of those years and presently Assistant Director. Laurie Wolsing, educational and special services coordinator, gets a special thanks for her incredible skills in organizing and supporting our efforts. Laurie helped develop intervention plans for the most challenging referrals, including firesetting and bus interventions for disruptive behaviors. Her positive relationships with parents, teachers, staff, and community members enabled many interventions to succeed. LeAnna Weber contributed case material. We wish we could list all of the teachers. The end result of our 1992 book also was aided by a magnificent critique by Mark Wolery, and many of his suggestions are maintained in this revision.

While building on the earlier work, the present edition was served greatly by a 6-year grant from the Ohio Department of Education, Division of Early Childhood. We would like to especially thank Jane Wiechel, Mary Lou Rush, Karen Sanders, Mary Peters, and Edith Greer at the Division for their support, and coworkers on the grant, including Lisa Barnhouse, Annie Bauer, Kristal Ehrhardt, Cindy Peters, Stephanie Stollar, Laurel Hannum, Linda Reifin, Candace Stone, Jackie Smith, Chris Gilkey, Amy Air, Kristen Helenbrook, Sabrina Petrelli, Kelly Maples,

Karin Nelson, Cathy Murphy, Linda Conway, Sheryl Siemoens, Kathy Westcott, and Kathy Scheidler. Susan Bell would like to thank the teachers and staff of the Arlitt Child and Family Research and Education Center for their assistance in understanding the issues that underlie inclusion of children with challenging behaviors in developmentally appropriate practice settings. Special appreciation is extended to Vicki Carr, assistant director, and Louise Phillips, disability and mental health coordinator. We appreciate the careful reading of the entire text by Natalie Vorhis, and sections read by David Kolko and F. Ed Lentz, Jr. Many others contributed to our presentation of material, including Amy Calla-Murdoch, Barb Siffel, Eric Dool, Amy Robinson, Marija Dunatov, Kelly Maples, and Amy Van Buren. In spite of all this help, all problems that remain are our own.

Preface

♦

The purpose of this book is to help educators and psychologists develop effective interventions for preschool children, ages 2 to 5, with learning and behavior problems. In our vision, assessment and intervention design is based on theory directly related to psychosocial change. Steps to achieve interventions are guided by a scientist-practitioner model that integrates research and deals effectively with realities of practice. This book is a revision of *Designing Interventions for Preschool Learning and Behavior Problems* (Barnett & Carey, 1992). The major changes include updated intervention research and an elaboration of the practices and procedures associated with naturalistic intervention design.

Most major intervention efforts have focused on serving groups of children and have been demonstration or research programs. This book examines specific interventions supported by research.

We highlight intervention design for enhancing roles of parents and teachers. Many interventions are based on studies of competence and on what parents and teachers do in teaching children developmental skills or resolving the challenges that children present. Thus, we emphasize a theory of psychosocial change embedded in developmental challenges faced by parents and teachers rather than developmental theories, and have organized the book by intervention design, and by the possible roles of caregivers in the natural settings of family and school.

Instead of identifying problem children or children described as disabled, we stress identifying *problem situations* for parents and teachers. Early intervention is important for children who present instructional or parenting difficulties, and for children who have limited positive experiences with peers—that is, young children who are difficult to parent, teach, or befriend. While some children traditionally characterized as disabled or at risk may fit this focus, intervention design requires an understanding of the ecology of the situation. In certain places, we have used traditional descriptors to help the reader, for example, in integrating children with disabilities into regular classrooms.

WHO SHOULD USE THE BOOK?

Designing Preschool Interventions: A Practitioner's Guide will appeal to professionals and graduate students in psychology and early childhood. It is written
for readers with prior background in applied behavior analysis, parent and
teacher consultation, and legal and ethical issues related to assessment and
intervention.

Throughout, we have attempted to identify sound interventions and
useful ideas contained in a technical body of research. Of necessity, details
of the studies have been omitted. In every case, we risk oversimplifying the
complexities of intervention design for readers not well versed in those areas mentioned earlier.

HOW TO USE THIS BOOK

The professional judgments involved in the delivery of preschool services
are considerable. The most important safeguards involve collaborative
problem solving, ecobehavioral and functional assessment methods, systematic consideration of valid intervention alternatives, and the evaluation of intervention outcomes. This book will be useful for examining assessment and intervention *plans* related to children's problem behaviors or
learning difficulties.

Intervention design is based on reflective and research-based strategies, and on a coherent model of service delivery. Thus, throughout, we
have attempted to find practical and creative ways to intervene with children and to specify intervention elements based on research.

Some of the situations and problem behaviors described are potentially dangerous. While we have tried to present reasonable approaches to
challenging problems, the ambiguities and unknowns are too great for
guarantees or promises. The ultimate responsibility for decision making
rests with individuals: knowledgeable professionals and well-informed parents.

TRAINING PRESCHOOL PROFESSIONALS

This book originated with David Barnett's experiences preparing psychologists to work with young children, their families, and teachers. The overall context of the training is important. At the University of Cincinnati,
practicum experiences with young children occur over three quarters, the
entire second year of graduate study. Most important, in addition to foundation courses in child development and assessment, the training in

preschool service delivery has been supported by many other applied courses: social cognitive interventions, applied behavior analysis, behavioral research and accountability methods and practicum (with an emphasis on single-case experimental designs), psychoeducational interventions, family interventions, and courses in consultation. Thus, in training students in preschool services we have been able to benefit from the perspectives of our respected colleagues in School Psychology at the University of Cincinnati and the functional training ecology they have helped to create. Currently, these individuals are Sarah Allen (Consultation), Janet Graden (Systems Change, Family Interventions), and Ed Lentz (Applied Behavior Analysis and Psychoeducational Interventions).

MORE RESEARCH IS NECESSARY

In every study reviewed, researchers could have concluded with the statement that more systematic research was necessary. Most often, they raised questions (or could have) about long-term effects, generalization, relative cost-effectiveness, and basic elements of design. In addition, since many studies appeared, more stringent research standards have been set and include such matters as procedural reliability and treatment integrity. To this we add criteria from naturalistic intervention design, which emphasize that natural interactions help establish a range of potentially acceptable interventions. We have decided to focus on creative and systematic efforts of researchers. For this reason, we also have emphasized the scientist-practitioner role, which includes evaluating intervention efforts on a case-by-case basis.

Contents

♦

DESIGNING PRESCHOOL INTERVENTIONS

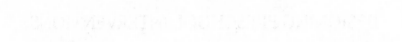

CHAPTER 1

◆◆◆

Critical Issues in Preschool Interventions

◆

Psychologists and educators, even those with very different theoretical and practical orientations, believe the preschool years are the most significant period for development. "It is unquestionably the period during which the foundation is laid for the complex behavioral structures that are built in a child's lifetime" (Bijou, 1975, p. 829).

Despite much-needed attention given to early intervention, many questions remain about how to identify children requiring services and how the interventions should be carried out. Core controversies include inappropriately labeling and assigning children to potentially ineffective intervention programs. In fact, a considerable amount of research shows that from a child's, parent's, or teacher's viewpoint, a referral to a professional is a chance encounter that may lead to a wide range of potential outcomes that are not always beneficial (Barnett & Macmann, 1992). Thus, intervention decisions merit close scrutiny.

One of the most significant issues is *who* should be served. Based on substantial research in applied developmental psychology, our response is that intensified efforts should be dedicated to young children who are difficult to parent, teach, or befriend. These children may or may not be the same as those traditionally classified as "at risk" or "disabled," since the focus is on *problem situations* and not necessarily characteristics of children.

A second issue is how children's needs should be determined. Many traditional assessment methods used to diagnose preschool children or identify their needs have come under increasing attack. The inherent problems with traditional test batteries of child-centered skills and behavior rating scales are much worse than imagined and greater than even the prevalent warnings would suggest. Problems include (1) even slightly different approaches to assessment or different assessment occasions often lead to different decisions concerning children, and (2) diagnostic profiles based on available developmental measures or behavior ratings may not lead to defensible psychological and educational interventions. Traditional tests and behavior rating scales thought to improve decision making may have unacceptably high error rates concerning risk or diagnostic status and lead to dead ends and wasted time with regard to intervention design. In the earlier edition of this book and in other writings, these concerns have been examined at length (Barnett & Macmann, 1992; Macmann & Barnett, 1999), and we have eliminated a repeated discussion of these issues. In contrast, assessment for intervention design is founded on ecological and behavioral principles, factors facilitating change, and sequential rather than diagnostic decisions—not by available tests or techniques.

A third issue is *how* children should be served. Assessment and intervention should be based on a theory directly related to psychosocial change, should be supported by research, and should deal effectively with the realities of practice through collaborative problem solving with caregivers.

FRAMEWORKS FOR ASSESSMENT AND INTERVENTION

Decision making begins with a strong personal model of practice. We discuss personal theoretical models, naturalistic intervention design principles, and functional service delivery whereby the emphasis is on expanding educational opportunities in typical settings.

Ethical Intervention: A Strong Personal Model of Practice

What factors guide professionals who must make decisions in complex real-life situations? "Professional judgment" is the pervasive term used to describe a personal process that "guides" practitioners in controversial and ambiguous circumstances. Professional judgment supposedly serves to bridge the gap between the knowledge base and actual strategies used to solve real-life problems. Whether obvious or not, these decisions are guided by theory and often private rules that are used to interpret theory.

Furthermore, professional psychologists and educators experience the normal difficulties of processing complex information. Messick (1983) commented, "[It is] impossible to measure all potentially important variables. . . . [I]n each instance a choice is made determined by value judgments and priorities" (p. 493).

Personal models of professional practice involve applying favorite theories, knowledge, and methods to unique situations (Schön, 1983). Thus, personal models lead to conceptualizations of problem situations and the detailed steps actually taken in the assessment and intervention process.

Both the *professional* and the *personal* practice issues need formal attention. Research is needed to identify and evaluate "professional practice" models linked to intervention decisions and outcomes. Professional psychologists and educators need to define adequately and describe their "personal models" of practice for informing parents and other stakeholders, and for accountability in developing plans for children.

With regard to intervention design, plans become ethically significant acts (Tversky & Kahneman, 1984). The questions that result include the following: What aspects of the child's experience receive attention and to what degree? Do the techniques that are selected contribute information or error to the understanding of psychological or educational problems? Do they contribute meaningful and cost effective information to the design of interventions? Where do intervention ideas come from?

Building a Personal Model of Professional Practice

Steps in early intervention follow from a personal model of practice. The stronger one's personal model of practice, the stronger are the professional judgments that result, the criteria being beneficial outcomes for children. Since it *is* personal, the readers will develop and apply their own. Here we clarify ours: social cognitive theory as a guide for professional actions, and applied behavior analysis as a guide for intervention plans.

Social Cognitive Theory

Strategies are needed to identify and clarify problem situations, to plan and implement interventions, and to analyze the changes that occur over time. One of the significant aspects of social cognitive theory is the concept of the *reciprocal influence process* as the basic unit of analysis. Bandura (1986) argued that "behavior, cognitive and other personal factors, and environmental influences all operate interactively as determinants of each other" (p. 23). The relative influence of specific factors in unique situations will vary with persons, situations, and behaviors.

Social cognitive theory has several aspects that are important in assessment and intervention design: the roles that cognitive processes play in decision making and actual performance; the stress on self-regulatory processes; the emphasis on self-systems and the analysis of life events, including those that are accidental; the self-efficacy of the consultant, in addition to that of child and caregivers, when faced with difficult tasks; and the criterion of behavior change in order to test the value of theory, including the personal theories of consultants. *Self-efficacy* reflects personal beliefs about competency, and thus has the potential for influencing decisions about interventions, and carrying them out. Self-efficacy helps determine the choice of activities, persistence in difficult tasks, thoughts, and emotional reactions. For our purposes, an important application of social cognitive theory is to help analyze planning strategies: the appraisal of current and potential systems resources, modifiable behaviors across numerous settings, implicit or explicit causal theories, the use of research on a case-by-case basis, and the interpretation of outcomes.

Applied Behavior Analysis

Our theoretical preference is social cognitive theory as a guide to professional behavior, but without question, the strongest documentation for positive early intervention outcomes is found in applied behavioral analysis. Among the critical dimensions of applied behavior analysis are obtaining high-quality data for decision making, selecting important behaviors for change, experimenting to identify factors responsible for behavioral change, and evaluating broad outcomes, including effective and replicable procedures and the generality of changes in behaviors (Baer, Wolf, & Risley, 1968; Wolf, 1978). One major advantage of applied behavior analysis is that the focus on observable events makes it possible to describe elements of the intervention with a high degree of specificity.

The combination of social cognitive theory and applied behavior analysis as theoretical foundations for early intervention consultation practice is not as implausible as it may seem. As professionals, we have direct access only to our own thoughts and behaviors, and to the behaviors of others—together these are the raw material of practice. The processes of psychosocial change involve the consultant's thoughts (and emotions), environments, and behaviors, all of which influence consultations with parents and teachers, and, ultimately, intervention plans. These plans are based on changes in children's environments and interactions with others. This is the focus of applied behavior analysis.

The Scientist-Practitioner

A significant foundation for practice is the scientist-practitioner tradition (Barlow, Hayes, & Nelson, 1984). The scientist-practitioner uses problem-solving techniques that stem from the scientific method and research to guide practice. The end result is accountability for professional decision making. We emphasize reflective, research-based, and empirical facets of being a scientist-practitioner.

Reflective practice is necessary because of the uniqueness of child and caregiver situations. Reflective practice is built on a series of problem-focused and creative steps guided by ecobehavioral consultation and problem solving appropriate to the individual situation. The stages of problem solving are followed within a consultant–consultee relationship. They generally include (e.g., Gutkin & Curtis, 1990) (1) problem identification, (2) problem analysis, (3) plan development and implementation, and (4) plan evaluation. In summary, reflective practices include strategies for problem structuring, problem solving, and creativity.

Research-based practices provide accountability. These practices include the use of empirically sound and relevant research to guide assessment and intervention plans, and the use of accountability designs to evaluate intervention outcomes.

One practice is to consider interventions that have some evidence of effectiveness for specific classes of problem behaviors. In response to the question "Where do practitioners get their intervention techniques?" (Barlow et al., 1984), the response should be based at least in part on studies whereby interventions are well defined, carefully executed, and adequately evaluated. Thus, a critical component of practice is the ability to generalize from intervention research.

Within the scientist-practitioner tradition, intervention effectiveness must be ascertained—this is an empirical facet of practice. Functional assessments and practitioner-oriented single-case accountability designs are suitable for this purpose. The basic strategy is the repeated measurement of behavior under conditions that enable the evaluation of influences on behavior and the effects of interventions.

Naturalistic Interventions

Interventions may be viewed on a continuum of intrusiveness. At one extreme, radical changes may be suggested for teachers, parents, or children. At the other extreme, interventions may fit, or may be adapted to, existing styles of parenting or teaching. A basic premise is that, when possible, we should use the least intrusive intervention that will accomplish the goals of change (Yeaton & Sechrest, 1981). Using principles founded in developmental psychology, naturalistic intervention design stresses the analysis of actual roles, routines, skills, and interests of children and caregivers.

We think that naturalistic interventions are a fundamental approach to intervention design and to applying developmental principles. They are a form of environmental intervention (Hart, 1985) and are founded on developmental studies of competent caregivers. In other words, naturalistic interventions are revealed by the teaching and interacting styles of successful caregivers.

Learning builds on planned and incidental experiences within the context of a caring relationship. The caregiver selects learning events, focuses the child's attention on those that are important, and also, following the child's lead, helps frame events and encourages curiosity and skills development. Incidental experiences are sparked by interest shown by children, and attention and elaboration by caregivers. Thus, caregivers intentionally provide some experiences but also capitalize on subtle or serendipitous events. In addition, valuable learning events may be both pleasant and, unfortunately, unpleasant. Perhaps most events provide the opportunity to teach cognitive, behavioral, language, affective, and motor skills to some extent. Attitudes toward oneself, social competence, and social responsibility (attitudes and acts toward others) are taught, modeled, and valued. They also arise out of interactions with others. Therefore, one task of an early intervention consultant is to help caregivers explore an expanded and deliberate role in cognitive and social modeling. Behaviors of caregivers that elicit and mediate children's responses also are targets of assessment and intervention.

Based on longitudinal research related to risk factors, Werner (1986) concluded that interventions for children may be conceived "either by decreasing their exposure to biological factors and cumulative life stresses, or by increasing the number of protective factors (competencies, sources of support) that they can rely on within themselves or their caregiving environment" (p. 25). In summary, many successful interventions are based on ensuring that a caregiver is accessible to a child and on planned changes in caregiver behavior.

An example of naturalistic intervention is the use of incidental teaching in facilitating language development (Hart, 1985). In typically developing children, incidental teaching capitalizes on natural routines and on brief but important exchanges between a child and caregiver.

Picture a parent and child walking down the street. The child points to a truck. The parent says, "That's a truck." The child says, "Truck." The parent says, "Yes, that's a red [or broken, etc.] truck!" Coming to a busy intersection, the parent says, "We better be careful here. Let's look both ways." In contrast, imagine a different caregiver who frequently ignores the child's gestures and simply pulls the child back from the busy street. The ultimate value of these experiences is based on the diversity and profound cumulative effect of natural opportunities to learn, expand, and practice affective, social, cognitive, and language skills (Hart & Risley, 1995). Thus, naturalistic interventions include those that may be incorporated easily into caregivers' routines, or those that extend or modify experiences that occur within the settings important to children.

For many reasons, naturalistic interventions are of critical importance. Naturalistic strategies stress the need for assessment and intervention to occur within significant settings and with caregivers who have the greatest opportunity to interact with the child. Natural settings typically hold the potential for providing frequent opportunities for learning new skills or alternative responses for maladaptive behaviors. In addition, naturalistic interventions may help establish the generality of behavioral change.

In making naturalistic intervention decisions for children, identifying functional objectives is especially important. A *functional* model is based on developing "skills that permit children to negotiate their physical and social environment in an independent and satisfying manner to themselves and others" (Bricker, Pretti-Frontczak, & McComas, 1998, p. 18). To accomplish these goals, principles of parent and teacher consultation are stressed because the caregiver's concerns and plans are central, including the objectives, problems, and actual interactive strategies. For many children, the emphasis should be on language competence, cognitive skills, and preacademic skills. Interpersonal problem solving and social competence also are likely targets of many change efforts, and these can be taught, guided, prompted, and practiced in countless natural activities.

Functional and Natural Service Delivery

The characteristics of functional and natural services include three important concepts. First, *normalization* has been the guiding principle. In a seminal work, normalization referred to the "utilization of means which are as culturally normative as possible, in order to establish and/or maintain personal behaviors and characteristics which are as culturally normative as possible" (Wolfensberger, 1972, p. 28). However, this concept has evolved to mean that to be truly integrated, society must perceive the roles of people with disabilities to be socially valuable, must provide them with services and educational opportunities that are valued by the society in which they live, and must confer affiliation and enable participation in communities (Wolfensberger, 1983).

Second, to meet children's and parents' needs, a range of services usually is required. Alternatives may include school-based parent education efforts and home-based programs for parents and/or children.

Third, intervention decisions are based on the analysis of (1) current situations of children and caregivers, (2) developmentally appropriate and functional objectives that stem from mutual problem solving and intervention-based assessments, and (3) evaluation. Services should be provided without unnecessary diagnostic labels. *Inclusion* of children with diverse needs should be a fundamental policy. During assessment and intervention design, care must be taken to maintain a balance between assimilation and accommodation in decisions regarding target variable selection for children with identified disabilities. Intervention plans should include reasonable goals for child skills attainment and behavior modification, as well as environmental supports to maximize child participation in an inclusive environment (Wolery & Wilburs, 1994).

Positive Behavioral Support

The reauthorization of IDEA helped introduce the concept of Positive Behavioral Support for children with challenging behaviors. Elements of this concept are found throughout this book. Key ideas include responding to individual needs, teaching more appropriate behaviors, and providing contextual supports or environmental modifications necessary for a child's success. Tactics include schoolwide, classroom, specific setting, as well as individual child support. At the child level, procedures reviewed in this book include functional assessments, social skills training, self-management, and direct instruction (Koegel, Koegel, & Dunlap, 1996; Positive behavioral support, 1999).

RESEARCH IN EARLY INTERVENTION

Change is the major characteristic of childhood (Bijou, 1995). Unfortunately, understanding and, especially, altering the developmental trajectories of children have special difficulties, both theoretical and practical. The core questions include understanding the natural continuity and discontinuity of personal and social development, the processes of psychosocial change, and the limits of change efforts (Brim & Kagan, 1980).

The Complexity of Developmental Changes

There are good reasons for the many unknowns in early intervention. The course of personal and social development is complexly determined by psychological, social, biological, genetic, and accidental events. These sources cannot be disentangled for individual children with confidence. The task of the professional is to identify and modify factors that have the potential for enhancing development and altering maladaptive behaviors.

There is impressive evidence that personality and social behaviors are determined early from genetic potentials and interactions with environment (Lewis, 1997; Plomin, DeFries, McClearn, & Rutter, 1997), and also that substantial changes occur throughout developmental periods, including adulthood (Kagan, 1996; Lewis, 1997). Thus, evidence exists for both coherence and continuity of development and implies significant change within limits that are not easily defined for individuals. Perhaps the most reasonable view is that of Rutter (1984): "The concept of continuity implies meaningful links over the course of development—not a lack of change" (p. 62). Sroufe and Rutter (1984) suggested that "disordered behavior generally does not simply spring forth without connection to previous quality of adaptation, or without changing environmental supports or altered environmental challenges" (p. 22). Some children seem to adjust well despite quite threatening early environments and experiences, but even their development can be facilitated by a range of environmental supports (Garmezy, 1985; Werner, 1986).

Given the complexities, intervention should be guided, at least initially, by factors that enhance the child's adaptation to natural, well-functioning groups. As a practical matter, this means supporting and expanding the caregivers' roles in both families and preschools.

Early Intervention Research

The central issues of early intervention are avoiding the consequences of biological or social adversities, minimizing the impact of such adversities, and enhancing the development of children with identified disabilities through early intervention (Guralnick, 1997). It is a surprisingly small, inconclusive, but complex literature, and it is important to note that research in intervention design is in its infancy.

Typically, evaluations of large-scale projects such as Head Start (Zigler & Valentine, 1979), Abecedarian (e.g., Ramey & Campbell, 1987), and High/Scope (Berreuta-Clement, Schweinhart, Barnett, Epstein, & Weikart, 1984) suggested that early intervention holds considerable *promise* of effectiveness (Ramey & Ramey, 1998), but some of the conclusions have been criticized. Overall, early intervention programs may be quite cost-effective, but generalizations are based only on a relatively few carefully designed and executed studies (Barnett & Escobar, 1988, 1990; Farran, 1990). The research also suggests the need to evaluate multiple outcomes over long time periods, to evaluate outcomes for specific populations of children (such as children raised in poverty; children with hearing impairments), and to evaluate specific methods and programs (Guralnick, 1997).

Programs for children characterized as *high risk* have the following outcomes (e.g., Bryant & Ramey, 1987; Consortium for Longitudinal Studies, 1983): Children in these programs may be less likely to repeat grades or be referred for special education; they may be more achievement oriented, more likely to complete high school and enroll in postsecondary educational programs; cognitive and academic gains may be documented; program participants may be more likely to be employed, less likely to commit crimes, and may have fewer teenage pregnancies. Also, parents may have higher educational and career aspirations for children. Early intervention results are not guaranteed and may not generalize across different samples of children or different early intervention programs.

Relatively minor variations on well-developed educational methods may not be very important if the basics are in place (Dunst, Snyder, & Mankinen, 1990; Ramey & Ramey, 1998). Early intervention programs must be well designed, coherent, and should continuously monitor progress. They need to address a wide range of personal and social competencies in a way that is well timed developmentally and persists beyond the preschool years. Systematic individualized interventions within special educational programs for at-risk populations and children with disabilities are important because the needs of these children will vary in significant ways. Major efforts also should include interventions within normal preschool settings. The programs should meet parental needs as well; an examination of the family ecology is an important foundation.

In response to the critics of programs such as Head Start, which tend to show more immediate gains that fade over time (e.g., Haskins, 1989) or high variability, note that many children move in and out of risk situations and require benign and sustaining environments throughout the developmental period. Thus, for a specific child, a preschool intervention or special program may be unlikely to have sufficient power to bring about developmental and social changes in the absence of future supportive and nurturing environments. Furthermore, research shows that environments prior to typical preschool programming may produce highly significant differences in entering skills (Hart & Risley, 1995). For many children, especially in programs such as Head Start, *earlier* intervention and "Follow Through" programs may be critical to maximize success (Hart & Risley, 1995; Zigler & Valentine, 1979).

In summary, the empirical foundations for preschool intervention design include the promising effects shown by only a relatively few large-scale demonstration projects. Guided by these outcomes, preschool program personnel must ensure that key organizational components are in place, that instructional objectives are developmentally appropriate and functional, and that progress is continually monitored.

Importance of Single-Case Research

Other significant sources for early intervention effectiveness are published accounts of single-case research from applied behavior analysis. These are important for several reasons. Children referred for psychological or special services have diverse needs. The diversity necessitates at least some degree of individual programming. Also, single-case designs add to our knowledge base. The current literature reveals many effective interventions for learning and behavior problems. It also reveals many gaps. In these instances, single-case designs provide needed methods for accountability to evaluate and to make necessary changes in interventions.

CHALLENGES OF PRESCHOOL PSYCHOLOGICAL AND SPECIAL SERVICES

To actualize the potential of early intervention efforts, those providing preschool services face many challenges. For each challenge, the opportunities associated with preschool services are great.

Preschools are typically the first settings where developmental difficulties that have social and educational significance emerge. If young children are initially evaluated in clinic settings, observations that include social interactions, complex adaptations required by classrooms, and the outcomes of instructional experiences will be neglected. The challenge is to give preschool personnel the instructional and intervention skills they need to successfully include children with various learning and behavioral problems, and early identified disabilities.

Second, the range of preschool educational philosophies and corresponding objectives and teaching strategies is considerable. Furthermore, the formal preparation of preschool personnel varies greatly, with corresponding differences in theories about child development and teaching strategies. As one example, there have been many debates concerning developmental versus behavioral approaches. However, there are no insurmountable differences between these approaches to early intervention (Bijou, 1995). In fact, developmental and behavioral approaches share three important foundations for early intervention: (1) A nurturing caregiver is available; (2) the curriculum is developmentally appropriate (Bredekamp & Copple, 1997); and (3) the goal is functional environmental adaptation.

Third, the potential significance of parental behavior and family environment for early development is well known. Specific parent–child links for various maladaptive behaviors or syndromes have been fairly well established as, for example, with conduct-disordered behavior. At the same time, the increasing complexity of family life and trends of single parents and working mothers make parental intervention components quite vulnerable. The challenges of parental involvement need to be reconciled on a practical level.

Fourth, while classification in one form or another may be unavoidable for service allocation, established tests and classification schemes do not answer service delivery issues for young children. The challenge is for agencies to enable professionals to focus on functional assessments and intervention design.

Fifth, the issue of cultural diversity requires our attention in most settings. We agree with Gibbs and Huang (1989): "Developmental, ecological, and cross-cultural perspectives overlap considerably and may be conceived . . . parsimoniously as three interacting dimensions of the child's experience" (p. 11). The challenge is to achieve effective cross-cultural intervention design.

Selecting assessment procedures and interventions for young children is difficult enough; doing so in the context of different cultural groups is formidable. One must allow for many cross-cultural variables: language, opportunities and experiences, adaptive and coping methods, and possible mistrust and prejudice. Furthermore, it is not always clear how directly the specific problems are linked to complex interactions of social, economic, political, situational, and individual factors. When problems stem from more profound economic or social systems concerns, individual interventions may not be adequate.

Despite these complexities, we believe that many techniques in this book will fit children and families of different cultural or ethnic origins if guidelines are followed to establish the *ethnic validity* of the intervention efforts (Barnett et al., 1995). This is a collaborative process using team members of the same ethnic background as the child and family to establish and "anchor" the cultural appropriateness of assessments and interventions. The principles are founded in ecobehavioral analysis and in collaborative problem solving and decision making.

We do not want to minimize the challenges. However, those who wish to address the individual needs of culturally different children and families can take several important steps: (1) Establish an advocacy role; (2) understand and accept cultural differences related to the population being served; (3) involve professionals and other community members of the same background as parents and children in the process; and (4) use consultative and behavioral approaches to intervention design.

POTENTIAL RISKS OF EARLY INTERVENTION

The potential benefits of early intervention are clear, but there are risks as well. First, there is the risk of ineffective interventions or interventions resulting in inconsequential gains. Placements in special education programs should be considered a type of intervention. To help with this potential risk, professional practice should be focused on meeting functional objectives, building inclusionary classrooms, and identifying robust interventions for parents and teachers.

Second, there may be psychological costs associated with interventions, even those that have some measure of success—for example, an intervention so intrusive and exhaustive that a parent is reluctant to continue it or a teacher is unwilling to use it later with other children. Intervention outcomes need to benefit all participants. This is one reason we stress naturalistic interventions.

Third, interventions may involve stigma. One obvious example involves early labeling associated with special classes. In addition, parents or teachers may be concerned with the effects of individualizing programs that make some children seem more different than necessary. These are further reasons for the emphasis on integrated services and naturalistic interventions.

Fourth, there are risks in failing to apply what is known about early intervention. This is why we emphasize in subsequent chapters the research base for early intervention efforts.

KEY EARLY INTERVENTION THEMES

Given the complexities, we introduce key intervention themes in Table 1.1. To help with early intervention efforts, we stress naturalistic intervention design, and the basics of parent and teacher consultation. The core elements of intervention design include the analysis of problem situations, the experiences provided to children, the roles of caregivers and peers, and needed supports. Outcomes are related not only to child and situational variables, but fluency of team members in applying problem-solving skills. Throughout the following chapters, many examples of successful interventions are described for a wide range of problem behaviors. We note one more theme—applying strong accountability methods—discussed in several places throughout the book.

SUMMARY AND CONCLUSIONS

This chapter reviewed a wide range of considerations that professionals must face when designing and conducting interventions for learning and behavior problems of young children. The frameworks for these decisions are based on a theory of psychosocial change, reflective practices related to problem solving, and research. Our emphasis is on identifying intervention strategies that can be used effectively in natural settings.

TABLE 1.1. Mapping Early Intervention Themes

Natural design

    Chapter 1 (naturalistic interventions; ethnic validity); Chapter 4 (intervention script development); Chapter 5 (in-meeting ethical and legal concerns); Chapter 6 (basics of natural design).

Inclusionary practices

    Chapter 1 (rationale; positive behavioral support); Chapter 5 (eligibility for special services); Chapter 10 (research on inclusionary practices; transitions).

Functional assessment and planned activities

    Chapter 2 (collaboration and consultation as contexts; record reviews; ecobehavioral interviews); Chapter 3 (observations; functional assessment and analysis; curriculum-based assessment); Chapter 4 (experimental functional analysis); Chapter 5 (functional assessment and eligibility determination); Chapter 7 (parents' planned activities); Chapter 10 (classroom ecologies and routines; curriculum-based intervention).

Examples of likely keystone behaviors

    Social competence: Chapter 4 (as a keystone; peers, teachers, siblings as mediators of change); Chapter 7 (overview of group and peers as change agents; basic methods); Chapter 10 (inclusion of children with disabilities; classwide interventions; teacher prompting and peer initiations; affection training; environmental arrangements); Chapter 11 (research on play; further examples of interventions for children who have a variety of problems of interacting; research on sharing; research on social withdrawal and children who are selectively mute)

    Communication competence: Chapter 1 (as an example of naturalistic intervention design); Chapter 6 (language interventions); Chapter 7 (communication-based interventions for troubling behaviors).

    Compliance with natural and developmentally appropriate requests: Chapter 4 (as an example of a keystone variable); Chapter 9 (compliance training for problem behaviors).

    Self-regulated behavior: Chapter 3 (applications; stages; methods); Chapter 4 (rule-governed behavior; self-directed change; correspondence training; script development; generalization); Chapter 6 (choice making; functional communication training); Chapter 7 (self-regulation; language and correspondence training); Chapter 9 (parent self-regulation); Chapter 11 (self-protection).

        Overall, the preliminary results of early intervention are encouraging. Meaningful social and academic benefits have been documented but should not be viewed as givens. Many innovations in intervention design lie ahead. Most important, intervention design is not restricted to qualities of children, but implicates the skills and motivation of caregivers, and qualities of environments, over long time periods.

CHAPTER 2

♦♦♦

Consulting with Parents and Teachers

♦

Assessment and intervention practices require ongoing problem solving rather than explicit responses to a set of "given" questions (Schön, 1983). Consultation is a systematic way of guiding the problem-solving process. The stages of ecobehavioral consultation generally follow a similar sequence: (1) problem identification and clarification, (2) problem analysis, (3) plan development and implementation, and (4) evaluation. In contrast to diagnostic decision making, assessment strategies for intervention design are used in a sequential and iterative fashion, based on the problem-solving model. "Sequential" implies that the focus is on identifying the most reasonable steps in planning. Assessments should lead to a better understanding of the problem situation and the effective ways that it may be changed. Assessment strategies also are used to help develop treatment goals and intervention plans, and to monitor intervention outcomes. "Iterative" means that steps and assessment strategies are repeated as necessary, and with progressive refinement.

School-based and parent consultation is based on systems theory. Systems theory generally deals with issues of "wholeness" and purposive behavior, and such related factors as the analysis of complex interactions, the orderliness of behavior, and systems regulation. Comprehensive intervention-based services require an appraisal of the systems within which the child interacts, and a mutual and reciprocal partnership with the child, parents, school personnel, as well as with other community agencies. In addition, consultation helps practitioners deal with complex legal and ethical considerations, and can help prevent or defuse some tensions inherent in problem situations because the focus is on mutual decision making.

CORE FEATURES OF CONSULTATION

A primary underlying assumption of consultation-based service delivery is the importance of providing assistance to caregivers rather than direct services to children (Gutkin & Curtis, 1990). It is founded on team members' mutual respect for one another. A collaborative atmosphere of openness and trust between participants is essential. Parents, school personnel, and other professionals are considered experts in their knowledge about a child and setting; the consultant demonstrates expertise in problem solving and intervention design. Thus, the consultant is able to provide structure and organization to the problem-solving process. The active involvement of caregivers is important for successful outcomes, although involvement alone does not guarantee success. Gutkin (1996) describes consultation as a partnership "in which both members have important leadership roles to perform, some of which are held jointly and others of which are unique to individual 'partners'" (p. 217). Another important premise is that caregivers' problem-solving skills can be enhanced by the experience of working with a skilled consultant (Curtis & Watson, 1980).

Witt and Martens (1988) critiqued consultation-based methods from an ecobehavioral viewpoint. They stressed the need to assess prerequisites such as environmental variables and teacher skills before implementing behavioral change programs, and to build on existing strengths. We believe many of their concerns are addressed by the use of naturalistic intervention design principles and strategies.

Teaming

A team perspective underlies consultation. Teams are appropriately composed for each problem situation. For children with severe learning or behavior problems, team members include parents, teachers, and often specialized consultants. Teams can function in different ways. They can be *multidisciplinary* (team members function independently), *interdisciplinary* (members work together in a coordinated effort), or *transdisciplinary* (members share roles and responsibilities) (Bagnato & Neisworth, 1990).

Some may perceive consultation as different from teaming; they may believe that a consultant provides the "answers" for others, who then implement the consultant's recommendations. Rather, problem-solving methods are used throughout the assessment–intervention steps, and "consultation" is the term used to describe this process with teams as well as individual consultees. Teams may be comprised of parents and a range of professionals in different combinations, but the core element is interactive problem solving between team members.

Problem-Centered and Developmental Consultation

Kratochwill and Bergan (1990) distinguished between two types of behavioral consultation; both have important implications for relationships with parents and teachers. *Problem-centered* consultation refers to situations where the problems are limited to "specific behaviors of immediate concern to the consultee" (p. 37). Examples would be relatively minor conduct problems in the classroom or home. *Developmental* consultation refers to situations where the focus is on one or more long-range objectives requiring repeated problem solving, combinations or sequences of interventions, and different change agents. An example would be improving comprehensively a child's social interactions.

Assessment Techniques for Consultation-Based Services

There are thousands of test instruments and assessment procedures, but we advocate only four to help guide problem solving: record reviews and functional developmental histories, ecobehavioral interviews, observations, and curriculum-based assessment. Conceptually, the reasons for advocating these four have to do with their intervention utility in contrast to the questionable utility and expense of adding other procedures, and the devastating results of studies regarding the reliability and validity of decisions based on many assessment procedures. Parents give permission for both assessment and later, intervention (Chapter 5).

RECORD REVIEWS AND DEVELOPMENTAL HISTORIES

There should be an extensive empirical literature on record reviews and developmental histories, but we could not find one consistent with a functional perspective. Yet both are critical first steps that help frame assessment and intervention decisions and potentially save professionals from embarrassment. While we have heard some argument that record reviews should occur after assessments are finished, we suggest that professionals do not follow this plan. The issue is balancing concern about becoming potentially biased from information contained in the records with the appropriate use of prior information found in record reviews. Prior information may be critical in judging the soundness of assessment and intervention plans.

What should one look for in a record review or ask in a developmental history? The answer is open-ended. Primarily we suggest ascertaining the degree to which health and family issues may be contributing to the reason for referral. Examples of health issues include hearing, vision, early identified disabling conditions, and medication. Under family issues, from an ecobehavioral perspective, problems with providing continuity in care and family stressors serve as examples. A child's educational and day care history also may be instructive in evaluating adjustments to school routines. Last, prior interventions should be considered.

Some aspects of record reviews and developmental histories are important in a professional sense, but their contributions to intervention design need to be carefully weighed. Examples include pregnancy history, birth anomalies, developmental progress (birth weight and early developmental milestones), or maternal health. Answers to these questions *may be* predictive to a degree and often are used to help define the need for intervention services, but they are related to actual intervention decisions for preschool children mostly to the degree that they influence significant daily activities and routines. Assessment practices related to intervention design should be dedicated to features of the environment or behaviors that may be changed.

ECOBEHAVIORAL INTERVIEWS

Ecological theory is based on the tenet that problems do not reside within individuals but instead are shared by members within pertinent systems (family, school, peer, community) and have even broader influences as well. *Ecobehavioral* interviews are useful for understanding ecological factors that affect behaviors, since parents, teachers, and other caregivers describe behaviors in context. Information is shared in a dialogue between team members within collaborative consultation, and the interview format helps structure the information for problem solving.

An important step in ecobehavioral consultation is "mapping" the world in which the family lives, including the networks of parental work, family and social relationships, community involvement, and preschool and day care settings. Ecobehavioral interviews generally may be used to initiate consultation with parents and teachers, and to plan for subsequent steps. An ecobehavioral approach provides alternatives for resolving problem situations: (1) modifying the problem behavior(s); (2) altering or clarifying the expectations of persons encountering the problem behavior(s); or (3) changing situations or environments. Often, elements of all three alternatives may be used to guide intervention plans. In addition, system strengths such as healthy adaptive coping strategies can be analyzed.

Waking Day (and Sleep) Interview

The waking day interview provides a detailed description of behaviors within settings. It is used to help select targeted variables, planned activities, daily routines, and environments to support interventions. Thus, behaviors and settings of greatest concern to the caregiver often are revealed during the interview. At the same time, it is used for identifying times and settings that are working well for children and caregivers, and may enable capitalizing on natural interventions for problem situations.

In the interview, the parent is asked to describe the child's typical day by focusing on planned activities, routines, and behavior from awakening until bedtime. Similarly, preschool teachers may be asked to describe behavior during transportation to and from school, entering school, specific class activities, transitions, lunch, and other events. Routines are a subset of planned activities that become highly predictable. Routines have set expectations and limits, and for these reasons may facilitate children's self-regulation.

As examples, from a parent's perspective, planned activities may include shopping, play, visiting, and routines such as dressing or bedtime. For teachers, examples of planned activities might include free play and small-group or individual instruction. Routines may include entering classrooms, transitions between activities, and behaviors associated with bus rides or mealtime.

A typical waking day interview is shown in Figure 2.1. The technique was suggested by Wahler and Cormier (1970). We have added questions concerning sleep disturbances because of their importance to child and family functioning (Durand, 1998). The interview typically takes from 20 to 40 minutes for each caregiver.

Studies have found high procedural reliability and acceptability with teachers (Hampel, 1991), and acceptability by parents (Bell, 1997). In Bell's study, parent responses to the waking day interview reflected appreciation of the open-ended format, which they thought was thorough and allowed them to share in more detail information they deemed most important. Because caregivers perceive the questions as relevant, the interview also has been helpful for rapport building. In summary, we consider the waking day interview as basic to parent and teacher consultation because of the information it provides for intervention decisions. Also, the interview is used to examine successful settings and events for children that may provide ideas for naturalistic interventions.

Problem-Solving Interview

A problem-solving interview has two functions: scanning problem behaviors and circumstances, and analyzing problem situations in depth (Peterson, 1968). The basic interview with modifications is used throughout the assessment, intervention, evaluation, and follow-up phases.

A 12-point framework for the guided interview, developed by Carey

WAKING DAY INTERVIEW
(Home Setting)

Child's Name _____   Date _____
Respondent's Name _____
Relationship to Child _____   Child's DOB _____
Consultant _____

Describe your child's behavior in the following settings or situations.

Home settings	Behaviors
Waking up time?	
Breakfast?	
Dressing?	
To day care/school/morning?	
Lunch?	
After day care/school?	
Dinnertime?	
After dinner?	
Bath time?	

FIGURE 2.1.   Waking day interviews for home and school settings.

Bedtime?

Sleep patterns?

Play?
  With siblings?
  With peers?
  Alone?

In the car?

Toileting?

Discipline techniques?

Chores?

Shopping?

Other community settings?

With visitors?

Family recreational activities?

Describe your relationship with the teacher(s)?

(continued)

FIGURE 2.1. *cont.*

WAKING DAY INTERVIEW
(School Setting)

Child's Name _____   Date _____

Respondent's Name _____

Relationship to Child _____   Child's DOB _____

Consultant _____

Describe the child's behavior in the following settings or situations.

School settings	Behaviors
On the bus?	
Entry in classroom?	
Organizational activities?	
Transition times?	
Lunchtime?	
Bathroom?	
Large-group activities?	
Freeplay time?	
Individual activities?	
Small-group activities?	
Out-of-classroom activities (i.e., gym, walks, special events, or trips)?	
Describe your relationships with parents (e.g., home–school communication)?	

FIGURE 2.1. *cont.*

(1989) and Vedder-Dubocq (1990), is presented in this section. It is based on the work of several authors: Alessi and Kaye (1983); Kanfer and Grimm (1977); and Peterson (1968). With modification, the interview format may be used with various caregivers such as parents or teachers.

Effective communication—both verbal and nonverbal—is basic to interviews. Some of the important factors include genuineness, listening and encouraging consultee verbalizations, empathy, questioning skills, clarification, summarization, and, at times, confrontation (Gutkin & Curtis, 1982).

1. *Explain the problem-solving interview and its purpose.* It is best to set the tone and establish guidelines for the interview by giving an overview of what is to be accomplished.

> *Example:* "The purpose of this interview will be to talk about problems related to parenting [or teaching] so we can develop goals to make parenting easier or more enjoyable. In order to accomplish this, we need to discuss the areas of difficulty which bother you most, when they occur, how often they occur, and what you think might influence these behaviors."

2. *Define problem behavior.* Question and probe as needed to determine the caregiver's view of the problem: what the child is doing, or not doing, and whether others see this as a problem. If the caregiver responds in generalities such as "my child is 'hyper'," ask the caregiver to describe the behavior more explicitly.

> *Examples:* "Please describe your greatest areas of difficulty related to your role as a parent. What exactly does [child's name] do when [he or she] is acting this way?"

3. *Prioritize multiple problems.* If the caregiver identifies multiple concerns, guide him or her in prioritizing these behaviors. It may be helpful to have the caregiver's perceptions about which behavior the intervention process might reasonably start with.

> *Examples:* "Which bothers you the most? Which of these concerns are most pressing to you? Tell me which of these problems you think you could learn to manage most easily or successfully?"

4. *Define severity of the problem.* Try to link estimates of severity with specific examples and trends of actual occurrences. This may require problem probing (Peterson, 1968, p. 121).

Examples: "How often do you, or does your child . . . ? About how many times a day, week, etc., does this problem occur? Would you say this problem behavior is starting to happen more often, less often, or is it staying about the same?" (adapted from Alessi & Kaye, 1983, Appendix B).

5. *Define "generality of the problem."* Question and probe to determine the length of time the behavior has been a problem, and the situations in which it is observed (Peterson, 1968, p. 121).

Examples: "How long has this been going on? Where does the problem behavior usually come up? Do you observe the behavior at home? How about when visiting friends or family, or shopping?" (adapted from Peterson, 1968, pp. 121–122).

6. *Explore determinants of the problem behavior* (Peterson, 1968, p. 122). This aspect of the interview is based on a functional analysis of behavior. In addition, beliefs about causality may be important in considering motivational issues and intervention alternatives.

a. *Conditions that intensify the problem. Example:* "I want you to think about the times when . . . [the problem] is worst. What sort of things are going on then?" (adapted from Peterson, 1968, p. 122).
b. *Conditions that alleviate the problem. Example:* "What about the times when . . . [the problem] gets better? What kinds of things are happening then?" (adapted from Peterson, 1968, p. 122).
c. *Caregiver's perception of the origin of the problem.* The causes should be accepted as stated, but when necessary, reframe the interpretation in order to discuss intervention implications. For example, ADHD or "hyperactivity" can be reframed as "frequent activity changes," "doesn't complete tasks," "difficulty with sustained play or attention," or "difficulty with self-regulation." Some perceived causes may require considerable attention, for they may reduce motivation for the intervention process (e.g., if the caregiver thinks that inherited qualities are responsible for aggressive behaviors). *Example:* "What do you think is causing . . . [the problem]?" (Peterson, 1968, p. 122).
d. *Antecedents, personal, and social influences. Examples:* "Think back to the last time . . . [the problem] occurred. What was going on at the time? Where were you? Were there any other people around? Who? What were they doing? What were you thinking about at that time? How did you feel?" (adapted from Peterson, 1968, p. 122).
e. *Consequences. Examples:* "What usually happens after . . . [the problem] occurs? Does this happen consistently?" *For social consequences:* "What did . . . [significant others] do?" *For personal consequences:* "How

did that make you feel? "What were you thinking about then?" (adapted from Peterson, 1968, p. 122).

7. *Determine modification attempts.* This topic may reveal information related to naturalistic interventions and self-efficacy.

Examples: "What things have you tried to stop this problem behavior? How long have you tried that? How well did it work? Have you tried anything else?" (adapted from Alessi & Kaye, 1983, Appendix B).

8. *Identify expectancies for improved behavior.* It is important to determine desired levels of performance or changes in roles and behaviors. These also help determine goals for intervention.

Examples: "In this kind of situation, what would you like . . . [your child, yourself, spouse . . .] to do instead of the problem behavior? If [child] were to improve, what would you notice first? What is the desired behavior you would like to see [your child, yourself] accomplish?" (adapted from Alessi & Kaye, 1983, Appendix B).

9. *Summarize caregiver's concerns* (Alessi & Kaye, 1983, Appendix B). Give a rationale for the summary and briefly summarize parent or teacher concerns, confirm caregiver's definition of the problem behavior, priorities, and goals for treatment. Summarization is used to integrate information and to facilitate continued exploration of a problem area.

10. *Explore the caregiver's commitment and motivation to work on the problem.* One of the reasons for natural design is to explore the least amount of change that may successfully resolve a problem situation.

Examples: "How would solving this problem make your day easier? Were this problem to go away, how would this change your day? If this problem were to get worse, how would this affect your parenting/teaching? What do you think the chances are of resolving this problem?" (adapted from Alessi & Kaye, 1983, Appendix B).

11. *Have caregiver summarize problems, treatment goals, and plans.* At different phases of the assessment/intervention process, caregivers may be asked to summarize the exchange of information. Having the caregiver restate meeting events gives an immediate and powerful check for the effectiveness of the communication and areas that may need clarification. It also may give caregivers an important opportunity to "own" plans. The consultant may facilitate summarization through careful wording of the request.

Example: "In order to make sure I understand your concerns and goals, would you like to summarize them for me? Please describe your impression or understanding of how the intervention will work."

12. *Discuss and mutually arrive at plans for the next steps.* The subsequent steps may include further consultation to review uncertainties about information revealed in the interview, plans for observation, referral to another agency, or a wide range of other mutually agreed upon outcomes.

In summary, the problem-solving interview is a basic technique for uncovering and clarifying caregiver concerns, problem settings, and possible contributions of individuals to intervention plans. It is used to help narrow the focus of the waking day interview.

Organizing Interview Information: Planned Activities

Plans for intervention design are derived from parents' and teacher's planned activities that have resulted in problem situations. This is the case because these activities constitute the complex settings, routines, and care provider expectancies where some dissatisfaction has given rise to a referral. An understanding of planned activities is built from the ecobehavioral interviews (waking day and problem solving) through consultation.

There are a number of benefits to building problem analysis by starting with observations of problem situations by parents and teachers. Many studies have shown that parents and teachers are able to provide sufficiently accurate information about children through structured interviews to begin problem solving. Moreover, initial use of parent and teacher information is required to meet the requirements of social and ecological validity. *Social validity* is defined by judgments about the significance of intervention goals, the appropriateness of intervention procedures, and the importance of outcomes (Wolf, 1978). *Ecological validity* has been defined in several ways, but the basic principles pertinent to intervention efforts include the following: (1) The realities that guide the behaviors of parents, teachers, and children are shared with the consultant; (2) the significant concerns of parents, teachers, and children are included in these problems that are eventually addressed; (3) intervention outcomes are consonant with setting expectancies; and (4) ecological principles are used to help establish appropriate intervention outcomes, including the evaluation of planned and unplanned results over long time periods (the origins of these definitions are described in Barnett, Lentz, Bauer, Macmann, Stollar, & Ehrhardt, 1997). Last, the concept of planned activities taps into the self-regulated behavior of parents and teachers important for collaboration and intervention design (Mischel, 1981).

MORE ON INTERVIEW TECHNIQUES

There are many other approaches to interviews. In this section, we review general considerations in interviewing preschool children and other interview approaches with parents.

Interviewing Children

Many factors influence child interviews: the child's motivation, developmental level, communication skills; possible manipulation by others (Poole & Lindsay, 1995); specific problem areas (e.g., abuse); and interviewer characteristics. Because of all these factors, it is difficult to conduct or analyze research regarding interviews.

At the same time, there may be compelling reasons for conducting child interviews. First, many young children can participate in the intervention process. Second, interviews may reveal information and emotions that are impossible to gain from other sources.

One of the classic descriptions of child interviews is by Yarrow (1960), and we borrow from his analysis. Although developmental ages may be misleading for generalization, some guidelines can be offered. Between the ages of 4 and 5, children become interested in exchanging information and describing persons, objects, and events. Also, at this age, they may be able to describe causes and the emotions of others. However, young children may have difficulties in understanding temporal relationships.

While direct interpretations of interviews often are difficult, the information does not necessarily need to be treated as factual to be of value. From the child's point of view, perceptions can be significant. Yarrow (1960) stressed that the interview may be important in "uncovering subjective definitions of experiences" (p. 561), assessing children's perceptions of significant people and events, and studying conceptualizations of life experiences.

Especially with young children, the motivation to communicate with an adult is "developed during the course of the interview" (Yarrow, 1960, p. 568). If information is not revealed under one set of circumstances, it may be offered at other times or to other individuals. Yarrow described many adaptations (such as toy phone and doll play) that may help with rapport or accommodate for expressive language development. Many strategies may be used to help with anxiety, such as having the child bring samples of pictures that they have drawn.

One of the most extensive discussions of interviewing children is by Garbarino and Stott (1989). We refer child care professionals who must interview children to their guidelines. They emphasize using familiar language and terms that the child will understand, and conducting interviews in everyday settings when possible. Another example is having the child try to repeat what is said instead of asking perfunctorily, "Do you understand?" (p. 190). Garbarino and Stott also review interview techniques related to specific problem areas such as sexual abuse.

Ecobehavioral versus Other Interview Approaches

There are many interview formats. An important criterion in judging the utility of interviews for professional practices is their contribution beyond the information revealed through waking day and problem-solving interviews to help with the development and evaluation of intervention plans (Carey, 1989). Examples of potentially important information are parental, family and school events, stressors, coping strategies, resources, and the family and school environments as they interact with or influence child behavior. Based on the preliminary ecobehavioral interview findings, professionals may want to examine these areas in more depth.

Our recommendation is to structure further ecobehavioral interviews (waking day and problem solving) and observations around core concerns in ways that assist with intervention decisions and use them iteratively with progressive refinement. Ecobehavioral interviews are flexible and powerful in this regard. For example, parents may reveal that they have poor health and a lack of support systems. Ecobehavioral interviews and observations can reveal the extent of parental functioning vis-à-vis child care responsibilities and specific plans, possible sources of support, and a range of intervention alternatives within actual parental capabilities. The periodicity of a disorder may be significant for a parent (as with sickle-cell anemia) and ecobehavioral interviews can help examine parental coping within the context of specific crisis situations. Other limitations in caregiver's ability or motivation to perform duties related to childrearing similarly may be examined. Many questions have been raised about the effects of a child with disabilities on the family, and this may be examined functionally through ecobehavioral interviews and observations.

Technical Adequacy of Interviews

The technical qualities of interviews have received insufficient study. Peterson (1968) warned that interviews should not necessarily be "regarded as the 'truth' about the individual and his environment, but as another form of data whose reliability, validity and decisional utility must be subjected to the same kinds of scrutiny required for other modes of data collection" (p. 13). One of the greatest problems with interviews is the reliance on self-report information. Important factors may be out of awareness (Bowers & Meichenbaum, 1984), not reflected upon, or not something a person desires to communicate perhaps due to embarrassment, legal threat, or lack of rapport with the consultant.

Earlier, we described parents and teachers as full participants in consultation, and as "experts" regarding their observations of children and behavior contexts. We now begin to raise possible questions about this facet of the assessment process. The most important factor is that many of the problem areas are pertinent not only for caregivers, but also potentially influence all participants who are engaged in problem solving. There are differences in roles between consultants and consultees, but there are commonalities: Both are subject to normal difficulties that surround inference and judgment. It is not surprising that a wide range of consultant and consultee variables may influence the outcomes.

In summary, ecobehavioral interviews contribute to the formulation of an overall professional practices plan and to its evaluation. When interactions and related activities are thwarted or are unsatisfactory for care providers, or fail in meeting developmental goals, they become problem situations and require problem solving. Parents' and teacher's planned activities serve as organizers for understanding these interactions.

Reducing Errors of Judgment

The iterative nature of the problem-solving process is the best safeguard for developing workable plans and reducing errors of judgment, because the outcomes of plans are evaluated and adjustments are made to plans based on empirical data. Another fundamental way to reduce error is to avoid the use of weak constructs and instead use clearly defined descriptions of behavior. However, professional judgment is a complicated topic. There are many other tactics based on research in information processing and decision making (summarized in Barnett & Zucker, 1990), but most of these have been studied in relationship to diagnostic decision making. We review several other strategies for reducing errors here.

1. Consider a range of alternative plausible hypotheses and hold them as tenable for as long as is reasonable in order to avoid premature closure. Spend energy looking for possible disconfirming as well as confirming information. As professionals, it is tempting to appear "quick and ready" with suggestions, but doing so means that one increases the chances for error-prone suggestions.

2. Reduce the reliance on memory. Memory loss may function to preserve preconceived notions the professional may have about children. Professionals use case notes to guide (and sometimes to defend) decision making. We use note taking based on the idea of decision frames. This

refers to the decision maker's "conceptions of the acts, outcomes, and contingencies associated with a particular choice" (Tversky & Kahneman, 1984, p. 25). The entries succinctly and objectively describe thoughts, events, and actions in the consultation, based on analyzing problem situations and establishing the reasonableness of actions. These should be fully elaborated in situations related to risk. Examples include professional–parent–teacher communications for fire setting or severe aggressive behavior.

3. Use formal decision aids. This increases the likelihood that questions necessary to structure problems adequately will be applied. Examples include the use of structured ecobehavioral interview guides presented earlier in the chapter (in contrast to "winging it") and the use of graphic data displays and accountability designs (Barlow et al., 1984).

4. Accept uncertainty. We can make limited predictions about child–parent–teacher behavior and intervention outcomes. Countless variables may alter intervention outcomes. Professional judgment errors are made when we go beyond our data. Even with data, only descriptive estimates of patterns of behavior can be made.

5. Avoid intervention biases. First, extending Kanfer and Grimm's (1977) discussion, consultants may guide intervention plans by considering interventions that come easily to mind or those that have been reinforcing for the professional through past successes. Our tactic for reducing these errors is the process of naturalistic intervention design based on an understanding of evident patterns of interactions as a starting place. Second, a goal to keep in mind is not to come up with "*an* intervention," but to help establish a range of plausible interventions that are then refined through problem solving and experimentation.

The Relationship between Interviews and Observations

Ecobehavioral interviews are used to clarify a wide range of issues pertaining to intervention design: problem behaviors and circumstances, settings, key persons, likely change agents, and significant time periods. Interviews also are used to examine intervention alternatives and possible barriers to the intervention processes, and to help evaluate intervention outcomes. Defining the problem situation by its physical and social characteristics is one of the first steps in problem solving, and interviews are essential in this regard.

Interviews also provide incomplete information. The results of interviews are dependent on the skills of consultants and the caregiver's observations. There are three potential problem areas for "participant observers"—parents and teachers. First, certain types of observations, such as those pertaining to broad ecological variables, participant–child interactions, and child–child interactions out of the caregiver's view, are problematic. Second, interviews typically stress the "verbal behavior" of the teacher or parent and not actual child, teacher, and parent behavior in specific contexts. Last, caregivers may serve as "untrained" observers (Kratochwill, 1985) and data may be variable or hard to interpret. Consultation may be needed to pinpoint what to observe and which strategies of observation to use.

Only through direct observation is it possible to closely examine the relationship between environment and behavior. Reliable observations are necessary for the analysis of home and classroom environments, specific skills, behaviors, interactions between persons, and sequences of interactions. In addition, observations are used to monitor interventions and to help determine the effectiveness of interventions.

OTHER CONSULTATION-BASED ASSESSMENTS

Telephone Contacts

In some situations, a professional's only feasible ongoing access to parents may be through the telephone. It also can be used as an adjunctive source of information sharing throughout the assessment–intervention process. Phone contacts may be relatively nonintrusive and may result in minimal reactivity. While further research is necessary, the research that does exist is promising.

One of the best examples is described by Patterson, Reid, Jones, and Conger (1975); telephone contacts with parents were used to obtain information on low-rate or infrequent problems. This feature is important because low-rate behaviors are more likely to be missed in direct home observations. They used a 34-item Parent Daily Report (PDR), a relatively simple structured interview, to collect data on specific behaviors. Because it deals with behaviors of concern to parents, another potential benefit of a PDR target behavior score may be its sensitivity to intervention outcomes.

To use the PDR, the professional reviews items at an orientation session and parents indicate the problems relevant to their child. During scheduled telephone calls, parents report the occurrence or nonoccurrence of the specific events during the past 24 hours. The phone contacts take about 5 minutes each. The PDR is reproduced in Figure 2.2. We have developed a similar form for Teacher Daily Reports that may be used via telephone or mail systems in schools.

Chamberlain and Reid (1987) described the PDR and reviewed its technical characteristics. The PDR yields two scores related to total problem behavior and targeted behaviors. Interrater agreement (obtained

Phase: baseline, intervention, termination, follow-up

Week beginning: (Mon) _____/_____ (Sun)

Behavior	*M T W Th F*
Aggressiveness	
Arguing	
Bedwetting	
Competitiveness	
Complaining	
Crying	
Defiance	
Destructiveness	
Fearfulness	
Fighting w/sibs	
Firesetting	
Hitting others	
Hyperactiveness	
Irritableness	
Lying	
Negativism	
Noisiness	

Behavior	*M T W Th F*
Noncomplying	
Not eating meals	
Pants wetting	
Pouting	
Running around	
Running away	
Sadness	
Soiling	
Stealing	
Talking back—Adult	
Teasing	
Temper tantrum	
Whining	
Yelling	
Police contact	
School contact	
Parents spank	

FIGURE 2.2. Parent Daily Report Checklist. From Chamberlain and Reid (1987). Copyright 1987 by Elsevier Science. Reprinted by permission.

through the use of an extension phone) was good (85% entry-by-entry agreement). Agreement between parents was marginal, similar to other interrater findings in many studies. Comparisons with direct home observations support the validity of the measure. Chamberlain and Reid noted the possibility of a "first day effect," in which the total behavior scores may be inflated for the first day. They suggest that seven telephone calls over a 2-week period will give adequate estimates of problem behavior if the first day interview is discarded.

Other examples of phone use related to early assessment and intervention are provided by Brown, Cunningham, and Birkimer (1983) and Frankel and Weiner (1990).

Home–School Notes

These also may be conceived of as home–school notes, indicating that either parents or teachers may initiate a system of communication. The use

Darren sat for

_____

minutes in circle today.

We talked about

_____

_____

I can sit in circle!

FIGURE 2.3. Example of a home–school note for circle time.

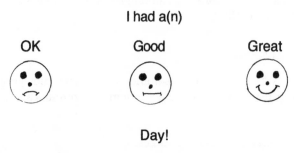

Mickey's Day at Head Start
(Circle all that apply)

I used my friendly voice.

I kept my hands to myself.

I walked inside the room.

I had a(n)

| OK | Good | Great |

Day!

FIGURE 2.4.   Example of a home–school note for compliance with classroom limits.

of home–school notes is a natural communication strategy used by many teachers and parents (Kelley, 1990). It also has countless forms, from daily "report cards," usually indicating specific descriptions of events or behaviors, to individual child journals. A system of home–school notes also may constitute an intervention and may be used for progress monitoring. Figures 2.3 and 2.4 show examples of home–school notes; procedures and cautions are discussed in Chapter 8.

SUMMARY AND CONCLUSIONS

This chapter introduced functional assessment for intervention design. Defining the purpose of assessment is critical. From ecobehavioral theory, a central purpose is to restore or improve the functioning of groups for the well-being of all group members. Thus, ecobehavioral analysis focuses on natural systems such as families and schools. Children are described as hard to teach, parent, or befriend because they are not participating satisfactorily in school, family, or peer groups.

A second consideration is "What is the service delivery system?" There are countless possibilities. We presented the core features of parent and teacher consultation as a service delivery system that is adaptable to many different programs, practices, and philosophies. The central process is mutual problem solving.

Ecobehavioral interviews help elucidate which environments and behaviors will be the subject of analysis. They enable consultants to consider a range of intervention alternatives, possible barriers to interventions, and potential resources. Planned activities help organize information from interviews into ecologically sound units of analysis for intervention design.

Interviews are not necessarily reliable or valid. We introduced several tactics to help reduce judgment errors. We closed by reviewing two potentially versatile intervention-based assessment techniques (home–school notes and planned phone contacts).

CHAPTER 3

◆◆◆

Principles and Techniques for Observing

◆

This chapter reviews principles and strategies for observing situations when children are referred for developmental, learning, or behavior problems. To conduct observations, basic decisions are necessary: *what* and *where* to observe, *who* is to observe, *when* to observe, and *how*.

PLANNING OBSERVATIONS

Two general strategies are recommended for developing observational systems for individual children. First, ecobehavioral interviews, parent and teacher consultations, and preliminary observations are used to help define important situations and target variables. Situations are defined in terms of physical and social factors, objectives or goals associated with settings, and the observable events that occur within the setting (Bijou, Peterson, & Ault, 1968; Bijou, Peterson, Harris, Allen, & Johnston, 1969).

Second, structured observations are conducted, based on the problem identification and clarification stages of consultation, preliminary observations, and an analysis of relevant intervention research. The selection of variables and methods for observation requires conceptual, empirical, practical, and ethical frameworks.

While many sources state that "informal" observations may be used as an assessment strategy, we do not think that they reliably produce effective results. To reduce sources of error, initial observations should be as "hypothesis free" as possible regarding potential target variables and interventions. Decisions regarding meaningful times to observe planned activities, including those that are satisfactory as well as those that are troublesome, are guided by prior information from interviews. Hypotheses about the child's behavior, setting and event characteristics, and interactions are then formed, based on the integration of the preliminary observations with the interview results, or, depending on confidence in the outcomes, the child may be observed further before hypotheses are formed. Theory and research also guide the development of hypotheses, strategies, and definitions of behavior.

What to Observe?

Practically speaking, it is impossible to record all that is occurring in most preschool situations or family environments, even through the use of video recordings (e.g., Fagot & Hagan, 1988). Naturalistic observation is so complex that observers must use "filters." The observer's decisions about the variables on which to focus constitute one kind of filter. Filters also are created by individual observer differences in selective attention, perception, and vigilance (Cairns & Green, 1979). Filters should be planned. When unplanned, or not noticed as such, they result in observations that are difficult to evaluate. This is a major criticism of informal observations. In considering *what* to observe, perhaps the greatest errors result from being guided solely by the most salient behaviors of the child, or behaviors that may be inconsequential for the purposes of intervention design.

Frequently, it is necessary to measure several different dimensions of behavior. For example, the play behavior of socially isolated children initially requires the measurement of frequency of interactions, and later, duration and quality (e.g., Hendrickson, Strain, Tremblay, & Shores, 1982). Different tactics children have for gaining entry into play groups, types of play interactions between children, and a variety of play behaviors may be targeted for observation (e.g., play initiations, refusals to share).

Perhaps the best guideline is that there should be a natural basis for behaviors that are observed and recorded. The natural units should meet at least the following criteria: (1) They should have unequivocal validity for describing significant interactions between the child and environment; (2) they should be capable of reflecting planned changes that result from interventions; and (3) they should be countable or repeatable (Johnston & Pennypacker, 1993). Determinations of validity are based on the importance of the behavior for the child's adaptation.

Where to Observe?: School, Home, Community, and Clinic

School Observations

For practical reasons, most observations related to interventions are conducted in preschool settings. As general strategies, we recommend the following steps: (1) record reviews and waking day followed by problem-solving interviews with teachers, (2) preliminary observations, and (3) depending on the outcomes of interviews and preliminary observations, constructing an observation plan. The plan includes times and conditions for observations, the length of observations, and strategies.

Home Observations

There are many significant reasons for conducting home observations. Observations in clinic settings may be too limited to be of value. Drotar and Crawford (1987) commented that home observation can be a positive factor for parents because it demonstrates professional commitment and facilitates productive communication. For understanding ecological and cultural influences, home observations are essential.

Many techniques described in this chapter may be adapted to home observations (e.g., real-time observation, antecedent–behavior–consequence analysis [ABC], multibehavioral codes). We summarize the major practical considerations:

1. A detailed rationale for home observations is important. Drotar and Crawford (1987, p. 343) offer the following:

> In our work with other children who have problems similar to those of your child, we have often found that a home visit can provide important information which can be used to understand and help your child. The purpose of this visit is to observe how your child behaves and interacts with you and your family at home. Because children are generally more comfortable interacting with their family in their home setting, this is often a good way to evaluate your child's problem in order to determine the best way of helping you and your child [we use the phrase *child's problem situation* to help avoid a child-related pathological bias]. In addition, we have found that the entire family is important to your child's development and that it is often helpful for us to work together to find ways to help him or her. For this reason, we would like to have you and other family members participate in the home visit.

2. We recommend the use of parent consultations, waking day, and problem-solving interviews to structure observations around specific planned activities that represent concerns and contrasts in behavior. From these activities, settings, events, and times for observation sessions are collaboratively decided. Problem-solving interviews are useful for prioritizing target behaviors and determining specific observational techniques. Preliminary observations (i.e., real time) may be used to further define classes of behaviors for structured observations.

3. It is necessary to observe the behaviors under natural conditions, or to structure observations in a way that facilitates specific interactions between family members without interruptions. Ground rules need to be covered carefully. Key family members should be present, guests may be discouraged, activities may be restricted to one or two rooms, and telephone calls can be limited to brief responses to incoming calls (Dishion et al., 1984; Reid, 1978). Rules, such as no talking with the observers during the session, also should be considered.

4. Given the complexities of interactions, the strategy used by Dishion and others (1984) is instructive. The Family Observation Code is made up of "coding segments" or "trials"; for each trial, one family member is selected as the focal person (child, mother, father, siblings). Coding is restricted to recording the interactions of the focal participant with other family members.

The potential difficulties in home observations are numerous. Home observations will not be readily accepted by some parents and may be difficult in some communities. Reliability and validity may be difficult to evaluate. The observations may be influenced by the presence of the observer (termed "reactivity") or unknown distortions. However, Thibodeaux, Gardner, Forgatch, and Reid (1984) summarized the research this way: "Though parents might be prone to attempt a 'look good' impression, the ability to effectively achieve that result is uncommon, especially in problematic families. . . . Habitual modes of acting exert a much stronger force on behavior than any attempt to 'fake good' or 'bad'" (pp. 1–2). In summary, home observations provide an *estimate* of behavior that would occur under natural or structured conditions.

Extreme poverty and family stress will be likely to induce professional stress. Drotar and Crawford (1987) wrote: "In some instances, naturalistic observation yields discouraging information concerning family constraints that interfere with a family's capacity to implement intervention" (p. 346). Safety concerns—for family members and professionals—may exist. We recommend that teams be used for reasons of safety and for estimating agreement in fast-paced and stressful situations. The economics of home observations may be the greatest perceived drawback; cost–benefit analyses are necessary.

Overall, we think that the use of home observations of young children is a significant strategy, especially in cases of severe behavioral problems. Likely applications include facilitating the natural teaching role of parents in situations associated with risk or children's developmental problems, programming the generalization of skills taught in preschools, and conducting functional analyses of severe problem behaviors (Arndorfer, Miltenberger, Woster, Rortvedt, & Gaffaney, 1994).

Community

Many times, parents will reveal concerns about children's behavior in public places or friends' or family members' homes. As examples, in later chapters, we review interventions for restaurants, shopping, and car behavior. In these cases, a system for observation can be developed with parents.

Clinic and Analogue Measures

Many interventions reported in the literature involve observations in clinic or *analogue* settings. These settings simulate natural conditions and are used when direct observation is not possible. The analogue conditions can include a wide range of structured events, role play, or approximations to natural behavior. Direct measurement is used in analogue settings, and thus similar reliability and validity considerations apply—with one important exception. Analogue measurement may not provide strong predictions of natural occurrences for many behaviors. Examples include procedures developed by Barkley (1987a), Forehand and McMahon (1981), Robinson and Eyberg (1981), and Roberts and Powers (1988) for noncompliance. Analogue procedures also have been widely used for social competence training. Analogue and clinic observations lend themselves to the use of equipment such as audio and video recording, one-way mirrors, and "bug-in-the-ear" communication devices to give private instructions or prompts to participants.

Who Is to Observe?

Four strategies may be used to answer this question. These are direct observation by a consultant, participant observation by a caregiver, co-observations by a teacher, teacher assistant, or parent, and self-observation or self-monitoring. They may be used advantageously in various combinations. We describe the different approaches briefly.

Consultant Observation

This refers to a trained observer who has no specific responsibilities with the target child (or group). The amount of time that may be dedicated to the observations is usually brief, but the advantage is the potential for observing complex interactions and behaviors out of the purview of parents and teachers.

Participant Observation

This strategy has been widely used in ethnographic research whereby the observer has two roles: "(1) to engage in activities appropriate to the situation and (2) to observe the activities, people, and physical aspects of the situation" (Spradley, 1980, p. 54). In anthropological studies, the participant observer also is the scientist. However, the term has been applied to a range of caregivers (Hay, Nelson, & Hay, 1980).

Participant observation with caregivers is widely used, and the range of techniques is quite broad. It is generally useful for consultants to help structure participant observations to reduce the complexities and to improve the interpretability of the data. It is especially important to ensure that observations will be sensitive to intervention outcomes. Examples may be marking numbers of tantrums or aggressive acts on a home or school calendar, or compliance with a bedtime routine.

Overall, participant observation can have important side effects or unique outcomes, some of which may be beneficial. When parents and teachers are observers, their behavior, as well as the children's behavior, may change. If the procedures are too burdensome, they will be ignored or errors will be substantial.

Examples of forms for parents to collect intervention-related data are included in Figures 3.1 and 3.2. The shopping intervention was set up like a checkbook for the child, and was also used for structuring rewards. Instead of recording minutes as the unit of analysis, the number of aisles could be recorded.

Co-Observations by a Trusted Colleague or Loving Spouse

Co-observation may be carried out by a teacher, teacher assistant, or in families, by a parent, when these persons are not directly interacting with the targeted child. Good relationships are necessary, and the tactic is built

Shopping Intervention

Time ___ minutes Date __/__/__ Store: _____	Arm's reach	Hands/Feet to self	Follow Mommy's directions
1.			
2.			
3.			
4.			
5.			
6.			

FIGURE 3.1. Intervention script and data collection sheet for community shopping incorporating compliance with basic rules, time spent shopping, observation date, and setting.

☆

Date: _____   Time to bed: Begin _____
People involved: _____   End _____
_____   Total number of requests _____

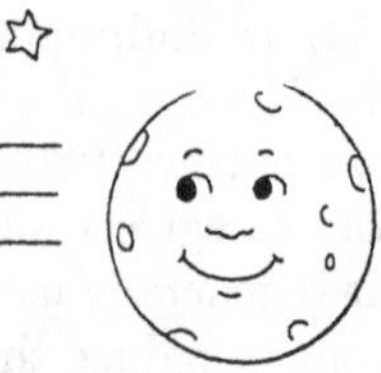

It's time for bed!

Bedtime Activity	Carol	Christine	Michael
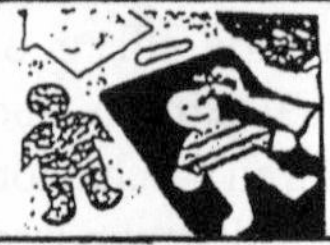			
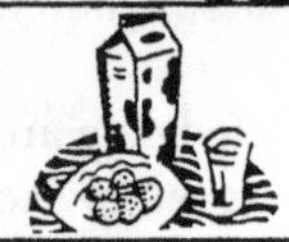			
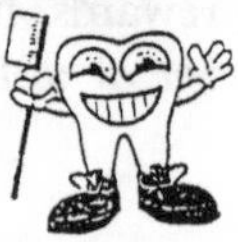			
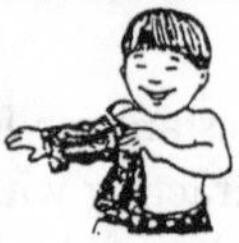			
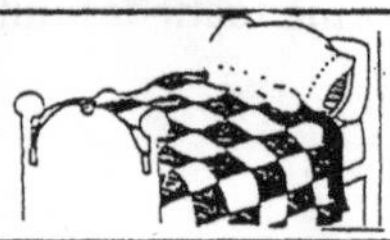			
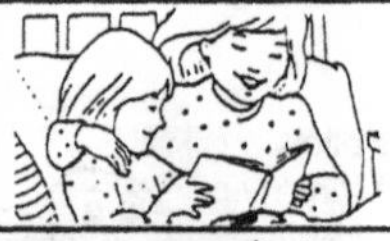			
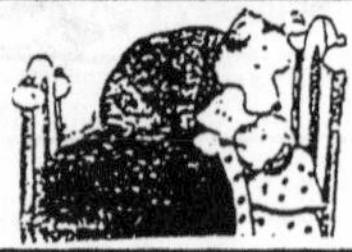			

FIGURE 3.2. Intervention script and data collection sheet for three siblings incorporating completion of bedtime activities, time to completion of bedtime routine, total number of parental requests, observation date, and intervention agent(s).

on premises of teaming, not group or marital therapy. Examples may include observing a spouse or teacher carry out an intervention, or, in language interventions, co-observing to provide estimates of the intelligibility of a child's speech. Specific training in how to give and receive feedback effectively may be important (Harris, Peterson, Filliben, & Glassberg, 1998) as is confidentiality.

Self-Observation and Monitoring

Self-observation is similar to direct and participant observation in method. Self-monitoring describes the two processes of observing and recording behaviors. These are viewed as separate, since each requires attention and effort. Especially for children, motivation or the presence of external contingencies or feedback may be critical.

Self-monitoring procedures may involve the recording of frequency, duration, or intensity of behaviors, and they are amenable to time-sampling procedures discussed later in the chapter. They can be used across the various functions of assessment and intervention, both with caregivers and children.

When to Observe?

Continuous observation is usually not possible, so the question becomes how to *sample* behaviors across periods of time. *Intersession* sampling has to do with deciding which "chunks of time" are used as observation sessions (Suen & Ary, 1989). Observation sessions represent only a small part of the time period of interest. Researchers or practitioners generalize from baseline sessions to the time period before intervening; observation sessions during and after interventions are used to generalize about intervention effectiveness (Suen & Ary, 1989).

How Long and How Often?

First, an appropriate duration for the observation session must be selected. Considerations are based on the results of ecobehavioral interviews and the qualities of the behavior to be observed. For example, behaviors with low rates have to be observed during longer time periods. Alternatively, high rates of behaviors require sustained vigilance, thus setting limits on the session length or suggesting sampling procedures. Highly variable or episodic behavior suggests the need to extend the length of observation sessions.

Second, decisions need to be made related to how often the observations will be conducted. Again, the solution is based on the qualities of the behavior being observed. Trends and stability of the behavior are of basic importance in making these decisions. Stable behavior, or behavior with an observable trend requires fewer sessions.

In summary, the length of observation sessions and the number of occasions must be determined for each situation. The guiding factors are that the samples of behavior are representative and the observations are accurate. The number of observation sessions needed is determined by the rate, variability, trend, and other characteristics of the data. The over- all considerations are based on the level of confidence and generalizations that are desired.

Recommendations for Sampling Planned Activities

We recommend organizing assessments by planned activities described through waking day interviews. Since all behaviors within all planned ac- tivities cannot be observed, critical decisions are necessary about what to observe and how to sample by focusing on significant settings and daily events. Carefully derived sampling plans are needed (1) to insure the eco- logical and technical soundness of assessment and intervention decisions, including generalizations that may be made about behavior and interven- tion results; and (2) to make observations efficient.

During the first phases of ecobehavioral consultation, typical prob- lem situations and activities are sampled from many planned daily activi- ties because they are disturbing to someone. Then, from a set of typical problem activities, those that are most impactful for the consultee are se- lected or sampled for further analysis. For a sampling strategy to be used for intervention design, the following conditions should be met: (1) Obser- vation sessions should occur during planned activities that are potentially significant with regard to learning or behavior objectives and thus are nat- ural times during which the problem may be addressed; (2) selected planned activities and times need to be equivalent in opportunities for be- haviors of interest to occur, and similar conditions must be maintained for observation sessions to be compared; (3) sufficient observations need to be carried out for decision purposes but should be thinned to the minimum to reduce costs; and (4) technical adequacy criteria as applied to interven- tion decision making should be met. This final criterion refers to the relia- bility and validity of information about targeted activities and behaviors, treatment integrity, and other factors related to the evaluation of interven- tion outcomes.

Based on interviews with teachers or parents, planned activities with- in the period of interest are identified to create "pools" of potential obser- vation times that are both important for intervention purposes and com- parable. Next, sets of planned activities representing the same activity/

time across days, or equivalent sets of planned activities (e.g., all large-group instructional activities) are identified as potential periods for observation/analysis. From these potential observation times, observation sessions are planned. In summary, the main objectives are to represent important dimensions of the problem situation and to obtain sufficient data points for decision-making purposes.

As an example, ecobehavioral interviews might reveal that all group instruction periods (A.M. and P.M.) constitute the planned activities of interest. Rarely would a professional (or researcher) be able to select every such instructional period for observation. It is only necessary to generate sufficient information for decision purposes to evaluate the stability of the data and ensure confidence in predictions. However, *explicit* comparisons between the actual observation plans and the ideal pool of possible observation sessions would enable judgments about the overall adequacy of the data and allowable inferences, and may help establish the need for alternative plans for data collection.

As a further example, perhaps observations should cover morning activities for a child, but this may not be possible due to the consultant's schedule. Observations by teachers may be used for mornings, or, at the very least, the absence of data on morning activities will be recognized as a gap in allowable inferences. As a last example, all trips in the car and shopping may constitute two critical planned activities to be sampled. Direct observation by the professional is not feasible, but selection of a random or semirandom plan for parent data collection may ease the burden of data collection overall and enable inferences about times when parents were unable to collect data.

In summary, sampling as described here has two related functions. It is used for supporting reasonable inferences and generalizations concerning behavior within the context of planned activities and for making the best use of limited consultant and care provider time and resources. Comparisons between the actual observation plans and the ideal pool of possible observation sessions allow for judgments about the representativeness of the data and may help establish the need for alternative plans for data collection. In our research, we have referred to these procedures as *strategic sampling* (Barnett, Lentz, et al., 1997).

OBSERVING AND RECORDING BEHAVIOR

There are two very different objectives that address the question of how to observe. First, observations may address natural behavior in specific settings. This involves "recording the stream of behavior, dividing it into units, and analyzing the units" (Wright, 1967, p. 10). The record of observation is a "detailed, sequential, narrative account of behavior and its immediate environmental context as seen by skilled observers" (p. 32) or samples of these behaviors and contexts.

Second, observations also may be structured for instructional and intervention purposes. In these cases, observation methods are guided by specific questions related to behaviors, skills, tasks or demands, environmental conditions and manipulations, and teaching strategies (Wolery, 1989).

Narrative Real-Time Observation

Observations conducted in natural environments provide an ongoing record of behavior as it actually occurs. We recommend that *preliminary observations* be done using narrative real-time methods (shortened to real-time) to help determine the features of behavior and environment that are important to record.

In conducting real-time observations, it is important to focus on the child's setting as well as the behavior. Examples of settings for behavior include school entry, lunch or snack periods, and free play. After describing the setting, actions of others (peers, teacher) toward the child, as well as the child's behavior, are noted in an ongoing manner. Each line (or sentence) should contain one molar (meaningful and complete) unit of behavior. Behaviors should be mutually exclusive (i.e., one activity is recorded) and exhaustive (all of the time is accounted for by recorded behaviors) (Sackett, 1978; Suen & Ary, 1989). Time notations are made at prespecified intervals. Wright (1967) suggests 1 minute; Bijou and colleagues (1969) suggest 2 minutes; we present a variation.

The procedure depicted in Figure 3.3 requires the recording of the exact times for the initiation and termination of behavior. In addition, changes in the setting should be noted (such as transition from free play to snack time). The child's activity changes are recorded by the time notations. In Figure 3.3, arrows may be used to incorporate the observer's judgments of the appropriateness (up) or maladaptive nature (down) of the behavior. Brackets [ ] can be used to record notes or interpretations. Real-time observations also may be used with preestablished behavioral codes (Sackett, 1978).

From real-time observations, the following data may be derived (Suen & Ary, 1989).

1. *Frequency.* This also is known as event recording. The frequency equals the number of times behaviors occur in a session. Frequency may be useful to describe behaviors such as hitting or swearing.

2. *Rate of occurrence.* The rate of behavior is the frequency of behav-

Setting: Preschool Classroom; Free Play   Date:
Time: 1:17 to 1:40   Child: Henry

1:17   Henry is observed in play area with three peers (boys). *H* is fighting with another child over cars.

1:19   *H* hits peer. Teacher intervenes: "Why did you hit *M*?" *H*: "That is my truck. I don't want to play with him!" Teacher: "What if he hit you, would you like that?" *H*: "I wouldn't care."

1:22   *H* leaves cars and moves to dollhouse. Plays with *P* (girl).

1:23   *H* tries to take doll from *P*.

1:24   *H* begins moving the furniture in the dollhouse that *P* has set up.

1:25   *H* to *P*: "Can we trade places?" *P* says "OK."

1:26   *H* begins knocking furniture around. *P* says "Stop." *H* continues to knock down furniture then stops.

1:28   *H* is playing better.

1:29   *H* leaves dollhouse. Says to another child, "Hey, big butt!" Other child appears not to have heard *H*.

1:30   *H* moves to puzzle area with two peers (one girl, one boy). Sits down and begins putting puzzle together.

1:32   Other children left area. *H* working alone. Trying to put clock puzzle together.

1:34   Gets another child to work with him. Another child comes. Both leave.

1:35   Works on puzzle. Chewing on sleeve of his shirt.

1:36   Leaves puzzle area. Did not clean up. Moves to sandbox. Tries to get other child to leave: "How much time have you been in? I'll be your friend if you get out." Child leaves sandbox. *H* gets in sandbox and plays.

1:38   Playing alone in sandbox.

1:40   End observation

FIGURE 3.3. An example of real-time recording.

ior divided by the length of the observation session. Using the rate of behavior enables comparisons of frequency across observation sessions of different lengths (e.g., activity changes in free play).

     3. *Bout duration.* Bout duration is the length of time that the behavior occurs. Duration of behavior may be useful for *states* (such as crying), on-task behavior during instructional periods, or activity engagement (such as sustained play). A state is a stable pattern of behavior that occurs over time.

     Sometimes it may be useful to record clusters of behaviors that occur together as a single bout (i.e., outbursts that occur as sequences of acts in close proximity such as hitting, kicking, or self-injurious behaviors). A decision rule is used that requires defining the behaviors of interest as a bout (i.e., rapidly occurring hits or a string of swear words) and setting an empirically derived interval that adequately separates bouts (i.e., 15 seconds).

4. *Prevalence.* Prevalence is the proportion of time that a behavioral state is found within a session. Durations of behavior are summed and are divided by the session length (expressed in the same time units). The result is multiplied by 100%. It is used to compare states of behavior across observation sessions of different lengths.

5. *Interresponse time (IRT).* This is the time between specific behaviors (or bouts), such as aggressive acts, and is calculated by recording the time period from the end of a behavior to the initiation of the next behavior. The mean IRT may be calculated by dividing the sum of all interresponse time durations by the number of nonoccurrences of behavior. One practical use of IRT is to help set the initial time span for an intervention based on differential reinforcement of other behavior (DRO). The IRT also is used to help set observation intervals, discussed in the subsequent section on time sampling.

Advantages and Disadvantages of Narrative Real-Time Observations

The most important advantage is that many classes of behavior, interactions, events, routines, and their natural sequences, may be recorded. Thus, real-time observations are most useful in provisionally determining the behaviors of interest and in clarifying problem behaviors that are difficult to define. Real-time observations serve as an important criterion for other assessment methods and for judging the adequacy of observational methods in general.

For young children, the technique may provide a recording of the stream of behavior, including (1) play activities; (2) peer relationships; (3) relationships with adults; (4) responses to learning tasks, routines, demands, and rules; (5) antecedent and consequent events for specific behaviors (such as disruptive play initiations); and (6) language samples. Real-time observations also may be used to describe successful and partially successful natural interventions from which intervention scripts may be at least initially derived or used as a starting place. Real-time observations may be used to analyze sequential or conditional behaviors (discussed in a later section). Another dimension—intensity—is infrequently used, primarily due to practical measurement problems.

Real-time observations can be quite demanding; the method is ill suited for participant observers. Also, the results may vary greatly by setting characteristics, behaviors, and skills of observers. The salience of certain behaviors may lead to others being ignored. Accuracy may be difficult to determine, and the results may be subjective. It may be difficult to achieve satisfactory levels of interobserver agreement because of the complexities of events. The technique is not suitable for rare or episodic behaviors. Despite these disadvantages, we view it as a fundamental technique.

Functional Assessments

A functional assessment of behavior has five outcomes: (1) a description of undesirable behaviors, including related behaviors (response classes), and sequences of behaviors that occur together; (2) a description of the "events, times, and situations" when the undesirable behavior(s) "will and will not occur across the full range of typical daily routines"; (3) "identification of the consequences" that maintain the undesirable behavior(s); (4) development of summary statements that link behaviors, situations, and outcomes or reinforcers maintaining them together; and (5) observation data that support the summary statements (O'Neill et al., 1997, p. 3). Functions of misbehavior may be classified in two ways: "to *obtain* something desirable and to *avoid* or *escape* something undesirable" (O'Neill et al., 1997, p. 12). Narrative real-time observations may be used for functional assessments, but they may benefit from adaptations, discussed next, to make them more specific and accurate.

ABC Analysis

ABC stands for *Antecedent–Behavior–Consequence*. Antecedents are events or stimuli that precede a behavior of interest and that may increase or decrease occurrences of the behavior. Examples include a teacher asking the class (or child) to clean up materials or to stand quietly in line. Consequences may be either reinforcing, punishing, or neutral; for example, praising for compliance or repeating a command ("I told everyone to be quiet").

The ABC method of recording behavior was described by Bijou (Bijou et al., 1968, 1969) and has similarities to real-time observation. First, as with narrative real-time observations, the setting is described. Second, observations are recorded on a three-column form (Figure 3.4). A column for time notations also is included. Recording time notations can create ambiguities. Two systematic ways are to make a notation at preestablished intervals such as every 2 minutes, or to record the times associated with activity changes.

Date: _____   Behavior of Concern: _____
                             _____
                             _____
                             _____
                             _____

Time	What was going on before	What was the behavior	What happened after

FIGURE 3.4.   An example of ABC analysis.

Advantages and Disadvantages of ABC Analysis

ABC recording is a basic strategy for the functional assessment of behavior. Many of the advantages and disadvantages of ABC analysis are the same as those described for real-time observation. Judgments of the technical adequacy of ABC analysis need to be determined on a case-by-case basis. Identifying antecedents and functional consequent events may be difficult in complex settings. Reinforcement intrinsic to the behavior (such as self-stimulation or automatic reinforcement) will not be detected through ABC analysis because the behavior is performed without observable antecedents or consequences. Also, behavior may be a function of environmental conditions and not discrete antecedents or consequences, or antecedents may be remote. Behaviors may be associated with multiple functions (e.g., crying).

Functional Analysis

Functional relationships are not necessarily revealed through observations of natural events; experimental procedures may be necessary (Iwata, Vollmer, & Zarcone, 1990). Functional analyses are used to test hypotheses about the control of behavior and behavioral change. Alternative methods, such as real-time observations or ABC analysis, are referred to as *descriptive*, since variables in the environment are not manipulated. Experimental methods for examining hypotheses about behavior through functional analyses should be considered when an ABC analysis proves to be insufficient or when problem behaviors may lead to aversive interventions. Procedures are discussed in Chapter 4.

Frequency (or Event) Recording

This method is based on real-time or continuous observations during a specified period of time, but it is simplified greatly, since only certain predefined behaviors or events are recorded. Frequency recording involves tallying the number of times the behavior of interest occurs in an observation session. Behaviors that may be successfully recorded this way are discrete behaviors of brief and stable duration, for example, activity changes, swearing or calling out, aggressive acts, and specific teacher–child or parent–child interactions. Rates of behavior are used to compare observation sessions of unequal duration.

Duration (or State) Recording

Duration recording—the elapsed time for each occurrence, and the total duration or prevalence of the behavior—may be used when the focus is on the length of time a child engages in a specific behavior. For some behaviors such as tantrums and play, it may be important to record both the frequency and duration of behaviors. Also, the *latency* of a response may be of interest. Latency is defined as the amount of time before beginning a task or initiating a behavior, such as the length of time it takes a child to comply with instructions.

Advantages and Disadvantages of Frequency and Duration Recording

A major advantage is simplicity. Also, these measures may be interpretable as basic dimensions of behavior. For low-rate behaviors, participant observers may be able to provide accurate records. The disadvantages are that behaviors have to be discrete (having clear beginnings and ends). Also, obtaining satisfactory measures of agreement requires that specific time intervals be recorded for the observation sessions. Recording multiple behaviors and bursts of behavior may be difficult.

Time-Sampling Techniques

Time sampling is an alternative to continuous observation of behavior. Professionals must decide when to conduct observation sessions (discussed earlier) and how to sample behaviors within observation sessions (termed *intrasession* sampling) (Suen & Ary, 1989). Time sampling also enables practical and systematic observations of several children or multiple behaviors (Thomson, Holmberg, & Baer, 1974), and facilitates assessment of observer agreement. Two strategies—momentary time sampling and interval sampling—have been widely used. There have been many debates concerning time sampling (i.e., Harrop & Daniels, 1993); we take the position that technical adequacy issues need to be resolved for the individual case.

Momentary Time Sampling

Momentary time sampling is most useful with continuous behaviors, when time is of primary interest (how long behavior is happening), and when behaviors have no clear beginnings or ends (Hartmann, 1984). These characteristics may be described as states of behavior. Momentary time sampling also is useful with behaviors having high rates.

To use momentary time sampling, an observation session is divided into smaller intervals. The occurrence or nonoccurrence of a defined behavior is recorded at the specific moment of an observation. Thus, within each session, at a prespecified interval (i.e., 15 or 30 seconds), the observer records whether or not the child is engaged in the behavior. The interval of interest is the time between discrete observations. For this reason, it is also referred to as "instantaneous time sampling" or "discontinuous probe time sampling." Figure 3.5 combines event recording with momentary time sampling. In the upper part of the observation form, the observer places a mark for each teacher prompt which occurs during the interval. In the lower part, at each time interval (i.e., 15 seconds) the observer notes whether or not the child is engaged in activities (making a "/" for yes and an "x" for no). Summaries of observation sessions using this format include rates of teacher prompting and percentages of engagement.

Advantages and Disadvantages of Momentary Time Sampling

Studies have demonstrated that momentary time sampling yields an unbiased estimate of prevalence (Suen & Ary, 1989). Depending on the interval length and behavior of interest, momentary time sampling may be time efficient and convenient (Hartmann, 1984). Relatedly, with very prevalent or high-rate behaviors, it may be acceptable for use by participant observers, such as teachers, because the time span for measuring can be set at long intervals. For accurate frequency estimates, Suen and Ary recommend that the interval length be less than both the shortest bout in a session and the shortest IRT.

Child: _____   Date: _____

Start Time: _____   Ending Time: _____

Planned Activity: #1 _____ #2 _____ #3 _____ #4 _____

(Circle the interval in which the change of Planned Activity occurs and note the specific activities above.)

Observer: _____

Interval # (15 s)	1	2	3	4	5	6	7	8	9	10	11	12
Event												
Teacher Prompt / (yes) x (no)												
Momentary Time Sampling												
/ (yes) x (no)												
Active Engagement												

FIGURE 3.5. Observation for combining event recording (rate of teacher prompting) and momentary time sampling (percent of active engagement).

Momentary time sampling is not useful for brief and low rate behaviors. The amount of error may be large if the interval size is great. Frequency is likely to be underestimated in such cases. As with other methods of time sampling, the coherence of behavioral sequences and interactions may be lost as interval lengths are increased.

Interval Recording

Interval recording has been used to record both events and states of behaviors. As with momentary time sampling, the observation session is divided into smaller time intervals (such as 10 seconds). However, here, the observer records the occurrence or nonoccurrence of behavior within each interval instead of at one precise moment. Observers must decide how to record behaviors within the interval and how to determine the length of the interval.

Two different strategies are used primarily. With *partial-interval sampling*, an occurrence is defined by the presence of the target behavior during any part of the interval. Each occurrence is only scored once even though behaviors may be repeated during the interval. Partial-interval sampling may be useful for behaviors of brief duration and when the goal is behavioral reduction (Cooper, Heron, & Heward, 1987; Hall & Van Houten, 1983; Wolery, 1989).

Whole-interval sampling requires that the behavior occurs for the duration of the interval. Whole-interval sampling may be most helpful for behaviors of relatively long duration and when the goal is to increase behaviors (Cooper, Heron, & Heward, 1987; Hall, 1984; Wolery, 1989).

Figures 3.6 and 3.7 illustrate different approaches to interval recording. In Figure 3.6, an observation session is divided into 15-second intervals. If the behavior is observed (e.g., disruptive behavior) during the interval, a slash or check is recorded [/]; if the behavior is not observed, a zero [0] or [x] is recorded. The percent of intervals where the behavior was observed is used to summarize each session.

The example in Figure 3.7 also uses 15-second intervals. If the teacher is monitoring the child's behavior during the entire interval, a slash or check [/] is recorded. If the teacher moves away from the child, orienting her visual attention elsewhere any time during the interval, a zero [0] or [x] is recorded. The percent of intervals where the behavior is observed for the entire interval is used to summarize each session.

Advantages and Disadvantages of Interval Recording. Interval sampling and recording has been widely used in behavioral studies because it is applicable to a broad range of responses and facilitates observation of several children or multiple behaviors. It also aids in estimating agreement

Child: _____ Date: _____
Start Time: _____
Planned Activity: #1 _____ #2 _____ #3 _____ #4 _____ Ending Time: _____
(Circle the interval in which the change of Planned Activity occurs and note the specific activities above.)

Observer: _____

Interval # (15 s)	1	2	3	4	5	6	7	8	9	10	11	12
Partial Interval Time Sampling												
/ (yes) x (no)												
Disruptive Behavior												

FIGURE 3.6. Observation form illustrating partial-interval time sampling (percent of disruptive behavior).

Child: _____ Date: _____
Start Time: _____
Planned Activity: #1 _____ #2 _____ #3 _____ #4 _____ Ending Time: _____
(Circle the interval in which the change of Planned Activity occurs and note the specific activities above.)

Observer: _____

Interval # (15 s)	1	2	3	4	5	6	7	8	9	10	11	12
Whole Interval Time Sampling												
/ (yes) x (no)												
Teacher Monitoring												

FIGURE 3.7. Observation form illustrating whole-interval time sampling (percent of teacher monitoring).

between observers. A practical strategy is to alternate observing with brief recording intervals.

A primary disadvantage of interval sampling is that estimates of frequency and duration are confounded. Also, systematic biases exist in estimating these dimensions. Partial-interval sampling tends to overestimate prevalence and underestimate frequency of behavior; whole-interval sampling is likely to underestimate both prevalence and frequency (Suen & Ary, 1989). Harrop and Daniels (1993) pointed out that partial-interval sampling still may have advantages under these circumstances, one being intervention sensitivity, despite these biases.

For accurate frequency estimates with partial-interval recording, Suen and Ary (1989) recommend that the interval length be less than the shortest bout and also less than half of the shortest interresponse time. For accurate frequency estimates with whole-interval recording, they recommend that the interval length be less than half of the shortest bout and also less than the shortest interresponse time.

Other Methods of Collecting and Analyzing Data

Many other observational strategies may be useful for preschool assessments. Some of these overlap with methods described earlier.

1. *Discrete skills sequences* are frequently used to record behaviors. Examples include problem-solving steps, social skills, dressing, and bathroom skills. Task analysis, discussed later, is a method to derive skills sequences.

2. *Category sampling* is used for behaviors that can be descriptively analyzed or categorized (Wolery, 1989). Examples include recording on-task or play engagement, or types of play. The categories should be mutually exclusive and exhaustive, so that observed behavior fits only one category and the categories together account for all of the behavior in the session. Occurrences of behaviors represented by the categories may be recorded through real-time, event, or time-sampling procedures.

3. *Permanent products* result from tangible effects of behaviors. Examples include work or puzzle completion, coloring, bedwetting. Also, audio and video recordings are classified in this way.

4. *Trials to criterion* involve maintaining a record of how many times a learning trial is presented before a child performs at a specified criterion (Cooper et al., 1987). This measure is helpful for comparing alternative teaching techniques for the same skills.

5. *Levels of assistance* is a method of recording the level of support needed for participation in activities (Wolery, 1989). The occurrence–nonoccurrence of behavior is recorded, based on different levels of assistance provided to the child.

6. *Probes* are brief, structured presentations of tasks (Wolery, Bailey, & Sugai, 1988, pp. 77–78) or brief measures of behavioral states. Probes are useful when continuous observation is not feasible or desirable, and when assumptions can be made with confidence that a behavior is relatively stable. They also may be useful when repeated measures result in reactivity. Carefully planned probes may help avoid "ritualistic" data collection whereby the performance level can be predicted accurately.

Preintervention probe *trials* may be conducted intermittently on behaviors that will subsequently be trained, and probes can be conducted later to measure outcomes of the intervention, including maintenance and generalization. Most probes have dealt with academic-related skills. James and Egel (1986) used probes in evaluating sibling play skills; they conducted free-play, generalization, stimulus control, and follow-up probes. For the free-play probes, siblings were brought to a play area and were instructed to play together while their behavior was recorded for 5 minutes. Data were collected an average of four times per week. Probes may be used to record brief samples of behavior in different time periods, conditions, or settings. When used to evaluate interventions, the criteria for consistent conditions applies.

7. *Discriminated (or restricted) operants* result when the opportunity for responses is controlled. This method is related to the ABC method described earlier but is used to study specific antecedents. To record these units, observers note the antecedent, interaction, and consequence. One example is that of parent or teacher commands; the antecedent is a request, the child's behavior is recorded (e.g., comply), and the consequence is recorded (praise). Compliance is typically represented as a percentage. The difference between this class of behaviors and others is that parents and teachers *create* the specific opportunities for children's responses (Baer & Fowler, 1984). For early intervention, the points of analysis are rich and multiple: As examples for noncompliance, the antecedents (requests or commands) may be occurring at high rates, may not be salient (the parent may be making requests from another room), or may not have a sufficient wait time (such as 3–15 seconds); the child may not have the appropriate skills; or the consequences may be inconsistent (such as repeat commands followed by ignoring).

Scanning: A Key Observation Skill

Parents and teachers naturally monitor children's behavior in settings by periodically scanning or "seeing" what is occurring in activities across a setting. This is an important skill that has received insufficient attention, and it is quite different than focusing on one child's behavior through techniques discussed earlier such as real-time observations. Increasing effective scanning is often a key to problem analysis and many intervention designs discussed in later chapters. For young children in diverse activities, caregiver scanning may include the behaviors of (1) moving to strategic locations depending on the activity; (2) visually sweeping the room (Paine et al., 1983) or setting (car, store, playground); and (3) spot checking activities based on predictions from past behaviors or risk appraisals. Scanning is a *foundation* of intervention design, since it sets the stage for altering antecedents (e.g., guiding a child away from an inappropriate act, giving choices) or providing consequences (e.g., attention). Interventions themselves may depend on *positive* scanning (such as noticing improvements in performance, looking for opportunities to provide attention, see Differential Reinforcement of Alternative Behaviors); *negative* scanning (ignoring positive behaviors while focusing on disruptive behaviors or rule violations, see Differential Reinforcement of Other Behaviors); or on altering *patterns* of scanning (e.g., reducing intensive monitoring by teaching self-regulated behaviors; increasing intensive monitoring in risk-related interventions pertaining to dangerous behaviors such as firestarting). Where aversives such as reprimands are overused, increasing positive scanning may be an effective intervention component (e.g., noticing three positives for every negative).

Observing More Than One Child

There are other occasions when it is necessary to observe more than one child within a group or classroom setting. First, the professional may want to compare the behavior of the referred child with other nonreferred children to help set goals. Second, and very different, more than one child may be referred for similar behavior problems. Classroom observers may use techniques building on methods of scanning, momentary time sampling, and interval recording by creating decision rules about how to sample individuals and behaviors, discussed next.

Micronorms

The term *micronorms* refers to accepted norms for a particular teacher, class, and activity. These judgments are focal points of referral and intervention decisions, either explicitly or implicitly. It is important to consider whether the behavior of an individual child differs significantly from other children in a specified way. The "comparison pupil method" and scan-checking (see below) are used to create micronorms. Walker and Hops (1976) credit Gerald Patterson and his colleagues as being the first to use samples of randomly selected peers as partial criteria for evaluating intervention effects for a target child.

Three important questions guide the process of creating micronorms. First, how should appropriate comparison children be selected? There are many possible answers to the question depending on the intervention decisions to be made. A reasonable approach involves random selection of teacher-nominated, adequately performing or typical children (not necessarily exemplary performers) of the same age and gender, who are engaged in the same task. Alternatively, the selection of marginally performing children yields an estimate of environmental and teacher tolerances of children that may be included in classrooms. Decisions regarding the number of comparison children observed must be made based on a consideration of (1) the availability of suitable comparison peers, (2) resources, (3) the potential risks in decision making related to the severity of the problem behaviors, and (4) the stability of the observation data.

Second, which observation and sampling strategies should be used? A general strategy for the measurement of peer micronorms is to move from concurrent, ongoing peer micronorms to discontinuous, more infrequent probes once the variability of the targeted behaviors or skills is ascertained. Within observation sessions, for many applications, interval or momentary time recording (discussed earlier) and *sequential sampling* (Thomson et al., 1974) may be used. In sequential sampling, the observation session is divided into brief intervals. The observer records the behavior of the first child in the first interval, records the behavior of the second child in the second interval, and so on. After all children have been observed, the rotation process then is repeated.

Third, what behaviors, skills, or instructional variables, or combinations of variables, should be observed? This decision follows a careful consideration of information from initial interviews and observations, and a review of related literature, and is made in collaboration with teachers and parents. As examples, variables that have proven likely for many referrals include (1) time spent by the teacher in monitoring or interacting with the referred and comparison children, (2) child time spent engaged in appropriate classroom activities, (3) specific instructional or prompting strategies used by the teacher to facilitate learning, or (4) child progress through identified curricular objectives.

Advantages and Disadvantages of Micronorms. The logic for the use of micronorms is clear; we view the technique as fundamental. Observations for the referred child can be compared with micronorms to give information about the need for further assessment plans, potential goals, and intervention outcomes (Alessi, 1988).

Alessi also presented potential problems with micronorms. First, micronorms may not predict norms in other classrooms or settings. Second, the micronorms for a classroom still may not be suitable for establishing goals if overall rates of targeted classroom behaviors are unusually high or low. In this case, other classes in the school or system may yield more adequate comparisons. Other problems involve basic sampling, reliability, and validity issues (Alessi, 1988; Barnett & Macmann, 1992). The sample of time may be inadequate or inappropriate. The comparison children similarly may not be reasonable (an ideal performer will exaggerate differences, or the comparison child also may have a behavior problem). As with other observations, the behaviors need to be well defined. Last, since the referral is dependent in part on teacher perceptions, misperceptions of the target child (and other children) will reduce the validity of the procedure. When used to establish goals or measure changes in behavior, the significance of differences may be difficult to determine (see special issue of *Behavioral Assessment*, 1988, *10*[2]). Ultimately, decisions about discrepant performances will be based at least in part on the judgments of teachers (or social validity), but micronorms can be used for data.

In summary, the use of micronorms is an important part of the decision-making process. However, it is also vulnerable to sources of error found in observations in general. For a more complete discussion, see Bell and Barnett (in press).

Other Group Observation Strategies

PLA-CHECK (Planned Activity Check) is a variation of time sampling (Risley, 1972). A group of children is observed at the end of a specified interval, and the number of children engaged in the behavior of interest is counted. The number is divided by the total number of children in the group to arrive at the percentage of children engaged in the activity. Alessi (1988; Alessi & Kaye, 1983) described a procedure referred to as *scan-checking*, adapted from PLA-CHECK procedures. At a brief interval (1 or 2 minutes), the observer scans the classroom and records the number of children who are behaving appropriately (reported as a percentage).

For large areas such as playgrounds or cafeterias, a *zone system* of sampling may be used along with time sampling (Sulzer-Azaroff & Mayer, 1991). The space is mapped and divided into zones, and the observer sequentially observes and records the behaviors of individuals within a zone. The observer makes several observations in one zone, then moves to the next.

Multidimensional Observation Codes

Interest in one isolated target behavior is unusual for several reasons. Children are often referred for more than one behavior. The likelihood of target behaviors occurring may be a function of setting events, behaviors of others, or may occur along with other functionally related behaviors (termed a "response class"). Furthermore, intervention design requires that intended and unintended outcomes be evaluated. For all these reasons, a broad range of behaviors should be considered. Examples of important multidimensional codes are Ecological Assessment of Child Problem Behavior (Wahler, House, & Stambaugh, 1976) and Ecobehavioral System for Complex Assessment of Preschool Environments (ESCAPE) (Carta, Greenwood, & Atwater, 1985).

Bramlett (1990) developed the Preschool Observation Code for use in preschool classrooms across intervention phases (baseline and intervention monitoring). The code categories (shown in Table 3.1) were developed from an analysis of real-time recordings of referred Head Start children over a 5-year span, a comprehensive review of interventions found in the literature, and empirically based constellations of behaviors such as conduct disorders and social isolation. The code is based on a State–Event model developed by Saudargas (1980). The code requires about 5 hours of training.

TABLE 3.1. Categories of the Preschool Observation Code

State behavior

Play engagement (i.e., putting a puzzle together)
Preacademic engagement (i.e., in group instruction)
Nonpurposeful play (i.e., playing with puzzle pieces without putting them together)
Unoccupied or transitional behaviors (i.e., wandering around room)
Disruptive behaviors (i.e., throwing objects)
Self-stimulating behaviors (i.e., rocking)
Other behavior (to be used for observations not included in code)
Social interaction–peer (i.e., talking to a peer)
Teacher monitoring/interacting (i.e., teacher is close to the child and is looking at child or child's activities)

Event behaviors

Activity changes (i.e., changing from puzzle to join another child in play)
Negative verbal interactions (i.e., name calling)
Positive motor behaviors (i.e., giving a toy to a peer)
Negative motor interactions (i.e., pushing)
Disruptive behaviors (same as above)
Child approach teacher (i.e., child asks for teacher's help)
Teacher commands—alpha (i.e., clear and direct commands)
Teacher commands—beta (i.e., vague commands)
Child compliance (the child performs the task required by the command within approximately 5 seconds)
Teacher approval (i.e., praise or a pat on the back)
Teacher disapproval (i.e., "You're in trouble now!")

Note. From Bramlett (1990).

Sequential Analysis

The sequential recording of behaviors adds a potential level of analysis to systematic observations. The primary questions are how behaviors are sequenced in time, and how behaviors are meaningfully related in time. At a basic level, examples of sequential analysis may be found whenever interactions are studied.

Sequential analysis involves comparisons of conditional probabilities of events. We use the example of a young child crying in school, which may seem to occur in relationship to home-setting events (e.g., lost sleep due to disruptions or illness). A simple probability is that he will cry on 15 days out of a 30-day span (probability = .50). A conditional probability may be calculated based on the days when disruptive home-setting events were present. If a setting event was present for 17 days, when the child cried at school, the conditional probability relative to crying and the disruptive event is 15/17, or about .88. Of course, the significance of the relationship would need to be determined. Other examples include the study of how behaviors vary by different antecedent or consequent events. Child compliance with parental commands may vary by different antecedents (types of commands) or different consequences (types of praise). Likewise, the probabilities of successfully entering a play group may vary as a function of different play engagement skills (i.e., gaining eye contact, making requests to share, and so on).

Sequential analysis can be much more complex and technical. Relationships between events can be studied both as immediately occurring probabilities and as a function of intervening events. *Lag* sequential analysis (see Bakeman & Gottman, 1986; Sackett, 1978) is a probabilistic approach to the analysis of relationships between events over time. "Lags are defined as the number of event (or time unit) steps between sequential events" (Sackett, 1978, p. 39). Lag 1 refers to probabilities of a target event occurring immediately after a given event. Lag 2 means that the probabilities are calculated after one intervening event. The current applications mostly are research oriented in describing or building models of social or family interactions, but the practical benefits may be great.

Applications of Self-Observation

Earlier, we described self-observation as one of four basic strategies that stem from the question "Who is to observe?" From a practical perspective, self-observation is significant because it is useful for behaviors that are inaccessible to direct observation. Self-observation is necessary for private or covert events such as emotions or thoughts. It also may be used for overt behaviors for which observations may be otherwise costly or inefficient.

Because of links to self-regulation, self-observation has been viewed as a keystone for behavioral change. In general, children are probably not accurate at self-monitoring (Nelson, Hay, Devany, & Koslow-Green, 1980). However, many conditions and innovations can be used to facilitate self-recording and improve its accuracy. Self-monitoring can be combined with other strategies, including caregiver monitoring of behavior and reward systems. Agreement or accuracy checks can be used to improve performance through the surveillance of behavior. For example, a teacher or parent can use a signal system to help the child monitor behaviors. The occurrence of behaviors can be unobtrusively signaled to the child, and the child can maintain tallies on a chart or color in small circles. Complete accuracy is not necessary to derive some benefits for assessment and intervention plans (Kanfer & Gaelick, 1986).

Self-monitoring may be a critical strategy for various aspects of caregivers' behaviors. Specific behaviors (such as giving approval or using types of commands) may be amenable to self-monitoring throughout the assessment–intervention process. Self-monitoring also includes indirect methods such as self-ratings.

Self-Observation as a Keystone Behavior

Keystone behaviors are those for which successful interventions are likely to result in beneficial effects *and* side effects. Koegel and Koegel (1988) wrote that "many researchers and theorists consider the absence of self-monitoring skills to be a pivotal deficit in normal development" (p. 53). Self-monitoring is fundamental to self-control or self-regulation (Bandura, 1978).

Self-Monitoring as a Multistage Process

Self-monitoring interventions require considerable planning and effort, but the external procedures are ultimately faded. First, the child must be able to discriminate the occurrence of the state or behavior and carry out intervention steps. Specific training may be needed. De Haas-Warner (1992) combined a story about a child having task-related problem behaviors with drawings depicting the behaviors, and a story that described the intervention. Children were asked to repeat the story and the procedures used by the child in the story to remain "on task." Modeling of procedures, rehearsal, and positive feedback were used as well. Second, the results of self-observations need to be recorded. As an example, De Haas-Warner used a tone signaling children to self-record by coloring in a box whether they were doing their work. Third, self-evaluation occurs based on the data produced. Self-evaluations may have the quality of reward versus punishment.

While there are differences of opinion related to some of the stages, response discrimination and recording are basic (Mace & Kratochwill, 1988). The most important aspects of implementing a self-monitoring system are clearly defined target behaviors, training, and uncomplicated recording systems. Self-, social, or other reinforcement may be helpful.

The following stages are adapted from Koegel and Koegel (1988, pp. 54–55), based on their work with speech disorders of children with autism, and the review by Mace and Kratochwill (1988, p. 505).

1. *Preparation for self-monitoring.* Inappropriate behaviors and target responses are defined. Decisions are made about the treatment and generalization settings. Functional rewards (social or tangible) are selected. Time periods sufficiently brief to ensure success are also decided upon.

2. *Training in self-monitoring.* The child is taught to discriminate between instances of correct and inappropriate behaviors. This may be accomplished through modeling and prompting. Clear definitions of the target behaviors are necessary. Pictures representing the target behaviors may be used. Following the training, the child is taught to self-observe, evaluate, and record the behavior. The child is trained to an individually established criterion. At this point, the child is prompted to perform self-monitoring under natural stimulus conditions still as a part of training.

3. *Evaluating and rewarding self-monitoring that occurs in the natural environment.* It is necessary to evaluate whether the self-monitoring activities occur in the intended environment. Strategies for this typically involve participant observation by parents or teachers. If it is not occurring, prompts or rewards may be used.

4. *Fading the formal self-monitoring activities.* Fading may be accomplished in several ways by (1) increasing the number of points necessary for a reward; (2) lengthening the time period of appropriate behavior required for a reward; (3) expanding the amount of "work" required for a reward; or (4) when appropriate, "simply telling the child that because he or she is doing so well the self-monitoring is no longer necessary" (Koegel & Koegel, 1988, p. 55).

Reactivity of Self-Monitoring

Although we have discussed it as an observational method, self-monitoring may result in behavioral changes as well; this is called *reactivity*. The changes in behavior may be consistent with treatment goals. Thus, self-monitoring may also be considered as either a supplementary or primary intervention (Mace & Kratochwill, 1988). Self-reinforcement frequently has important social qualities that may be critical to the efficacy of self-monitoring in altering behavior. Thus, the social consequences of self-recording may be important determinants of intervention outcomes.

When studied as an intervention, the results of self-monitoring have been variable. However, many factors may influence the reactivity of self-monitoring: the type of behavior (pleasant or unpleasant thoughts, verbal or nonverbal behavior); the type of recording strategy and its obtrusiveness; the time period for self-monitoring and recording; other competing tasks and responsibilities; the monitoring of behavior by an independent observer; the instructions and training given to the client; and motivational factors. Behaviors with a negative valence have a potential for unintended negative outcomes. Thus, it may be important to reframe some target behaviors (depression) so that positive behaviors are monitored (pleasant exchanges or activities).

CURRICULUM-BASED ASSESSMENT

One of the most useful approaches for making educational decisions involves the systematic and ongoing assessment of children within the contexts of a well-constructed curriculum and instructional techniques. As we saw earlier, developmental measures have frequently been criticized. Curriculum-based assessment circumvents many problems because developmental sequences are tied to ongoing measurement related to instructional efforts and skill progression rather than a "profile" of skills at one point in time, and the results are used in iterative problem solving rather than conclusions such as developmental delay.

Characteristics of Curriculum-Based Assessments

To enable decisions about interventions, a curriculum must have (1) a wide range of functional, developmentally sequenced tasks; (2) ongoing measurement of progress; and (3) a variety of teaching and learning strategies. Curriculum-based assessment enables ongoing observations of the child's performance in preacademic, social, and other developmental areas. The observations are used to delineate the classroom environmental conditions necessary for competent performance (LeBlanc, Etzel, & Domash, 1978). Analysis of the child's level of skills development provides information about the appropriate level for instruction and allows for the continuous evaluation of the child's progress. A range of research-based teaching strategies that match instruction to skills development and the needs of individual children are essential to ensure progress. Children who remain at a particular level of a skills sequence, or who are unable to complete a task, may require a change in instructional strategies in order to progress to the next step. Appropriate instruction may reduce avoidance and disruptive behaviors.

Through ongoing assessment of the classroom environment and the curriculum, information about the conditions necessary for learning can be obtained. By assessing current performance, altering instruction strategies, and adapting materials for a child, teachers can develop goals, and educational techniques can be designed that may help the child develop competencies within a specific target area. The information gained from a curriculum-based assessment includes (1) current level of performance or functioning; (2) rate of learning new skills; (3) strategies necessary to learn new skills; (4) length of time the new skill is retained; (5) generalization of previously taught skills to a new task; (6) observed behaviors that deter learning; (7) environmental conditions needed to learn skills (individual, group, peer instruction); (8) motivational techniques used to acquire skills; and (9) skills acquisition in relationship to peers.

Currently, there are numerous preschool curricula. Some may be adapted by parents and professionals for use in home situations (Chapter 10).

Task Analysis

Task analysis "involves breaking a complex skill or series of behaviors into smaller, teachable units" (Cooper et al., 1987, p. 342). It has been widely used with people who have severe developmental disabilities, but its potential for broader clinical applications is promising (Hawkins, 1986). Task analysis requires attention to behaviors and settings. "Not only are the behaviors relatively specific, but so are the situations in which they are to occur" (Hawkins, 1986, p. 339).

The first step in a task analysis is to identify how a task is competently performed. The component steps that lead to the overall performance are identified; these are usually sequential steps, but concurrent and alternative performances may be important as well. Hawkins (1986, p. 361) gives an example of a concurrent response where the suggestion of a joint activity, such as play, is "accompanied by a smile or other positive facial expression." Alternative behaviors, such as training in the use of different ways to approach peers in play, may be important for many interactions.

Several practical methods can be used to help construct and validate a task analysis sequence.

1. Observations of competent performers may be made.
2. Experts can be consulted regarding the skills that need to be learned.
3. The task may be self-performed by the person developing the task analysis, or the steps may be logically constructed.
4. Sequences may be based on steps observed through skills acquisition.
5. A task analysis can be sequenced by task difficulty and levels of assistance.

TECHNICAL ADEQUACY OF OBSERVATIONS

The technical qualities of observation strategies have generated an enormous amount of discussion and research. Some argue that the traditional notions of reliability and validity do not readily apply to behavioral assessment (Hayes, Nelson, & Jarrett, 1986); others believe that the traditional concepts have value (Barnett & Macmann, 1992; Barrios & Hartmann, 1986). Regardless, it is important to consider the overall quality of measurement procedures and to evaluate their impact on decision outcomes.

Reporting Agreement between Observers

The basic strategy for determining agreement involves comparisons between observers who are coding the same sample of behavior. The quality of data obtained from observations may reflect upon the skills or training of the observers, characteristics of the behavior to be observed (difficulties include bursts of behavior, episodic behavior, covert behavior), the clarity of definitions for problem behaviors or units of analysis, different occasions for observations, and characteristics of different settings. If interobserver agreement is low, these facets represent possible points of analysis. We review several basic methods for determining agreement.

Total agreement refers to an overall summary of agreement about the number of occurrences of behavior within an established time interval. This type of index does not measure agreement on specific instances of behavior, and there may be substantial disagreement on occurrences of behavior even when total agreement percentages are relatively high (Page & Iwata, 1986). Even so, it may be useful when other agreement indices are not applicable. To calculate total agreement, divide the smaller estimate by the larger. For example, a teacher may report seven aggressive acts during the day, while the teacher assistant may report five. The total agreement may be expressed as 71%. Similarly, duration may be expressed by dividing the smaller estimate of duration for a behavior (e.g., crying) by the larger estimate and multiplying by 100 to arrive at the percentage agreement (Cooper et al., 1987).

Interval agreement involves analyzing specific occurrences of target behaviors within time intervals. The units of analysis are discrete opportunities in which the observers agree or disagree that the target behavior occurred.

Interval agreement takes into account both occurrences and nonoccurrences of behavior to arrive at a measure of *overall* agreement. It is calculated by adding the numbers of agreements and disagreements, and dividing that sum into the number of agreements (Hopkins & Herman, 1976). However, one significant problem is that results vary widely by the rates of behavior. To circumvent that problem, Page and Iwata (1986) suggested reporting three agreement indices for a data set. Through the same basic equation, occurrence agreement, nonoccurrence agreement, and interval agreement may be reported.

Another practical strategy is simply to coplot the data for the second observer along with the other observation data. This may be valuable because agreement can be directly linked to decision outcomes, such as the need to intervene or to change interventions.

Agreement estimates are necessary to examine the effects of observers, the adequacy of target behavior definitions, and observational systems. Estimates of agreement also are important over different occasions of measurement and across settings. Measurement occasions include different phases or conditions of the child study such as baseline, intervention, and follow-up. Interobserver agreement indices also are used to determine if the intervention is being carried out as planned. General procedures from research provide the foundations for practical considerations related to technical adequacy. In research applications, agreement indices are reported usually for about 20–25% of the observation sessions. While desirable standards or criteria for reliability indices related to decisions are usually set from between .80 to .90, they generally have not been linked to individual decision outcomes. When observations are used for educational decisions (e.g., eligibility for special services) or other serious decisions, it may be important to provide basic evidence for behavior similar to traditional standards of reliability and validity.

Agreement and Accuracy

Agreement stresses the consistency between raters; accuracy shifts the emphasis more stringently to the relationship of observations with objective indices of actual performance. The assessment of observer agreement provides an *estimate* of accuracy (Foster & Cone, 1986). To determine accuracy, observations are compared to a criterion measure. An exact index of the behavior is necessary. These may be provided by scripts, video, or audio recordings. The approaches to estimating agreement also are used for assessing accuracy. Although accuracy is desired, most investigators "settle" for agreement (Kazdin, 1982b).

Many factors influence the quality of observations (Repp, Nieminen, Olinger, & Brusca, 1988). One is *observer drift*, which means unintentionally adopting idiosyncratic definitions of target behaviors and changing the measurement operations. Another is *expectation bias*, meaning that observers may "see" improvements (or lack of gains) that do not exist. Also, the location for preschool observers may be critical. For example, observers who remain in a fixed position are likely to miss important interactions during free play. For all these reasons, training and frequent agreement checks are critical.

Validity of Behavioral Assessment

Relative to reliability, surprisingly little has been written about the validity of behavioral assessment. Validity may be defined in this case as the appropriateness of the behavior for change. There is no direct correspondence between the accurate description or salience of behaviors and their intervention design implications. The issues surrounding validity are examined in the next chapter, where the emphasis shifts from measuring behavior to selecting target variables.

The Interpretation of Behavioral Observations

The final step in conducting behavioral observations is to analyze and interpret the data. The most basic way to interpret observational data is to graph the results (Parsonson & Baer, 1978, 1986). We continue this discussion at the end of the next chapter in considering how to evaluate interventions.

SUMMARY AND CONCLUSIONS

The foundations of assessment for intervention design are record reviews (including educational, developmental, and medical histories), problem-solving interviews, observations, and curriculum-based measures. The context for these four strategies is critical. Consultation offers a coherent service delivery model based on problem-solving strategies. The focus is on providing needed services to parents and teachers in natural settings.

Observations are fundamental to the analysis of behavior. Other assessment methods are used to simplify, structure, or give meaning to observations. However, many decisions are necessary: what, where, who, when, and how to observe. Each facet of planning and interpreting observations requires professional judgment influenced by one's personal model of practice.

CHAPTER 4

♦♦♦

Designing Effective Interventions

♦

Intervention design should be guided by factors that are likely to facilitate change: (1) parent and teacher collaboration and involvement, (2) an understanding of problem situations, (3) the analysis of intervention research, and (4) step-by-step or *sequential* (rather than diagnostic) decision-making strategies. The targets of assessment and analysis may be different from those revealed by developmental theories or traditional measures because the goal is altering developmental patterns or reducing risk status rather than understanding normal development or "defining" deviancy. Intervention plans are built on design factors, but designs must be transformed into practical and acceptable actions (or scripts).

GUIDELINES FOR SELECTING TARGET VARIABLES

A targeted variable is the focal point of consultation—it is the variable predicted to change a problem situation in a desirable way. However, many children have more than one area of difficulty; alternative target behaviors have to be prioritized or meaningfully grouped together, and the sequence and loci of intervention efforts must be decided. The selection of target variables is followed by evaluating resources and plans.

Traditional discussions have used the term "target behavior" even though reference is made to a wide range of variables. We use both terms but not interchangeably. The term "variable" is introduced to shift emphasis to a broader range of targets of change consistent with ecobehavioral analysis. Examples of target variables are changing the manner in which free play limits are made known to children (e.g., practicing posted limits or rules), or changing the setting, such as the introduction of new

71

play or activity centers into a classroom. Examples for parents may include modifying routines for dressing, shopping, or bedtime.

The term "behavior" is maintained for specificity in discussing more narrow targets for change and when traditions or common usage call for it. Examples of targeted behaviors are sharing to increase play engagement, or making functional requests such as "I need to go to the bathroom."

Guidelines for target variable selection are based on pragmatic, conceptual, and empirical factors. Furthermore, it is accomplished "progressively and with continuing refinement" (Kanfer, 1985, p. 15). Many decisions are necessary.

Evaluate the Basics: Health, Impairment, and System Functioning

A preliminary question is the degree to which a behavioral intervention is necessary (if at all). Children should be screened for medical problems that may be contributing directly or indirectly to the behavior. For example, a child with hearing loss or middle-ear infection may be described as inattentive or noncompliant. Sleep patterns, diet, and medications that might influence behavior should be considered.

Also, children may be referred for behavioral interventions when it is the classroom or family that is in chaos. In the schools, teacher consultation for classroom management, curriculum design or modification, and teacher and administrative support for change efforts may take precedence over consultation for individual child misbehavior. Likewise, parents may refer children for misbehaviors when their lives are disrupted by separation or divorce, family illness, involvement with the criminal justice system, or other personal or social factors. We have had children referred when both parents were holding down two jobs and were rarely home with the child. Basic rebuilding of family and parent–child relationships, or helping to create some stability for at least one parent or alternative caregiver, may be necessary to evaluate the effects of family functioning on child behavior. Thus, it is important to determine the degree to which the environment is contributing to disturbing child behaviors and the degree to which the environment will support needed child-related interventions.

Determine Physically Dangerous Behaviors

Health-related behaviors, safety, and injury prevention take immediate priority over other concerns. Key ecobehavioral factors include parental situations, motivation, skills, and stressors—all of which may affect monitoring and responsiveness to child care needs. With children, one of the initial goals may be to ensure a safe environment while behaviors are being monitored and interventions planned. Aspects may involve abusive and neglectful parental relationships or elements of home and community safety. For example, in a consultation with parents concerning an aggressive 4-year-old boy, initial assessment targets involved the parental monitoring of play behaviors, baths, and stair behaviors (to eliminate pushing and shoving on concrete steps) to protect a toddler sister. Thus, risk assessment is an important initial step.

Evaluate Empirically Based Constellations of Behaviors

Constellations of behaviors or syndromes refer to "multiple characteristics that co-occur and encompass different behaviors, affect, cognitions and psychophysiological responses" (Kazdin, 1985, p. 36). Some believe that appraising the degree to which empirically based syndromes fit an individual child is an important point of assessment. In fact, a considerable research base exists for certain classes of behaviors and some medical syndromes (conduct disorders, social withdrawal, autism, Down syndrome). The syndromes may be predictive of difficulties in adjustment and contribute to prioritization of target behaviors. Constellations of behavior, such as those related to autism and selective mutism, may link the practitioner to very specific intervention research.

The traditional procedure involves making comparisons of the similarities between a child's "profile" based on diagnostic instrument results and the *prototypical* or distinctive features of empirically based or medical syndromes. Child and setting characteristics, treatment components and alternatives, the magnitude of expected changes, and the possible utility of specific observation systems and measures all can be logically compared to the problem situations associated with the referred child. The use of an empirically based constellation of behaviors may lead to uncovering behaviors, factors, or circumstances that otherwise would have been missed. Many excellent sources for interventions are organized by syndromes (e.g., Guralnick, 1997; Kratochwill & Morris, 1991; Mash & Barkley, 1997, 1998), and, collectively, these represent "best practices" for specific referral problems.

However, the high error rates from the use of profile analysis based on developmental and behavior rating scales prevent labeling *individual* young children with confidence for many syndromes. Errors related to profile analysis have many sources (Macmann & Barnett, 1999), but the most important sources for variable descriptions of syndromes result from correlated skills (i.e., cognition, language) and situational analyses of behavior (required by intervention design). Other potential vulnerabilities include pressures to diagnose or the politics associated with the use of diagnostic categories, and stigma and unintended or deleterious outcomes introduced when syndromes are used as labels. Thus, we are asking the reader to walk a very fine line by being guided by empirically based syndromes for assessment and intervention planning, while not necessarily labeling a child with the name associated with the syndrome. This is a fine line, indeed, because parents need to be made aware of information used in intervention plan development—that research pertaining to a constellation of behaviors is partially guiding plan development. Also, in some settings, labels or diagnostic categories are necessary, and that is why we mention the politics of practice. Still, error rates need to be communicated to parents as decision reliabilities (Barnett & Macmann, 1992), and for many child labels, these reliabilities may be only slightly above chance levels.

Evaluate the Social and Economic Impact of Behaviors

Behaviors that have potentially damaging social or economic consequences for caregivers also receive high priority. For example, selecting targets for severely disruptive child behavior may include evaluating the impact on the caregiver's economic realities. Initial consultations may be directed to day care settings and, later, home and community settings. In other circumstances, parents may be discouraging visits from friends and family because of child behaviors that are embarrassing, disruptive, or harmful. These parents may be losing needed support systems.

Consider Values, Goals, and Beliefs

Belief systems are direct and indirect sources of the learning experiences that are provided to children (Sigel, McGillicuddy-DeLisi, & Goodnow, 1992). They also play a significant role in plans for changing behaviors. Parents and professionals may have different priorities for change efforts. Ecobehavioral assessment practices are based on elucidating these priorities and considering caregiver priorities in intervention design. Services that more closely match caregiver needs may be associated with beneficial outcomes for families and children.

Caregiver beliefs also may undermine intervention effectiveness. For example, we have worked with mothers of noncompliant children whose fathers were in jail for violent acts. To the degree that mothers may believe that such behaviors are the direct result of "bad genes" instead of learned, they will invest little in interventions related to improving parenting skills. Questions about beliefs should be included in ecobehavioral interviews even though beliefs that guide actions may be difficult to communicate or out of the caregiver's awareness.

Plan for Expanding Positive Behaviors

Whenever possible, target behaviors should specify desirable goals rather than inappropriate behaviors. Increasing the amount of time spent behaving appropriately will decrease the time spent behaving inappropriately. The *fair pair* rule states that "any behavior reduction objective should be accompanied by an objective designed to teach an appropriate skill that replaces the behavior targeted for reduction" (Wolery, Bailey, & Sugai, 1988, p. 54). Because of the time-consuming process involved in sequential decision making, attention should be given to "enabling" behaviors that are likely to have powerful overall effects on adjustment, or "access" behaviors that allow entry into beneficial environments.

Improve Coping as an Intervention Goal

In many situations, such as those involving children with severe developmental disabilities or degenerative disorders, goals related to improving caregivers' coping skills and examining their sources of satisfaction are appropriate. An important focus may become the involvement of care providers in the implementation and revision of change programs over the developmental period through adulthood.

Plan for Sequences of Behavior Change

Some target behaviors may be prerequisites for other changes, primarily because they may influence later, more significant or "pivotal" behaviors (Kanfer, 1985). Behaviors that are viewed as aspects of a normal developmental progression and linked to functional adaptation, and that may result in cumulative deficits if not mastered, are given high priority. Sequences of behaviors are established through developmental studies and comparisons of skilled versus nonskilled performances on specific tasks.

For example, before learning preacademic tasks, some children need to be taught *preattending skills:* looking at materials, listening to instructions, and sitting quietly during instruction. Reading to young children is a naturalistic method to teach and improve preattending skills. Template matching, discussed later in this chapter, is a method that enables the evaluation of specific skills necessary for success in current or future environments. Task analysis, presented in the last chapter, breaks complex tasks into a series of easily performed steps.

Organize by Planned Activities

Within the ecological approach to early intervention, the basic unit of problem analysis and intervention is derived from settings that are meaningful to parents and teachers, and within which problems occur. In the previous chapter, we stressed that the relevant ecological units may be further defined as *planned activities*. Components of plans include (1) goals and standards for achieving goals that are personalized and valued, and (2) self-statements, including self-instruction, self-managed contingency rules, and self-praise or other self-produced consequences, that mediate or guide behavior through steps to achieve goals. Thus, planned activities define instructional or intervention periods involving goals and behaviors important to adults and children. Practically speaking, plans are explored and analyzed during ecological consultation to reveal what care providers would like to accomplish within specific settings and activities.

Parents' plans refer to ways of organizing their behavior related to social, economic, and personal well-being, and child care. Parents' plans include both natural plans and, ultimately, constructed plans that follow from intervention design. Adult plans for children may have a wide range of intended developmental outcomes that include social and personal competence, independence and mastery, and satisfaction of curiosity (Sroufe, 1979). Effective adult child-related plans are at least partially dependent on benign, if not interesting and nurturing, environments. Unfortunately, adult plans may be ineffective or even nonpurposeful for important parenting activities, and children may be referred for how they respond to these situations. Examples of problems that are clarified by the analysis of existing parents' plans or activities include (1) parents who may be "trapped" at home or in apartments because of their child's dangerous behaviors in cars or community settings, (2) parents who have experienced loss of friends or other social support for reasons related to challenging child behavior, or (3) parents who have missed considerable sleep due to their child's disruptive sleep patterns. In these cases, intervention-related assessment may focus on the revision or construction of plans for transportation, behavior in community settings, visits from friends, and sleep.

Research in *teachers' plans* has addressed two kinds of decisions: planned decisions that take place before an activity and "in flight reactions." Interventions in plans and their related routines are significant techniques that teachers have for regulating their own behaviors and classroom management linked to learning (Paine, Radicchi, Rosellini, Deutchman, & Darch, 1983). Attention to comparatively unremarkable activities, such as consistent participation in classroom routines and following directions in groups, may enable children with disabilities to be integrated into regular preschool settings (Sainato & Lyon, 1989).

Evidence suggests that strong plans may reduce the need for ineffective in-flight decisions (Paine et al., 1983). Routines are used to help carry out plans. Routines may take the form of social scripts that describe the detailed actions that facilitate activities. Effective routines free teachers to attend to other significant elements of teaching, such as content, process, or student behavior.

Consider Keystone Variables

An emerging strategy for target variable selection is the evaluation of keystone variables (Evans & Meyer, 1985). The defining characteristic of these strategies is selecting a relatively narrow target variable that has widespread positive consequences. "The keystone behavior is the one on which all the others appear to depend" (p. 31). This is an important idea because children may be described as having a multitude of problem behaviors that can be organized meaningfully. Keystone variables are those that, if changed, are likely to impact positively the largest set of other significant behaviors, perceptions, or problem environments to most efficiently provide long-term resolution of problem situations (Evans & Meyer, 1985). Keystone variables as targets for change have the following elements:

1. Keystone variables are prerequisite skills or pivotal behaviors (Koegel & Frea, 1993; Koegel & Koegel, 1988) or events associated with response classes of maladaptive behaviors that can positively influence other important child behaviors. Response classes are natural groupings of behaviors that originate and evolve from natural forces that control behavior (Johnston & Pennypacker, 1993). They may occur together as a function of a stimulus or event and can serve the same *function* for an individual. Thus, a response class is a group of behaviors that vary together; a change in one involves changes in the related behaviors. Keystone targets are based on these interrelationships or structural relationships of behavior (Wahler, 1975) that contribute theoretically to a syndrome and are consistent empirically with a syndrome (Nelson & Hayes, 1986). Theory is important to enable predictions about key constructs for assessment and intervention design.

2. Variables targeted for change are selected to have maximum positive collateral effects (Voeltz & Evans, 1982). Thus, keystone variables lead to other beneficial child behaviors and other benefits for those with significant child care responsibilities. The key factor here is that a collateral behavior does not have to be a member of a response class of a child's behavior. As an example, selecting a keystone variable for change may have

the potential for decreasing extensive parental or teacher monitoring of behavior, reducing "expensive" ongoing behavior management, or, as a very different example, ameliorating depressive ideation concerning child care responsibilities. All of these outcomes would have widespread benefits for problem situations. Sometimes these collateral behaviors have been termed "side effects," but their importance may in the long run be equal to main effects. Firestone (1976) found reductions in verbal aggression and teacher attention, and increases in cooperative play following a brief intervention for aggressive behaviors.

3. Keystone variables may be foundation skills necessary for subsequent adaptation to natural environments or for positive behavioral changes being entrapped (Baer & Wolf, 1970) by natural environments so that they are maintained. Keystone variables hold significant potential for improving maintenance and generalization of behavior change efforts (Voeltz & Evans, 1982). Stokes and Osnes (1989) wrote, "Perhaps the most fundamental guideline of behavioral programming . . . is to teach behaviors that are likely to come into contact with powerful reinforcing consequences that do not need to be programmed" (p. 341). This "entrapment" of the target child into more normal maintaining environments is a critical notion within the keystone strategy and may be especially important when prosocial behaviors are being taught.

As an example, compliance may be a likely "keystone behavior" for children described as disordered (Loeber & Schmaling, 1985; McMahon, 1987; Patterson & Bank, 1986; Wahler, 1975). Compliance training has a broad base of support with respect to effective practices and implications for adjustment. Also, social behaviors have been widely studied for collateral effects. One of the best examples of this line of research is for children described as autistic (Koegel & Frea, 1993). We should note that in our research, we have sometimes identified more than one keystone variable for individual children with comprehensive or severe problem behaviors or developmental disabilities (Barnett, Bauer, et al., 1996). There may need to be more than one intervention, or intervention targets may need to be sequenced.

Evaluate Rule-Governed Behavior

Another example of a possible keystone variable is that of *rule-governed* behavior. Rules are guides for conduct or behavior in specific circumstances based on caregiver directives or expectations for behavior. As learning occurs, they lead to self-regulated behaviors. Initial targets for assessment and intervention for disruptive behaviors may frequently be classroom and family rules: how they are introduced and taught, and what the consequences are for appropriate and inappropriate behaviors.

Evaluate Social Competence

Children's play and social behaviors often are critical assessment targets for intervention design with broad implications for development. Guralnick (1987) wrote, "Establishing successful relationships with one's peers is one of the most important accomplishments of early childhood" (p. 93). Potential targets for assessment include facility with functional social routines (such as taking turns), strategies for gaining access to play, communication skills, and toy-play skills. Promising research has examined the effectiveness of peer-mediated (Hecimovic, Fox, Shores, & Strain, 1985; Hendrickson et al., 1982), teacher-mediated (Fox, Shores, Lindeman, & Strain, 1986), and sibling-mediated (James & Egel, 1986) strategies to extend play and social behaviors, although more research is needed, particularly with respect to generalization effects.

Plan for the Next Educational Environment

Part of current plans for a child also call for attention to next environments. As a guiding framework, Brown, Nietupski, and Hamre-Nietupski (1976) proposed *the criterion of ultimate functioning* to stress the need for functional assessments that might improve environmental adaptation for children with severe disabilities. Vincent and colleagues (1980) wrote, "Traditional special educational programming may be incompatible with child success in least restrictive programs" (p. 326). They argued that at least some instructional time should be dedicated to "survival skills" necessary for independent functioning in complex educational environments. They termed this *criterion of the next environment* (CNE). In a later paper, Salisbury and Vincent (1990) challenged early childhood professionals to transcend the instruction of survival skills to "work collaboratively with parents and regular educators to identify content and practices that will be meaningful and developmentally appropriate for all children in primary education classrooms" (p. 83). Their current position is that CNE is used to prioritize educational and developmental goals, and to identify supports necessary to facilitate inclusion in regular education settings.

Related to social validity and functional assessments, strategies to establish needed skills include temporary placements to determine skills deficits, consultations with receiving teachers, and observations in the next environments. Template matching, discussed next, is a research-based procedure to help with transitions.

Template Matching

Template matching is a promising target behavior selection strategy with origins in person–environment research (Bem, 1982). Essentially, template matching includes several different experimental procedures to assess discrepancies between client performance and the performance of "successful" individuals in transition or target settings. The discrepancies are used to (a) predict the likelihood of adaptation in specific settings, and (b) identify target areas for intervention in order to facilitate transitions to less restrictive settings.

The general strategies developed by Cone (as reported in Cone & Hoier, 1986) are straightforward and can be represented by four steps: (a) "The behavioral requirements of situations are conceptualized in terms of behaviors (template items) important to the social context of the particular client child"; (b) "behaviors most characteristic of exemplary performers . . . in that context are identified"; (c) the behaviors are "collected into templates against which the client is compared"; and (d) "discrepancies between the client's repertoire and the template indicate targets for intervention" (p. 15). For example, a child's behavior in the current setting (such as a special education preschool classroom) and adaptive behavior in the transition setting (regular education kindergarten classroom) are compared (Hoier, McConnell, & Pallay, 1987). "Index children" (those who are successful) are identified in the receiving classroom to create a template, which is a profile of child and teacher–child behaviors necessary for successful adaptation in the new setting. Discrepancies between the transitioning child's characteristics and the template reveal targets for intervention.

Applications include assessing social skills and the skills needed for successful transitions between settings (Le Ager & Shapiro, 1995). Under the rubric of transenvironmental programming (Anderson-Inman, 1981), Walker and associates (Walker & Rankin, 1983; Walker, Reavis, Rhode, & Jenson, 1985) have used a different approach to the construction of templates. Rather than observe the performance of successful students per se, they developed profiles of caregiver tolerance that are intended to reflect behavioral standards and expectations in specific settings. Teacher skills and tolerance are important factors in considering transitions.

In summary, planning for educational transitions is a critical aspect of assessment and intervention design. Template matching may help professionals identify probable transition settings and the selection of target behaviors to help with transitions. Template matching also has been applied to selecting target behavior related to social skills. Barnett and Macmann (1992) review the technical adequacy of template matching.

Target Variable Decisions

Target variables are selected based on pragmatic, conceptual, and empirical factors. Hawkins (1986), among others, recommends the conceptual use of a "behavioral assessment funnel" whereby the first step involves broad

TABLE 4.1. Decisions Concerning the Selection of Target Behaviors

1. The question of whether to develop new behavioral repertoires or to reduce troublesome behaviors and how to introduce self-mediated change.
2. The relative focus on child's versus caregiver's behaviors or environments.
3. The reliable and valid development of skills hierarchies and sequences.
4. The analysis of complex relationships between behaviors.
5. The decisions about changing the level of analysis from discrete behaviors to more global classes of behaviors (e.g., combining hitting, name-calling, and breaking objects into a category of "destructive tantrums").
6. The identification and prioritization of keystone target variables including the determination of *access* behaviors that enable entry into environments likely to enhance development.
7. The criterion for effective performance.

screening, followed by a narrowing focus, and, ultimately, the specification of target behaviors. Kanfer and Grimm (1977) developed what is considered to be a classic framework for selecting target variables. Many of their considerations have been built upon in this section and in Table 4.1.

INTERVENTION DECISIONS

Intervention stages are (1) defining and clarifying a problem situation and targeted variables, (2) designing an intervention, (3) executing the intervention, and (4) modifying, fading, or terminating the intervention based on intervention outcomes. Intervention plans are based on at least five considerations, all of which require professional judgment: (1) applications of change theory and the use of various assessment techniques in the process of problem solving; (2) child, caregiver, setting, and service delivery characteristics; (3) analysis of possible and likely interventions; (4) acceptability of interventions; and (5) relative costs and estimated potential benefits of interventions.

Interventions may include (1) changes in parent, teacher, peer, sibling, and child behaviors; (2) changes in physical environments and routines; (3) instruction to teach new skills or expand existing skills; and (4) techniques for increased self-regulation. Generally, interventions are selected based on a combination of strategies, including the analysis of situations and potential target variables through problem solving with caregivers, observation, and the evaluation of the research base for interventions. We emphasized organizing this information by planned activities and keystone variables.

Assessing the Research and Empirical Bases for Interventions

There are several broad reasons for this step. First, parents, teachers, and administrators generally expect that intervention decisions are guided by available and pertinent research. These expectations have significant legal, ethical, and professional foundations, as discussed in Chapter 5.

Second, research may be used as a general guide for both assessment and intervention design. As an example, caregiver behaviors and setting expectations, in addition to child characteristics, should be a focus of assessment and intervention plans for children described as "conduct disordered" (McMahon, 1987; Patterson & Bank, 1986).

Third, preschool consultants should be aware of valid and, ideally, replicated intervention strategies that have been successfully applied to specific behavior problems of interest. The process involves making logical generalizations from research to individual cases. This is not a "cookbook" recommendation; functional analyses are necessary to assist with making generalizations.

Avoiding Use of Aversive or Punishment Procedures

Many procedures that have been used for intervening with children's behavior problems are aversive. Self-injury, self-stimulation or stereotypical behavior, acting out, or psychotic behaviors have been associated with decisions concerning aversive techniques (Matson & DiLorenzo, 1984; Repp & Singh, 1990). Well-established interventions such as time out and overcorrection also are classified as aversive interventions. Because of the many controversies, decision making related to aversives includes evaluating risks to the child and others, the potential of positive procedures to work efficiently and effectively, and protections for the child. Established safeguards should be employed when these procedures are used, and these are reviewed in later chapters. Some interventions that are described in later chapters were perhaps more aversive than necessary, but they still may include useful components. Functional assessments and positive procedures can be added to reduce the need for aversive procedures.

Dealing with Uncertainty

Numerous gaps exist in the intervention research base for certain behaviors, child characteristics, or applicability of interventions to different settings. Also, creative parents and professionals will want to try out new ideas. These unknowns are of critical importance to professionals and parents in making decisions. In such circumstances, empirically based procedures are especially important, as is accountability based on single-case experimental designs, discussed in the next chapter.

Empirically Examining Hypotheses Concerning Behavior[1]

Functional analysis is an empirically based approach to examining hypotheses related to intervention design. The general strategy is to examine and, if necessary, alter environmental variables (positive reinforcement, negative reinforcement, stimulus control) to determine their *function* in modifying or maintaining behaviors (O'Neill et al., 1997; Skinner, 1953; Umbreit, 1995; a special issue on this topic appeared in the *Journal of Applied Behavior Analysis*, 1994, *27*[2]). Impressive validity evidence exists for these procedures for self-injurious, aggressive, disruptive, and stereotypical behaviors. The ABC analysis presented earlier is one technique designed for this purpose, and observations of natural events may help pare down competing hypotheses concerning functional relationships between environmental events and child behavior. However, due to limitations in events that may be observed through naturalistic observations, environmental events may need to be systematically manipulated (Lerman & Iwata, 1993). Data from a descriptive analysis (such as real-time or ABC observations) might not be precise enough to help practitioners accurately identify functional relationships.

Martens, Witt, Daly, and Vollmer (1999) describe three practical reasons why it is important to understand the principles governing behavior on an individual basis as accurately as possible. First, by identifying the controlling principles that are functionally related to the behavior (e.g., social attention, demands, pleasurable consequences), it is possible to design treatment programs that weaken the contingencies maintaining the problem behavior in the natural setting. Second, care providers are often unaware of their effects on child behavior. By examining functional relationships directly, care providers are likely to be more consistent in implementing intervention programs by virtue of understanding the systematic relationships between their behavior and child behavior. Finally, because problem behaviors often develop over long periods of time, there may be greater resistance to change. The *precision* of functional-analytic data in evaluating hypotheses for change is likely to minimize the extensiveness of the intervention, because the intervention program is based on the smallest possible number of variables shown to affect child behavior, thereby increasing the likelihood that the intervention agent will implement the intervention consistently. The fewer the intervention steps or variables, the more efficient and easier an intervention will be to implement, leading to greater intervention acceptability and use. In summary, the result of functional analysis is a data-based method to evaluate possible causes of behavior and ways to test intervention hypotheses. In fact, by

---

[1]Edward J. Daly III contributed to this section.

failing to discriminate functional relationships accurately, care providers may be at risk for implementing interventions that actually reinforce the problem behavior (e.g., using time out when the child is engaging in disruptive behavior to escape a demand).

Conducting a functional analysis is complex and can be time consuming. The costs of advanced planning and execution of a functional analysis have to be weighed against the high quality of the data provided by a well-done functional analysis. Even if a child displays high rates of severely disruptive behavior, a functional analysis may reveal simple mechanisms that support problem behavior and lead readily to environmental modifications (reducing aversive properties of instructional demands, changing contingencies for teacher attention).

The first step in conducting a functional analysis is to identify a setting where variables such as social attention, task demands, and other available reinforcers can be controlled. Approaches to functional analysis can be divided into (1) those that involve manipulations of antecedents (e.g., kinds of tasks, length of tasks, location of task), (2) those that involve manipulations of consequences (social attention, other reinforcers, escape from task demands), and (3) those that involve manipulations of both. The next step is to choose an experimental design to compare the results across conditions (such as the alternating treatment design; see Chapter 5). The most likely hypotheses should then be chosen, which requires (1) identifying those variables empirically linked to problem behavior in the experimental literature, and (2) using interview and naturalistic observation data to come up with a smaller number of possible conditions (cf. Lerman & Iwata, 1993). Next, the conditions have to be specified in such a manner that they provide high rates of the variables associated with that condition (e.g., attention, demand) contingent on the target behavior while holding other variables constant. It is important that the child be able to discriminate available contingencies, hence the necessity of high rates of possible reinforcers and holding constant other potential reinforcers. Finally, conditions are implemented until a clear pattern emerges in the results, suggesting that the behavior is functionally related to one or more of the conditions. Data are graphically displayed (expanded in Chapter 5).

Sequenced Interventions and Consequence Hierarchies

Earlier, we introduced the idea of sequences of intervention targets. Here we want to point out that sequenced interventions may serve as a general planning format for many situations. For example, a referral and functional assessment for classroom disruptions may lead to the following sequences and hierarchically arranged intervention steps, given an interesting and well-managed classroom: (1) re-teaching classroom rules as positive expectations for behavior; (2) reconsidering features of classroom design such as placements of activities or assigned carpet places; (3) giving specific directions and choices for activities; (4) practicing, prompting, guiding, and reinforcing appropriate rule-following behaviors in actual contexts; (5) when rules are broken, applying a specific series of consistent consequences (e.g., clear communication of expectations for behavior, two warnings, contingent observation or "sit and watch," or bonus response cost, such as loss of sticker for an added activity).

As an extension of functional analysis, Harding, Wacker, Cooper, Millard, and Jensen-Kovalan (1994) had parents try out a series of likely preselected behavioral interventions with their children in an outpatient behavior management clinic until an intervention produced improvements in child compliance. The series of interventions began with antecedent manipulations (specific directions followed by offering choices) and continued with manipulations of consequences (praise, offering contingent help, offering preferred activities, and guided compliance whereby the adult guides the child hand-over-hand), ordered from easiest to most difficult to implement. When an effective intervention was identified, they replicated the last two conditions (the last unsuccessful condition and the first successful condition) to demonstrate functional control over child compliance. An especially significant feature of the study is that intervention agents actually tried out interventions before full-scale implementation. It was also time efficient, because the conditions lasted about 6 minutes on average.

When the Change Target Is a Setting Event

To understand critical influences on behavior, it may be necessary to evaluate more distal setting events. *Setting events* are sources of behavioral influence that are remote in time or space. They are defined as specific but indirect antecedent events related to the likelihood of occurrence of a stimulus–response interaction (Wahler & Fox, 1981). Wahler and Fox warn about the bias toward brief temporal associations between stimulus and response, and they make the point that "no a priori assumptions can be made concerning ideal or even necessary time spans between suspected setting events and a particular target behavior" (p. 332).

Prototypical examples of setting events affecting school performance are hunger (Bijou & Baer, 1961), the presence versus absence of another specific person or favorite toy, or prior activity (Krantz & Risley, 1977). Other examples may be natural rates of approval or disapproval (Strain, Lambert, Kerr, Stagg, & Lenkner, 1983), parental history for using time out (Harris, 1985), or the overall reinforcement contexts that serve as consequences of behavior (Herrnstein, 1970; Martens & Kelley, 1993). Examples pertaining to home may result from stressors such as divorce or parental depression, both of which may affect monitoring of children's behavior and variability of family routines (such as sleep, household conditions prior to attending preschool, erratic use of psychostimulant medications), or social factors such as insularity (Wahler, 1980), or even physical or sexual abuse.

Occasions when setting events should be examined include (Kennedy & Itkonen, 1993; Wahler & Fox, 1981) (1) when other analyses (ABC) reveal that behavior is not a potentially powerful function of temporally close antecedents or consequences, (2) when the setting where the behavior is reported to occur is not readily accessed by the consultant, (3) when contingency management is not possible or is rejected, (4) when relatively stable performance within a phase appears to be disrupted by a covarying event.

To evaluate setting events, the same measures (i.e., of child-related disturbance) are maintained. Parents and teachers are asked to hypothesize about other circumstances related to behavior. Their anecdotal comments then may be systematically examined through an ABC analysis or through basic single-case experimental designs. These can be corecorded along with time series data, or reanalyzed as alternating, multielement, or periodic conditions (Barlow et al., 1984).

Assessing the Availability of Resources

A careful analysis of resources for reaching treatment goals is necessary. Interventions require an appropriate environmental context, the availability of caregivers, and a range of specialized personnel. Teachers may require planning time and support services. The roles of babysitters and extended family members may be significant. It is important to differentiate between currently existing resources, those that are accessible, and those that may be creatively identified.

Assessing the Acceptability of Intervention Alternatives

Acceptability refers to broad-based judgments by consumers (participants and caregivers) concerning "whether treatment is appropriate for the problem, whether treatment is fair, reasonable, and intrusive, and whether treatment meets with conventional notions about what treatment should be" (Kazdin, 1980, p. 259; see also Wolf, 1978). The general premise is that for many problem behaviors, a range of alternative interventions is likely to be effective. Those viewed as more acceptable are more likely to be "sought, . . . initiated, and adhered to" (Kazdin, 1980, p. 260). Wolf (1978) wrote, "If the participants don't like the treatment then they may avoid it, or run away, or complain loudly" (p. 206). Unless participants view the intervention as acceptable, important technological advances will not be used. Also, by considering a range of intervention alternatives, professionals help reduce the possibility of intervention biases (Kanfer & Grimm, 1977).

One of the major issues is how acceptability ratings may be altered through planned sequences of interventions. Witt and Elliott (1985) hypothesized that acceptability, use, integrity, and effectiveness of the intervention are sequentially and reciprocally related.

Fawcett, Mathews, and Fletcher (1980, pp. 508–511) argued that interventions that are contextually appropriate are more likely to be adopted. Based on their analysis, desirable interventions are (1) "effective," (2) "inexpensive," (3) "decentralized" and controlled by local groups, (4) "flexible" enough to permit input by participants, (5) "sustainable" with local resources, (6) "simple" or comprehensible, and (7) "compatible" or harmonious with existing perceived needs, values, and customs of the setting.

Assessing for Motivation

Acquiring significant behavioral change for children may require substantial behavioral change on the part of the caregivers. In the context of behavioral intervention, motivation refers to "the probability of an individual emitting the behaviors necessary for successful intervention" (Haynes, 1986, pp. 400–401). While there are no panaceas, active involvement by parents in assessment is likely to increase participation in intervention decisions (Brinckerhoff & Vincent, 1986), as are principles of naturalistic design.

Reducing rather than increasing caregivers' demands may be an important assessment and intervention goal in some situations. Caregivers may spend a considerable amount of time monitoring and responding to the disruptive behavior of young children. Preschool consultants need to assess the impact of interventions on caregiver–child interactions, and the caregiver's other roles and responsibilities. When possible, successful interventions should lighten burdens for conscientious, effective, but drained caregivers. Practical examples include reducing teacher monitoring and prompting necessary to manage a child's classroom behavior, and reducing the level of parental assistance that a child requires in self-care skills such as dressing or feeding.

Assessing Potential Effects of Child Behaviors
on Caregivers' Behaviors

Children's severe problem behaviors reciprocally alter qualities of environments. A major consideration in intervention design may be the effects of severe behaviors on adults who have responsibility for child care and, ultimately, intervention implementation (Carr, Taylor, & Robinson, 1991). Natural teaching attempts may be punishing, having the net effect of reducing teaching efforts. Intervention design for challenging children also is guided by the most effective and least punishing intervention for parents and teachers who are implementing interventions.

Estimating Probable Success

Intervention strategies must be realistically appraised with respect to their likelihood of success in changing selected target variables. Probable success rates are determined in part through a review of interventions found in the literature, intervention trials that follow a functional analysis, an analysis of settings and resources, and from judgments by persons carrying out intervention plans. More complex interventions, or those involving multiple change agents, are more vulnerable to intervention failure.

Intervention or *treatment strength* "refers to the ability of a given treatment to change behavior in the desired direction" (Gresham, 1991, p. 28). A preferred intervention, given cost and all other considerations, is the *weakest* that leads to successful outcomes (Yeaton & Sechrest, 1981). *Resistance to intervention* is defined as "the lack of change in target behaviors as a function of intervention" (Gresham, 1991, p. 25). Resistance must be analyzed by behavioral factors—severity, chronicity, generalization, and teacher tolerance of the behavior—and intervention factors—strength of treatment, acceptability, treatment integrity, and treatment effectiveness.

The analysis of resistance to intervention has many practical implications. Interventions must have sufficient "strength" to change the behavior. This means that interventions must be carefully planned and procedures specified, the length and intensity of the intervention must be determined, and change agents with appropriate expertise must be identified. Behaviors that are resistant to change require a functional analysis and replanning with respect to target variables, interventions, and appropriate services and support for caregivers.

In addition, Gresham (1991) has argued that behavioral disorders may be conceptualized in terms of resistance to intervention. The implications are important. First, the framework shifts professional decision making away from dichotomous classifications (disturbed vs. not disturbed), and psychometric approaches whereby the number of symptoms or behavioral profiles are considered, to functional assessments and intervention decisions. Second, and more basic, no classification decision is made unless the child's behaviors remain unaltered by well-planned and well-executed interventions. The classification logically leads to stronger interventions. Classifications of resistance to intervention also have applicability to severe learning problems.

The concept of "intervention strength" may lead to possible misinterpretation, especially related to aversives (giving louder commands for noncompliance, increasing time outs). Fundamentally, intervention strength has to do with the probabilities of interventions changing a problem situation. Principles from physics have been used to help explain resistance to intervention (Nevin, 1996; also see criticism by Houlihan & Brandon, 1996).

Self-Mediated Change

Earlier, we described self-monitoring as a keystone behavior, but surprisingly, research on self-directed change for children has been promising but inconclusive (Billings & Wasik, 1985; Bornstein, 1985; De Haas-Warner, 1992). In large part, this is due to experimental design considerations in determining the extent of self- versus "other" directedness. Because children are guided through the intervention, self-directed change is actually based on the efforts of caregivers.

However, despite the controversies, several methods may be used to encourage and facilitate self-regulation and independent problem solving. These include the basics of modeling, prompting, and reinforcing behaviors, and creating sufficient opportunities for practice. As one example, Stokes, Fowler, and Baer (1978) successfully taught preschoolers to appropriately elicit teacher attention. Overall, external means are important in developing self-regulation.

An example of a "self-mediated" intervention technique is that of "correspondence training." A number of studies have demonstrated the effectiveness of reinforcing children's verbalizations as a way to control behavior. The method, along with other self-mediated change strategies, is reviewed in later chapters. Another example, based on a series of investigations spanning three decades, is *delay of gratification*. Mischel has proposed this concept both as a significant psychological process fundamental to self-control and as a basic personal competence. Delay of gratification refers to "the ability to purposefully defer immediate gratification for the sake of delayed, contingent but more desired future outcomes" (Mischel, 1984, p. 353).

Estimating Cost-Effectiveness

The relative efficiency and cost-effectiveness of alternative interventions are additional considerations. Cost analyses in practice are complicated (Noell & Gresham, 1993; Yates, 1985) and not typically done, but they are always implied. Consumers assume that professionals help guide the process by the notion that the most effective–least expensive interventions deserve primary consideration. For many reasons, determining costs in a monetary sense may be too challenging and even misleading. Time in carrying out an intervention frequently may be used as a major cost variable.

Agreeing on Roles and Responsibilities

After intervention alternatives are evaluated and an intervention plan is selected, the responsibilities of the consultants and caregivers must be agreed upon. Gutkin and Curtis (1990) commented that this is often an overlooked but critical step. We elaborate on this topic in the next section on treatment integrity.

Assessing Treatment Integrity

Treatment integrity is an important idea in intervention design, and we approach it in two different ways: through a discussion of intervention implementation, and through the practical notion of scripts. Treatment fidelity is a broader term that refers to whether or not an intervention was conducted as intended (referred to as treatment integrity from here on), and whether an intervention differs and is as distinct as intended from other intervention procedures (Moncher & Prinz, 1991). If not evaluated, the question of treatment integrity casts doubt over intervention efforts. "Real treatments are often complex, are sometimes delivered by poorly trained or unmotivated people, and can be totally disrupted by events in the real world" (Sechrest, West, Phillips, Redner, & Yeaton, 1979, pp. 15–16). Interventions often are altered intentionally or unintentionally, or are not carried out as planned.

While changes in plans frequently are required to ensure that the child receives an appropriate intervention, the needed changes should be identified, planned, and mutually agreed upon. A common error is changing to a more restrictive or intrusive intervention because the outcomes appeared ineffective, when instead, the original plan lacked treatment integrity. The intervention may not have failed. Rather, it may not have been adequately implemented.

Factors related to treatment integrity and evaluation methods have been outlined by Gresham (1989) and Ehrhardt et al. (1996). These include naturalness of intervention steps, complexity, time requirements, materials and resources needed, number of treatment agents, perceived effectiveness of treatment, actual effectiveness of treatment, and motivation of treatment agents. Evaluation of treatment integrity includes specification of components and tolerable deviations. The occasions for the treatment and the occurrence–nonoccurrence of the components may be analyzed as percentages of steps completed and graphed along with data on behavioral change (Ehrhardt et al., 1996).

Using Scripts as Treatment Integrity Measures[2]

Scripts are defined as personalized and detailed guidelines for providing instructions and/or managing behaviors to meet specified goals. Scripts, written in care providers' natural language, provide a means for examining intervention steps in the context of problem situations. Other terms used to communicate intervention plans include "steps," checklists, or flow diagrams (i.e., Sulzer-Azaroff & Mayer, 1991). The difference between these terms and scripts is the emphasis on natural language and specific actions developed for problem contexts, in contrast to a more general portrayal of the intervention steps. Sample scripts are included in Figures 4.1 and 4.2.

Creating and Using Intervention Scripts

Using ecological and consultation-based approaches when designing interventions enables the professional to identify likely change agents and allows the individual who will be responsible for implementation to be aware of the conditions necessary for success. Scripts are built through consultation, problem-solving interviews, and from natural interactions derived by narrative real-time observations. Through training, modeling, role playing, and guided practice, individuals can become competent in the intervention techniques before they are actually implemented. A usually practical strategy is to construct the intervention steps through the use of written scripts and to role-play the complete intervention as needed to refine the script. Planning a trial implementation may be helpful. A provisional treatment integrity script will enable changes to be noted and carefully evaluated on subsequent trials. The script can be evaluated and revised as necessary. The caregiver contributes to the intervention design, the sequences of events or steps, and the wording of the steps. Observers also can help by collecting data on the intervention procedures administered in the natural environment. In addition, other teachers or family members who come in contact with the child may need to be informed about intervention programs so that they may be supportive of intervention goals.

After consultation and training in the intervention technique, the caregivers can be given enough copies of the treatment integrity script to

---

[2]This section is adapted from Ehrhart et al. (1996).

When John comes to the table for meals, snacks, or table-top activities:	Date: Time:						
1. Prepare food so that it is in bite-sized pieces, which will make it easier to scoop from the bowl and to load his utensils.							
2. Remind John of the lunch time rules by cuing him to repeat them (e.g., "John, where do your feet, hands go? How do we eat?").							
3. Seat John in close proximity to an adult so that she can prompt him to follow the lunch time rules (e.g., serving, passing, using utensils, napkins, keeping fingers from bowls) and how to hold the utensils correctly.							
4. Slide John's food away briefly when he stands or kneels in his chair, reminding him to sit.							
5. Praise John's sitting correctly, serving, waiting, and using utensils (e.g., "Good job using your fork").							

Lunch time or table top rules:

1. John needs to sit in the chair, feet on the floor, hands in lap until his food is passed or the activity is in front of him.
2. John needs to use the serving spoon (no helping fingers) to transfer food from the bowl to his plate.
3. John needs to use fingers for finger foods only (watch the teacher), and spoon or fork for other food.
4. John needs to follow the clean up routine following lunch.

Number of rules that John followed with two or less reminders:
Date   Number of rules

FIGURE 4.1. Script for John during meals.

use until the next scheduled consultation. The consultant and caregiver may co-intervene for the first few days of the intervention. While the consultant carries out the intervention, caregivers follow the script to help learn the intervention steps and to become familiar with the regimen. Teams may be formed within classrooms to help with monitoring interventions. The caregiver may bring in the script with checks for completed steps as a part of the ongoing consultation. It is critical that it be viewed as a helpful process, similar to feedback that is received in learning any new task.

	Step completed?
1. Plan ahead for shopping trip.	
a. Identify a shopping partner.	Y/N
b. Prepare grocery list and check.	Y/N
c. Review script with partner.	Y/N
2. Review rules before entering store.	
a. Stay within arm's length.	Y/N
b. Follow directions.	Y/N
c. Keep hands/feet to self.	Y/N
3. Set timer and remind Katie she can earn check marks for positive behavior.	Y/N
4. When timer goes off:	
a. Review successes and give check marks OR	Y/N
b. praise positive behavior, provide corrective feedback, remind Katie to try again.	Y/N
c. If Katie tantrums, ask shopping partner to finish shopping AND take Katie to the car. No rewards.	Y/N
5. After shopping, review Katie's success and tell her how many check marks she earned.	Y/N
6. Home reward for positive behavior in store.	Y/N

FIGURE 4.2. Home script—shopping.

Advantages of Scripts

Potential difficulties with adherence to intervention plans underscore the possible need to clarify exactly what is expected by interventions and to identify flexible ways to enable caregivers' modifications based on realities of situations as interventions are carried out. Parents and teachers have found intervention scripts to be highly acceptable (Barnett, Bell, et al., 1997; Barnett, Air, et al., in press). Here are some of the reasons.

1. Scripts may be used for describing significant instructional or problem situations for parents and/or teachers in terms of characteristic interactions.

2. Scripts may help identify interventions used by care providers or research-based interventions that may be useful to care providers such as modeling or types of correction procedures (Kamps, Leonard, Dugan, Boland, & Greenwood, 1991). Scripts can be compared through content analysis to other interventions found in research to facilitate the process of logical generalization.

3. Scripts may be used for teaching new behaviors or ways of responding to particular situations, including simple or complex routines. Scripts may be helpful in learning new roles because they address (a) skills or construction competencies ("how to do it") and (b) efficacy expectations by inviting participation ("I can do it") (Mischel, 1981). In script form, intervention steps may be shared across settings as needed for individual children and for replication by others.

4. Scripts may help create desirable situations and expectations for creativity, feedback, and coaching "to try out a new role." They focus on behaviors, not inadequacies. Changes may be easily made and recorded on scripts.

5. Scripts may be used to improve many aspects of experimental design in intervention research by clarifying the independent variable. Kara and Wahler (1977) described a preexperimental phase that serves several purposes, including establishing specific ways for adults to interact with children in carrying out a research plan. Through the specification of intervention steps, scripts may serve as important criteria for treatment integrity and for obtaining estimates of intervention integrity across intervention sessions (or as probes of sessions).

6. Treatment integrity may be increased through the use of scripts because acceptability may be enhanced in the script-building process.

7. The use of scripts in intervention design may facilitate behavior change and promote maintenance by encouraging self-regulation. Self-regulation may be defined as "the *gradual* assumption of control by the individual over cuing, directing, rewarding, and correcting his or her own behavior" (Kanfer & Karoly, 1982, p. 576) guided by rules for behavior in specific situations.

8. Scripts may promote behavior change through the possibility of reactivity as a supplementary intervention. Reactivity may occur for several reasons. Through ongoing consultation, script development based on observations of care providers' interactions in problem situations may result in greater awareness and monitoring of interactions. Also, the use of scripts by care providers to implement interventions in problem situations and to assess their treatment integrity could be considered a form of self-monitoring. Furthermore, assessment of treatment integrity with scripts by independent observers gives care providers information regarding the accuracy of their monitoring. Thus, reactivity of care providers to scripts may produce desirable changes in their interactions with children in problem situations, and may be a critical element in self-regulation.

9. Scripts may enhance the ethnic validity of interventions for care providers because they are tailored for use in natural settings to address problem situations identified by the care provider and written in the care provider's everyday language.

10. Scripts have been used to present more general patterns or models of communication that form the basis of interventions. Perhaps the best example, with considerable research support, is found within milieu teaching for language interventions. The difference between script usage in incidental teaching and other uses is that the intervention plan may include guidelines for incidental teaching, but since the child's interest serves as a stimulus for the parent or teacher, examples of scripts rather than specific scripts are used to convey the intervention plans.

11. Scripts are helpful in fulfilling the ethical requirement of informed consent, whereby all relevant aspects of interventions that are required for decision making are described without jargon.

Sampling Script Usage

Scripts are part of the collaborative evaluation of treatment outcomes that includes integrity of implementation, script acceptability, and behavioral change. The waking day interview serves as a guide for sampling script usage and to help set mutually agreed on plans for co-observing the script if possible.

Poor treatment integrity without behavioral gains may indicate that the intervention is unreasonable for a situation and that reconsideration of the steps or redesign of the intervention is necessary. Treatment integrity with desired behavioral gains, but with missing intervention steps, may indicate a need to simplify the intervention or a progression toward fading intervention plans. Serendipitous changes also may result in improvements.

Assessing Unintended Outcomes or Side Effects

Interventions may have positive, mixed, or negative outcomes; short term good may be followed by long-term harm (Willems, 1977). In addition to the specified targeted variables, other features of the social environment may be altered unintentionally for better or worse. It is important to evaluate potential negative outcomes. While there are no standard procedures for measuring unplanned outcomes, general procedures involve extending measurement or probes into longer time periods, measuring multiple behaviors, and assessing the behaviors of others in the social environment.

Making Data-Based Changes When Necessary

Interventions require data-based modifications. Time-series methods based on single-case research designs are appropriate for this function. Time-series methods may be used to monitor trends in behavior, and the effects of interventions. Guidelines for data-based decision making are included in the final section of the chapter. A practitioner-oriented overview of single-case designs is presented in Chapter 5.

Planning for Generalization

Many interventions necessarily begin with a limited set of objectives, are limited by setting or circumstance, and are characterized by a relatively high degree of control. Strategies for generalization frequently need to be a part of assessment–intervention plans from the outset, and special care must be taken when intervention planning does not occur within natural settings.

In this section, we review principles of generalization programming, drawing on the work of Stokes and Osnes (1986, 1988, 1989), which updates the classic paper by Stokes and Baer (1977).

According to Stokes and Osnes (1989, p. 338),

> Generalization . . . refers to the outcome of behavior change and therapy programs, resulting in effects extraneous to the original targeted changes. This occurs in the absence of comprehensive programming across stimuli, responses, and time. In therapeutic activities, these effects are sought across clients, stimulus conditions and settings, and behaviors.

Maintenance of behaviors is indicated by the durability of intervention outcomes over time. It is not enough to intervene and hope for effects that generalize and are maintained. For professionals, the issue is how to identify or plan for functional variables in the natural environment that will enhance generalization programming.

Stokes and Osnes (1986, 1988, 1989) discuss three principles and 12 tactics to promote generalization.

1. *Take advantage of natural communities of reinforcement.* Preschool and family environments have considerable potential for establishing the generality of skills development. Thus, target behavior selection is guided by the degree to which changes in behavior are likely to achieve "entry into the natural reinforcement community of the child" (Baer & Wolf, 1970; Stokes & Osnes, 1986). This principle focuses the analysis of generalization to settings (Stokes & Osnes, 1989). The principle requires an understanding of the arrangement of antecedents, responses, and consequences that influence behavior in "natural communities" of reinforcement.

a. *Contact natural consequences.* Stokes and Osnes (1989) stressed that *relevant* behaviors be taught. The rationale is that useful and adaptive behaviors are more likely to be maintained or elicited by natural communities of reinforcement. "Perhaps the most fundamental guideline . . . is to teach behaviors that are likely to come into contact with powerful reinforcing consequences that do not need to be programmed by a . . . behavior change agent" (p. 341).

b. *Recruit natural consequences.* Training may focus on both the frequency and skill of behavior, but, also, individuals in the environment may need to be recruited or trained to "notice and pay off" the appropriate behavior (p. 342).

c. *Modify maladaptive consequences.* Maladaptive consequences may be maintaining inappropriate behaviors; if these are eliminated, appropriate behaviors may be more easily developed and maintained. Environments may be supporting maladaptive behaviors and may need to be modified. An example is misplaced positive social consequences for inappropriate behavior.

d. *Reinforce occurrences of generalization.* Any occurrence of generalization should be noticed, valued, and followed by consequences that may reinforce the behavior. Plan for the conditions to facilitate generalization, but also take advantage of unplanned examples of appropriate behavior.

2. *Train diversely.* Changing to less rigid programming with greater variation in training and antecedent stimuli, responses, and consequences, may have a greater impact on generalization.

e. *Use sufficient stimulus exemplars.* A stimulus exemplar is a training condition. The tactic involves factors such as using multiple trainers and settings or locations.

f. *Use sufficient response exemplars.* These exemplars are different, appropriate child behaviors used in training. It is often necessary to train for response classes of behaviors rather than specific behaviors, in order for generalization to occur. Examples include teaching a variety of appropriate greetings, play entry skills, and play behaviors.

g. *Make antecedents less discriminable.* Also referred to as "loose training" (Stokes & Baer, 1977), this suggestion involves varying the conditions of training. An example is incidental learning based on interactions that the child initiates naturally.

h. *Make consequences less discriminable.* Strategies for increasing the likelihood for generalization include using intermittent reinforcement schedules, increasing the delay for presenting the consequences, and making the therapist's presence less predictable.

3. *Incorporate functional mediators.* Mediators are stimuli that facilitate generalization. They need to be easy to produce or must be present under relevant conditions. Stokes and Osnes (1989) give the following examples:

i. *Incorporate common salient physical stimuli* (or objects). A strategy to help with generalizing behaviors includes the presence of the same or similar stimuli in both the training and generalization setting. Posting pictures of rules for activity centers in preschool classrooms is an example.

j. *Incorporate common salient social stimuli.* This tactic involves using specific people or gestures to facilitate generalization through appropriate behaviors that become associated with their presence. Peer training in social skills serves as an important example. Another is the use of brief, preplanned signals between caregiver and child as a prompt for behavior.

k. *Incorporate self-mediated physical stimuli.* This strategy involves the use of a stimulus that is maintained and carried by the child as a reminder for specific behaviors. Self-monitoring techniques may be used in this way.

l. *Incorporate self-mediated verbal and covert stimuli.* These strategies generally relate to verbalizations and thought. Correspondence training, discussed in later chapters, is an example.

Behavioral fluency as a criterion of performance increases the potential for maintenance, transfer of skill to new situations, and positive affect related to mastery of a skill (Binder, 1996; see Chapter 5).

In summary, planning for maintenance and generalization is a requirement of intervention design. Another related skill is that of *adaptation*. Adaptation changes the focus from the use of a skill in different settings, and over time, to being able to modify the skill "to meet the requirements of changing demands or conditions" (Wolery et al., 1988, p. 61).

Naturalistic Interventions

Beyond establishing a research foundation, there are several basic reasons for examining naturalistic interventions. First, interventions vary greatly in the demands that are made upon participants. For parents and teachers, the more closely an intervention fits the caregiver's current situation, skills, and plans, the more effective and acceptable it is likely to be.

Second, frequently, interventions are accomplished in specific training environments, which may be considerably different from nontraining environments. To facilitate generalization to other settings, new activities and caregiver behaviors will need to be introduced. In designing interventions with generalization as an objective, Stokes and Osnes (1989) wrote, "Generalization programming seems to be well served by providing the least artificial, least cumbersome, and most natural positive consequences in programming interventions. Such programming most closely matches naturally occurring consequences and their entrapment potential" (p. 341). Introduced earlier, "entrapment" refers to the process whereby relatively simple behaviors lead to general behavioral change because they are "trapped" by reinforcement that occurs in existing environments (Baer & Wolf, 1970). Assumptions are that techniques in natural settings will parallel those used in training settings, and that trainers and caregivers will work collaboratively to plan and evaluate interventions. A prototypical example is that of naturalistic language training (Hart, 1985).

Third, naturalistic intervention design also stresses existing caregiver competencies and thus may serve to enhance their feelings of efficacy. Children who are hard to teach or parent may have devastating effects on a caregiver's self-confidence.

Plans for naturalistic interventions are based on the analysis of caregivers' actual roles, routines, skills, and interests. Assessment plans can identify (1) a range of treatment options based on research and functional analyses; (2) naturally occurring parent or teacher intervention strategies that are likely to be successful as implemented, or with changes, guidance, and feedback; or (3) interventions that may be adapted to evident styles of parenting or teaching.

Of interest to the consultant are successful naturalistic strategies, partially successful strategies, and skills that may be built upon, and the interventions that may readily fit caregiver's situations. For example, interviews and observations may reveal that caregivers use techniques that are consistent with other successful interventions. However, they may not be aware of the importance of their behaviors. Therefore, a role of the consultant may be to evaluate emerging skills of caregivers that can be further enhanced through consultation, practice, and feedback. Planning can be directed to the naturally occurring approximations to successful strategies. Naturalistic intervention design includes modifying or extending caregiver interventions or identifying interventions that may be easily incorporated into the routines of caregivers.

Data-Based Decision Making

Interventions require data-based modifications. Single-case accountability or research designs may be used to monitor trends in behavior and the effects of interventions. They can be applied broadly to philosophically different interventions and may be used to track behaviors when decisions are made not to intervene. This topic is resumed in Chapter 5.

"'Decision rules' are procedures which guide the evaluation of information to determine if changes in methods and/or content are necessary" (Liberty, 1988, p. 55). Wolery et al. (1988), building on the work of White and Haring (1980), and Haring, Liberty, and White (1980), provide guidelines for altering instructional strategies using data-based decisions.

If the guidelines discussed below are to be used, four requirements must be met. First, the goal for intervention and a date by which the goal is to be attained must be specified. "A well-specified goal is stated as a full behavioral objective, including the acts to be performed, the conditions, and the standards or levels of accomplishment" (Sulzar-Azaroff & Mayer, 1991, p. 290). Second, intervention effectiveness is determined by analyzing trend lines or "lines of progress" and "minimum 'celeration lines" drawn from the present level of performance to the point at which the goal is reached. The line describes the rate of change or progress needed for the child to reach a desired goal. Third, as the data are graphed, intervention effectiveness is monitored frequently by comparing the data to the minimum 'celeration line. Fourth, treatment integrity of the intervention must be ensured.

Once these initial requirements are met, data-based decision guidelines can then be used to determine whether intervention modifications are needed. Guidelines described by Wolery et al. (1988, pp. 133–137) can assist the practitioner in monitoring trends in behaviors and the need for instructional or procedural changes.

1. If correct responses are increasing and errors are decreasing or stable, no modifications are necessary, and the intervention should be continued (with modification of definitions, various behaviors or skills may be monitored in a similar fashion). The minimum 'celeration line is used to check progress toward goals.

2. If only some (e.g., 20–50%) of the tasks are performed consistently, the intervention is having limited success or progress is stalled. The intervention should be "sliced back" to skills the child is able to perform, while teaching one or two new steps in the sequence at a time. High error rates along with some successes also may reveal the need to try a different instructional procedure.

3. If correct responses are near zero, the intervention is having no success. The task is too difficult. The decision should be to step back and teach earlier, prerequisite skills.

4. If correct responses are highly variable or decrease significantly, the assumption is that the child can complete a task but does not. Compliance training may be needed.

5. If correct responses are stalled at a fairly high level (say, 80–90% correct) but rate is not improving, different contingencies or incentives and additional practice time may be required. The child may be bored, and it may be necessary to consider moving to a new phase of learning to build fluency.

6. If a child has met the specified criteria for accuracy and fluency (or rate), it is time to introduce a new skill. The learned skill may serve as a foundation for subsequent skills, and continued practice may be necessary.

The use of formal decision rules to improve practice for children with severe instructional and behavioral problems is gaining substantial attention. For further reading, we recommend Evans and Meyer (1985) and the edited book by Haring (1988).

Putting It Together: PASSKey

Ecobehavioral components including planned activities and strategic sampling of these activities have been combined in an assessment–intervention package termed PASSKey, which stands for *Planned Activity, Strategic Sampling,* and *Keystone Variable.* Presented earlier, waking day and problem-solving interviews, observations, curriculum-based measurement, and collaborative consultation are used to uncover significant planned activities and keystone variables within these activities. Keystone variables have the potentially widest range of positive consequences with regard to significant response classes as well as collateral behaviors. From observations, (in natural situations and possibly through a functional analysis) and within the consultation process, intervention plans are developed into scripts that detail intervention steps in a natural language and problem context. Validity evidence for PASSKey procedures may be found in Barnett, Bell, et al. (1997) and Barnett, Air, et al. (in press). Features of the model are summarized in Table 4.2.

TABLE 4.2.   Overview of PASSKey

1. *Planned Activities* in school, home, or community settings.
   * Use the Waking Day Interview and the Problem Solving Interview.
   * Examine the daily schedule important to family or classroom routines.
   * Consider the predictability or stability of daily activities.
   * Look for especially difficult *and* successful activities or times of the day.

2. *Strategic Sampling* of child behaviors and activities.
   * From Planned Activities, decide when to specifically observe the child's behavior.
   * Choose methods for observing and recording behavior (and other variables).
   * Observe the situation sufficiently to determine patterns of behaviors or interactions.

3. *Keystone Behaviors (or Variables)*
   * To keep the child safe.
   * Prerequisites for further progress.
   * Help socialization and help the child avoid rejection.
   * Behaviors which are important to parents' and teachers' roles.

4. *Scripts or Intervention Plans*
   * Written or pictorial personalized and detailed guidelines.
   * For providing instructions or managing behaviors or routines.
   * Based on natural caregiver–child interactions.
   * Designed to meet specified goals.

5. *Accountability*
   * Is the script or intervention plan being implemented as intended?
   * Is the plan comfortable and feasible?
   * Are there desired changes in targeted behaviors or variables?
   * What changes or revisions need to be made?

SUMMARY AND CONCLUSIONS

This chapter focused on conceptual and research-based strategies for selecting target variables and intervention methods. The selection process goes beyond the technical aspects of assessing behavior; it requires judgments that may range from straightforward to complex. At the focal point are general planning guidelines for practitioners. Specific attention also is required for the maintenance and generalization of behavior. Evaluating interventions for both intended and unintended results is critically important.

Intervention design is guided by the results of assessment. Since assessment results may be fallible, so may intervention design. We stressed the basics: ecobehavioral principles and collaborative problem-solving methods. While not fail-safe, these methods facilitate the analysis of problem situations, decision reliability (the convergence of decisions across reasonable approaches to assessment), and decision validity (which emphasizes the personal and social outcomes of decisions). The acronym PASSKey was used to emphasize organization of the process by parents' and teachers' planned activities, the identification of keystone variables, since most problem behaviors can be described or organized in many ways, and strategic sampling of planned activities because the sampling dilemmas have received insufficient attention in practice.

CHAPTER 5

◆◆◆

Evaluating Intervention Design and Outcomes

◆

Effective and accountable practice is guided by the ongoing evaluation of intervention design and outcomes. We approach evaluating interventions with young children in four ways. First, concepts from measurement theory that apply to intervention-based assessment are reviewed. Second, we link those concepts to the problem-solving process. Third, we address accountability through the use of single case experimental designs. Last, we review ethical and legal frameworks for intervention practice.

THE RELIABILITY AND VALIDITY OF TARGET VARIABLE SELECTION

The questions addressed by the reliability and validity of target variables include the amount of agreement between observers on the measured behaviors and if the behaviors selected are the most useful as targets for change. Overall, many factors influence target variable selection, and the quality of the assessment must be established for the individual case.

Reliability of Target Variable Selection

Research has demonstrated the potential for considerable differences when selecting behaviors for change. For example, Wilson and Evans (1983) sent descriptions of childhood disorders to a sample of members of the Association for Advancement of Behavior Therapy. The profiles described children experiencing fearful and anxious behavior; conduct disordered and disobedient behavior; and withdrawn, shy, introverted behavior.

For the major research questions, the psychologists were asked (1) to judge if treatment appeared necessary, (2) to indicate the child's major difficulty, (3) to identify treatment goals, and (4) to indicate and rank order intervention targets. Agreement on the decision to intervene was high while agreement on specific target behaviors was generally quite low (38.6% across all conditions). Although the study was not based on actual problem behaviors, it does serve to warn professionals of potential disagreement in selecting target behaviors.

Validity of Target Variable Selection

The *effects* of selecting different target variables fall under the topic of validity. There is not necessarily a direct correspondence between the accurate description of a particular behavior and its implications for intervention. Target variable selection is guided by the likely probability of changing a current or future problem situation (Kanfer, 1985). Challenges include understanding complex setting and behavior interactions, covariations of responses, sequences of events, and selecting appropriate treatments for target variables.

Construct Validity

Many constructs, such as conduct disorders and social skills, now appear in the behavioral literature; thus, construct validity has increasing relevance to target variable assessment. Messick (1995) views construct validity as unifying other validities. Foremost for the present discussion, it is important to select appropriate measures to help define and describe a problem area—an issue of construct validity (Hayes & Nelson, 1986).

When the assessment is focused on an individual child, the *personal constructs* used by the caregivers and psychologists also are important. Personal constructs (Kelly, 1955) are those that individuals use to "perceive, think, interpret, and experience the world" (Mischel, 1981, p. 486). For example, the degree that interventions fit parents' or professionals' beliefs about interventions, presumed causes of behaviors and the possibility for change will influence effort in carrying out interventions (e.g., learned vs. inherited and inevitable behavior). This underscores the importance of understanding the values, beliefs, and attributions related to hypothesized causes of behaviors of caregivers and consultants.

Content Validity

"Content" pertains to adequate sampling of a behavior. Content validity has been termed the cornerstone of behavioral assessment (Linehan,

1980; Strosahl & Linehan, 1986). Content validity requires the consideration of the following: (1) "specification of the behaviors of interest"; (2)
settings where the behaviors are likely to be of interest; (3) tasks, expectations, and instructions for the situation; and (4) "self-generated" stimuli
that may influence the performance (Strosahl & Linehan, 1986, p. 34).
One example is in the assessment of noncompliant child behaviors
(Barkley, 1997; Forehand & MacMahon, 1981). Examining content validity of an assessment technique for noncompliance may include (1) behaviors—whining, having tantrums, ignoring parental commands; (2) settings
and situations where the behavior is evident, such as home, car, shopping,
or school; (3) qualities of commands or requests that are reasonable, developmentally appropriate, clearly stated, given in close proximity to the
child, with appropriate consequences (praise, positive attention, effective
reprimand, discipline), and given at a contextually appropriate schedule or
rate; and (4) management of potentially interfering factors such as
parental anger, depression, or helplessness.

Criterion-Related Validity

Traditionally, criterion-related validity refers to the correlation between a
measure (e.g., ratings of play behaviors) and a criterion of performance
(e.g., observations of play behaviors). Criterion-related validity has been
applied both to current (concurrent validity) and future status (predictive
validity).

   The intervention implications of this type of validity were examined
by Kazdin (1985). Concurrent validity includes relationships between the
target behavior and other measures of the problem, other behaviors related to possible syndromes, and the impact of the target behavior on the
child's daily functioning. Predictive validity addresses effectiveness of target behaviors over long time periods.

   Examining the social skills of young children provides an example of
the questions addressed by criterion-related validity. Many converging
lines of research point to the significance of social development in the early years and its impact on overall development. However, deciding upon
specific strategies to improve social skills requires considerable planning
and falls under the validity of target variable selection. An unlimited number of potential social skills variables may be measured (e.g., eye contact,
greeting others, aggressive behaviors, specific play skills), and concurrent
validity would help answer the question of the relationships between various measures and criteria related to social behavior. Behaviors linked to
improving social skills should have as criteria changes in everyday functioning with peers across a variety of tasks and situations. Thus, as examples, criterion measures for intervention design may include successfully

joining peer play and increasing the length of successful play bouts. Behaviors related to discrete social skills (such as improving greetings) may be important, but their relationship to improved overall success in play for a specific child is a question that must be answered empirically by applying valid criteria.

Not all interventions related to social skills pertain to social behaviors of the target child. Some important variables related to social acceptance, such as physical attractiveness (Strain, 1985), require very different interventions. Also, for many reasons discussed throughout, social skills change efforts frequently involve peers.

Social Validity

This is concerned with defining socially significant problems for behavioral change, and establishing and obtaining goals through procedures acceptable to the immediate social community (Kazdin, 1977; Wolf, 1978). Practically speaking, parents and teachers contribute to selecting targets for change, interventions, and measures of intervention success. Furthermore, they help determine the significance of outcomes. Ideally, these judgments inform practice throughout intervention design and evaluation (Schwartz & Baer, 1991).

There are two general methods that stem from this approach. First, social validity involves social comparisons. For example, peer group (or individual) performance of the target behavior may help differentiate adept from inadequate performance and may suggest behaviors for change. This is essentially a normative approach to target behavior selection (see discussion of template matching and micronorms in previous chapters).

Second, social validity involves subjective evaluations or opinions by others who are in a position to judge the adequacy of functional skills or behavior, acceptability of methods, and improvements in such behaviors. Parents, teachers, and community members all serve in this capacity.

In summary, technical adequacy concepts applied to intervention design are not well developed. However, implicitly or explicitly, considerations regarding reliability and validity of target behavior selection are a part of every intervention design. No assessment strategy guarantees selecting reliable and valid target behaviors or intervention goals. We believe that the technical questions of reliability and validity are best addressed through the foundations of ecobehavioral analysis, collaborative problem solving, and functional assessments. Ultimately, questions of target variable and intervention validity are assessed through the evaluation of intervention outcomes.

THE TECHNICAL ADEQUACY
OF INTERVENTION DESIGN[1]

For legal, ethical, and professional reasons, the technical adequacy of the entire decision-making process requires scrutiny. We recommend sequential decision making based on problem solving, in contrast to diagnostic or classification decisions. Sequential decisions focus on the most reasonable steps in the assessment–intervention process.

   Reliability in problem solving refers to the consistency, or dependability of decisions made about plans or interventions. Reliability affects the interpretations and confidence given to information considered in the decision process, the stability of decisions, and predictions regarding future behaviors. *Validity* refers to whether or not the decisions made are likely to lead to beneficial changes for the child, parents, or other caregivers over long time periods in significant areas of behavior and/or development (Messick, 1989; Wolf, 1978). In the discussion that follows, we use these concepts to illustrate potential points of analysis for each step of the problem-solving process.

Problem Identification

Key Tasks

The primary focus of problem identification is defining and clarifying concerns in specific terms. To accomplish that goal, the problem situation(s) should be described in concrete, behaviorally descriptive terms that are both observable and measurable. Problem descriptions should include expected behaviors, current levels of performance, and characteristics of settings that impact the problem situation. Because problem situations often are complex and multifaceted, it may be necessary to break the problem into component parts, and, subsequently, to prioritize or sequence objectives.

Technical Adequacy Issues

Questions about the reliability of problem identification focus on likely sources of variability in decisions, including alternative sources of assessment information (such as different persons, interviews, observation techniques) and the strategies used to integrate information and develop coherence across multiple sources. Major points of analysis include the

---

[1]This section is adapted from Macmann et al. (1996). Copyright 1996 by Division 16, American Psychological Association. Adapted by permission.

following: (1) Do the results of interviews, raters, observations, and other data sources agree or disagree on concern(s)? (2) Do each of the participants agree on prioritization? Numerous strategies are available to clarify concerns and deal with disagreements, such as collecting additional data in order to help define problem areas and actively negotiating mutually agreed upon goals and rationales for target selection across participants.

The reliability issues have implications for validity. For example, failure to achieve consensus on problem identification suggests that the outcomes of the process may be differentially acceptable to all participants. Even when consensus is achieved, targets that can be reliably measured may not accurately reflect the broader ecology of caregiver concerns. Errors in problem identification can influence the outcomes of the entire problem-solving process (Bergan & Tombari, 1976). Basic questions related to validity include: (1) Do the problem areas represent significant concerns that interfere with parenting or teaching? (2) Does the child's behavior(s) or developmental progress place him/her at risk with regard to adaptive functioning and transitions to less restrictive and future environments? (3) How well have the theoretical and empirical foundations of problem identification been incorporated in the decision-making process?

Problem Analysis

Key Tasks

In the second phase of problem solving, the focus shifts away from description to questions about factors contributing to the problem situation and how the problem situation is structured. In attempting to understand the contextual variables that are contributing to the discrepancy between current and expected levels of performance, all factors that may influence the problem situation—both directly and indirectly—need to be analyzed.

Consideration should be given to factors serving as obstacles inhibiting desired performance and also to those that might serve as supportive factors or resources in problem resolution. The information collected during problem analysis is used to make decisions about possible areas for intervention planning (such as changes in caregiving environments that are likely to lead to desired results).

Technical Adequacy Issues

The central question for reliability is: Do all participants agree on the significant elements contributing to the problem? Different personal causal theories may lead to significantly different plans and outcomes. Thus, the reliability issues have implications for validity as well, and it is critical to have participants focus on the features of problem situations that are both amenable to modification and likely to produce desired changes.

The primary validity question raised is: What evidence exists that the identified factors contribute to the problem? The quality of the evidence may vary (ranging from armchair speculation to empirical analyses of functional relationships). Additional validity questions pertain to the contributions of problem analysis to plan development and treatment outcomes.

Plan Development and Implementation

Key Tasks

At this phase of problem solving, the focus turns to developing and implementing an intervention plan (or sequence of plans) in order to resolve the problem situation. Several specific tasks are undertaken in this phase, including exploring alternative strategies, selecting intervention(s), clarifying intervention plans, and implementing the chosen intervention(s).

In deciding what can be changed to resolve the current problem situation, consideration must be given to the acceptability of intervention plans and to the accessibility of resources, or feasibility of developing resources (e.g., caregiver training, materials), needed for implementation. Moreover, to be effective, interventions must be logically and empirically related to the identified problem and to the reasons that the problem situation exists. Therefore, the exploration and selection of intervention strategies must be based on specific information derived from problem analysis. Emphasis is placed on the selection and development of the most natural, least intrusive, and most effective strategy for accomplishing change.

Prior to implementation of an intervention plan, clarification of every component of the intervention plan and the responsibilities of each participant is needed. Specifically, it must be decided who will do what, when, where, and how.

Technical Adequacy Issues

Regarding plan development and implementation, the major reliability question is: Do all participants agree on the details of the plan? Different communication strategies, or combinations of empirical strategies, may be effective in developing consensus, including replanning, trial periods to work on plans, and further data collection.

As for validity, the following issues emerge. Is the plan likely to bring about desired changes? Is the plan workable? Is the plan linked to intervention research? Because the answers to each of these questions may vary across participants, reliability issues are embedded in the analysis as well.

Plan Evaluation

Key Tasks

The plan evaluation phase of problem solving focuses on determining how well the intervention plan is working and outlining subsequent steps. First, data collected through ongoing assessment should be examined to determine if the progress made toward goals is adequate. In order to fully understand the outcome, it also is necessary to evaluate the implementation of the intervention plan to determine if plans were carried out as intended (referred to as treatment integrity). Side effects and collateral behaviors should be evaluated as well. Last, decisions must be made regarding the desirability and feasibility of conducting experimental analyses (such as removing and then re-establishing an intervention in order to evaluate the effects of intervention). Depending on the extent to which the current intervention strategies have been successful in bringing about desired changes in the problem situation, participants may need to decide whether and how plans need to be changed. Accountability methods from single case designs serve as the building blocks for plan evaluation.

Technical Adequacy Issues

A major question is the reliability of treatment implementation: Is the intervention being carried out as planned? To answer the question, parents and professionals must look at (1) the occasions when the intervention is implemented, and (2) the steps described in the intervention or plan (Gresham, 1989; LeLaurin & Wolery, 1992). In those situations where occasions for implementing the intervention are missed, or individual steps are skipped or added, it may be important to determine whether the plan needs to be revised, resources need to be added, or motivation or other factors are issues to be examined. Parents and teachers may need to make revisions or changes to intervention plans, but changes need to be communicated to all team members.

Reliability issues pertain to the measurement of intervention outcomes. For example, do observers agree on occurrences (successful play bouts with other children) or nonoccurrences (aggression) of the targeted behavior? The primary validity question relates to treatment outcome: Is the plan leading to the desired changes? Ecological considerations suggest that the adequacy of plans needs to be evaluated over long time periods, including an analysis of collateral outcomes for others within the child's settings. For many reasons, outcome measures may not converge on conclusions about intervention effectiveness. Also important, measures selected may be differentially sensitive to change (Lipsey, 1990).

DETERMINING INTERVENTION OUTCOMES: ACCOUNTABILITY DESIGNS

Two basic reasons for selecting single-case research designs are to evaluate the effectiveness of interventions and to compare the effects of alternative treatments.

Key Features and Designs

Single-case accountability designs generally have at least three important facets: (1) measures of stability, level, and trend of behavior; (2) an introduction of a well-specified intervention while maintaining the measurement procedures; and (3) the evaluation of intervention outcomes over substantial time periods. The outcomes of observations are graphically represented. The visual presentation of data is used to help overcome the natural limitations of interpreting complex assessment information.

Conditions and Design Notations

"Conditions" refer to stable procedures for different phases of the assessment–intervention process. The data in each condition are used to (1) provide information about current performance, (2) predict future performance, and (3) test predictions from previous phases or evaluate interventions (Kazdin, 1982b). Throughout an intervention, specified conditions must remain consistent if comparisons are to be made over time.

   "Baseline" is the term used to describe behavior *before* the intervention is implemented (or when the intervention is temporarily withdrawn). Another important and realistic view is that baseline data reflect the intervention that is in effect in the environment before a new intervention begins. Level, variability, and trend are used to describe behavioral patterns. Level refers to frequency or prevalence of behavior; variability refers to relative differences in level among observation sessions in the same condition. For example, a child may have three tantrums on Wednesday and eight on Thursday. Trends are noted across observation sessions and may reflect improving, stable, or deteriorating situations, or observations may be too variable to be characterized by trends. In graphing baseline and intervention phases, the horizontal axis represents time (days or sessions) and the vertical axis represents a quality of behavior (frequency, rate of behavior, prevalence). In some cases, a baseline may be *reconstructed* using archival records such as attendance or discipline notes (Bloom & Fisher, 1982). *Retrospective* baselines result from histories given by caregivers (Gelfand & Hartmann, 1984). Reports of specific acts such as firesetting or bedwetting may serve as retrospective baselines. Because of errors of memory and verbal reports, retrospective baselines should be used only with discrete and salient acts or behaviors having zero (e.g., *"never* sleeps throughout the night") or 100% rates of occurrence (e.g., *"tantrums* every time we shop" or "wets every night").

The baseline condition is called Phase A. Different intervention phases are labeled B, C, and so on. Combined treatments are noted through letters depicting discrete components (e.g., B-C may stand for differential reinforcement plus time out). The use of a prime (B′, B″ B‴) indicates that slight deviations from the B intervention were used. Evaluating these systematic changes are basic for designs that look at the duration and frequency of an intervention. Examples include varying the length of time out, or the time interval used for a DRO (Differential Reinforcement of Other behavior).

If an intervention was ineffective, it serves as a baseline for the next intervention. However, when baseline phases are alternated with intervention phases, the second and subsequent baselines may be altered by the effects of interventions and they are not exactly comparable to the preintervention baseline.

Preexperimental Phase

Researchers hardly ever describe this phase, but an important consideration in planning interventions is making the intervention as natural as possible and simplifying and refining the steps as much as possible (Kara & Wahler, 1977).

B-Only Designs

This represents an intervention case study, not a true design or even a quasi-experimental design, but it can be used for intervention decisions and for accountability. The B notation indicates that a treatment was monitored throughout the intervention, but a baseline condition was not established. This might be done when intervening in crisis situations or consulting with a teacher or parent when an intervention is already in place. In fact, it may be highly unusual that a child is experiencing difficulty and nothing is being done. The B design may help evaluate naturalistic interventions, and while not acceptable from a research standpoint, it is still much more desirable than not evaluating an intervention. Conclusions can be made about behavior, but not in a way that specifically can be attributed to intervention effectiveness, because the natural course of the behavior is unknown. In other words, the child's behavior may have improved regardless of the intervention.

A-B Design

The A-B design is viewed as a cornerstone of accountability (Barlow, et al., 1984). It represents a baseline followed by an intervention condition. This is not a strong design for a research study to demonstrate validity for an intervention, but it is sufficient when the primary goal is to ascertain improved adaptation or skills development. There are many threats to interpretations for A-B designs because of potential unknown factors that may bring about change in behavior. At the same time, accountability designs have potential benefits. As an example, A-B and B-only designs were used in the Ohio Early Childhood Intervention Project to help document outcomes for individual cases and for overall project efficacy (Barnett, Bell, et al., 1997; Barnett, Air, et al., in press). Questions about behavior and interventions pertaining to the next designs may emerge in practice. A-B-A-B designs, alternating treatment designs, and design combinations, are frequently used to evaluate conditions for a functional analysis.

A-B-A-B or Withdrawal Designs

A-B-A-B designs are a part of the family of *within-series* designs that include A-B and B designs. The reason for using the A-B-A-B design is that it provides two chances to observe treatment effects and thus to strengthen conclusions (Figure 5.1). More complicated designs employing additional phase changes have been used to compare treatments or components of treatments. A related, strong practitioner design is represented by B-A-B (Bloom & Fischer, 1982). Sometimes researchers use the term "reversal" rather than withdrawal, but this has a different meaning (it applies to deliberately changing the direction of the intervention, such as reinforcing social interactions with children versus adults).

Some concerns about the withdrawal phase may be voiced, and so we summarize some of the attractive features of the design that fit the realities of professional practices. First, when the intervention is withdrawn and the behavior does not drop to baseline levels, there is evidence that

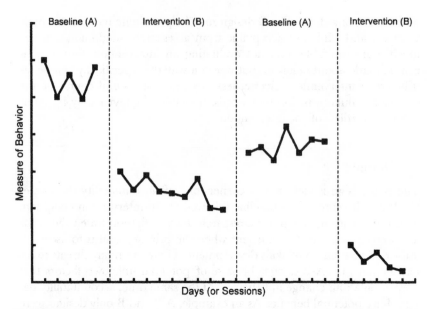

FIGURE 5.1. An example of an A-B-A-B or withdrawal design. From Barnett et al. (in press). Copyright 1999 by PRO-ED, Inc. Reprinted by permission.

the intervention effects may be durable. In this case, it is important not to provide unnecessary treatments. Second, the subsequent baseline does not have to be long. A possible misconception is that the withdrawal of the intervention is to "produce deterioration"; rather, it is to permit evaluation of treatment effects. Sometimes, a good rationale for caregivers is to "take a break" from the intervention and to "see where things are going." Also, since interventions cannot continue indefinitely, it is important to plan for withdrawals. Last, withdrawals may occur naturally due to illness or other circumstances. While they are not as convincing as planned withdrawals, these breaks still may help with the evaluation of interventions.

Changing-Criterion Designs

One logical way to view changing-criterion designs is that they are A-B designs on a repeated basis (Barlow, et al.,1984). They are useful when it is reasonable to specify a desired pattern of behaviors, and to change the objectives in a stepwise, gradual, or progressive fashion. Changing-criterion designs may be used for goal setting to accelerate or decelerate behaviors and to shape desired levels of performance. Shifts in criterion serve as replications of intervention effects (Figure 5.2). The design may be useful without a baseline condition.

Sainato, Strain, Lefebvre, and Rapp (1987) used a variation of a changing-criterion design applied to levels of teacher questions and the rate and quality of preschool children's group responses. Also, changing-criterion designs may be very useful for caregivers or children who feel initially overwhelmed by the magnitude of behavioral change needed. For example, the design may be useful for self-monitoring programs for parents to reduce shouting or excessive reprimands, or to set goals for children who are socially withdrawn. However, one potential problem is that set criteria may impede the potential for more rapid improvements (or make the study look bad) if progress is more rapid than set goals.

Multiple Baseline Designs

These designs often unfold naturally when the same intervention is considered across (1) settings (or instructional time periods), (2) different behaviors of a child, or (3) different children. Because concurrent measures are taken, the designs also can be used to study generalization (across settings, behaviors, or children). A basic assumption is that the target behaviors are independent but will respond to the same treatment. Two baselines are useful for practice; for research purposes, at least three are recommended.

An example of a multiple baseline design across settings is depicted in Figure 5.3. Such a design could be used to identify an effective treatment for a behavior in one setting (a resource room), to study the effectiveness of the intervention in another setting (the classroom), and to carry

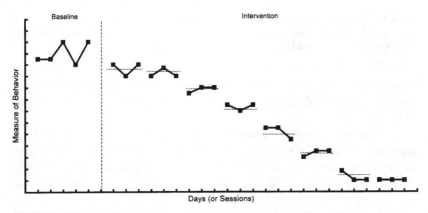

FIGURE 5.2. An example of a changing-criterion design. From Barnett et al. (in press). Copyright 1999 by PRO-ED, Inc. Reprinted by permission.

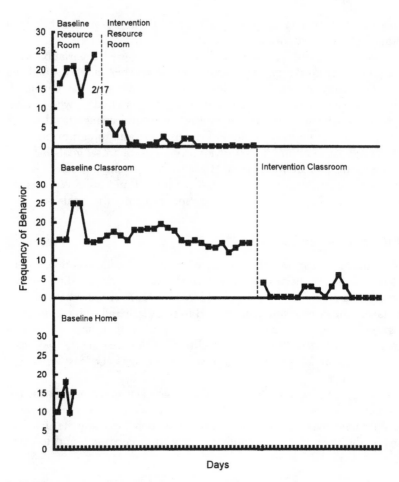

FIGURE 5.3. An example of a multiple-baseline design (across settings). From Poth and Barnett (1983). Copyright 1983 by the National Association of School Psychologists. Reprinted by permission of the publisher.

over the intervention to a third setting (the home environment). Poth and Barnett (1983) used this design to identify an effective treatment for a ticlike behavior.

Examples of multiple-baseline designs across behaviors may include separate baselines for whining, tantrums, and aggressive acts. Russo and Koegel (1977) used this design to evaluate the integration of a child with autistic behaviors by modifying, in turn, social behaviors, self-stimulation, and appropriate responses to verbal commands.

Multiple baselines also may be conducted across children. Several children in classes may have similar types of problem behaviors (such as social withdrawal). After a baseline period, an intervention may be implemented with one child, followed by other children who have similar problem behaviors. The Classroom Manager intervention (Sainato, Maheady, & Shook, 1986) provides an example of a multiple baseline across children described as socially withdrawn.

The *multiple-probe design* is an important variation of multiple-baseline designs (Horner & Baer, 1978). The major difference is that continuous measurement is not required. Instead, brief probes or data points are used to monitor baseline conditions and treatment effects. These practicalities are well suited for evaluating instruction, and when frequent measures are not feasible or may themselves result in unintended changes in behavior. An important assumption for the use of a multiple probe design is that the child's behavior or performance is stable and is unlikely to change without intervention. One application includes evaluating instruction for complex skills sequences.

Alternating-Treatment Designs

This design is useful for evaluating different interventions, since it involves the rapid, usually semirandom alteration, of two or more treatments. The question of relative effectiveness of interventions is ubiquitous in practice but is frequently associated with differences of opinion or judgment rather than data. The logic is that different levels of behavior will be associated with different conditions or interventions. Other designs used to compare interventions may be more cumbersome and lengthy (such as A-B-C-B-C).

Conditions may include treatment components, dimensions of treatment, time of day, settings, or behavior change agents. The rapid alteration can be based on natural units such as comparing interventions across similar morning versus afternoon conditions (e.g., free play, snack time, or bus behavior). Each time the child is scheduled for an intervention condition, it is alternated.

Another feature of the alternating-treatment design is that it can be used with or without a baseline condition. A modified baseline can be incorporated into the intervention by comparing an intervention condition to the data from an alternating nonintervention condition. (While useful, this baseline condition is not the same as a preintervention baseline or natural baseline.) The design also may be used with highly variable behavior. After comparing interventions, the alternating-treatment design ends with the more effective treatment (see Figure 5.4).

In this design, as with others, there are limits and potential problem areas. There may be confounding or interference between the conditions or interventions. Also, the conditions may be too brief to examine intervention outcomes. The design may need to be counterbalanced over

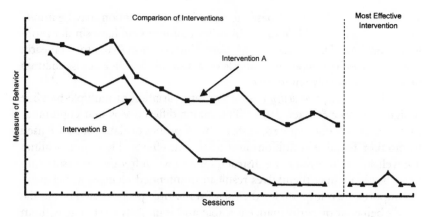

FIGURE 5.4. An example of an alternating-treatment design. From Barnett et al. (in press). Copyright 1999 by PRO-ED, Inc. Reprinted by permission.

many variables, such as teacher or time of day. For this reason, we recommend natural conditions as units of analysis.

Sherburne, Utley, McConnell, and Gannon (1988) used an alternating-treatment design, along with a withdrawal phase, to evaluate two interventions aimed at reducing violent and aggressive play. One condition included a contingent statement (a brief reminder and warning) and time out. The children were allowed to participate in violent theme play (involving guns, death, sounds of exploding bombs) only on a small rug identified for such use. Time out was used for occurrences of hitting, biting, and so on. A second condition, without the rug present, employed verbal prompts, inappropriate play was interrupted, and a suggestion was made to engage in alternative behavior. The two intervention conditions were counterbalanced across two free-play periods. While both procedures were successful when compared to the baseline condition, the first condition was more effective.

Interpretations of Data

Intervention Success

There are standard ways of visually evaluating the effectiveness of interventions, but even rather simple data sets can be complicated in their analyses (Parsonson & Baer, 1978). First, it is important to consider the number of data points in each phase and their adequacy for making conclusions. Within phases (e.g., baseline and intervention), it is important to look at level and trend changes, and the variability of data. For example, within a baseline phase, presumably without an intervention in effect, a child's performance may be increasing, decreasing, stable, or variable. Evaluating a child's variable performance, or a performance not predicted by the condition (e.g., improvements during baseline), may be an important step in intervention design. Procedures for evaluating variable performance within phases, assuming adequate measurement, include analyzing potential setting events discussed in the last chapter.

Similarly, changes that occur between phases or conditions are analyzed for level and trend differences. Immediate- and large-level and or trend changes during intervention, in the expected direction, demonstrate greater evidence for intervention effects. An intervention phase may show immediate positive effects that are not sustained, or variable intervention effects. Both lead to further consultation about intervention design or implementation.

Visual data analysis also has resulted in controversy (Furlong & Wampold, 1982; Greenwood & Matyas, 1990; Grigg, Snell, & Loyd, 1989). The major problem pertains to judgmental differences in interpreting data, and differences that stem from alternative ways data may be graphed.

Trend lines may help with interpretation, but there are different methods that may lead to slightly different results (Parker, Tindal, & Stein, 1992). Based on recommendations by Parker et al. (1992, Tukey II, p. 302), we outline the steps for drawing a trend line for individual phases: (1) Divide the data points in three equal parts with two vertical lines; (2) for all three parts, find the median value for the vertical axis (i.e., rate of performance) and the median for time (horizontal axis) and mark their coordinate points; (3) connect the first and third points; and (4) adjust the line up

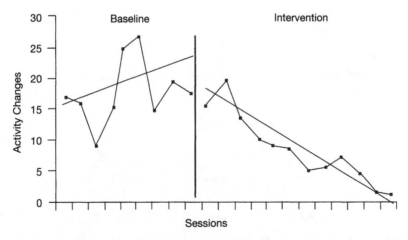

FIGURE 5.5. An example of drawing trend lines. From Barnett et al. (in press). Copyright 1999 by PRO-ED, Inc. Reprinted by permission.

or down by keeping it parallel to the intersect line one-third of the distance toward the middle coordinate point. Separate trend lines are drawn for each phase. Examples of trend lines for two different phases are presented in Figure 5.5.

Confidence in the Outcomes

Having confidence in outcomes rests on several foundations. Primary considerations are the measurable effects of an intervention on a child's behavior and the integrity with which an intervention is carried out. Figure

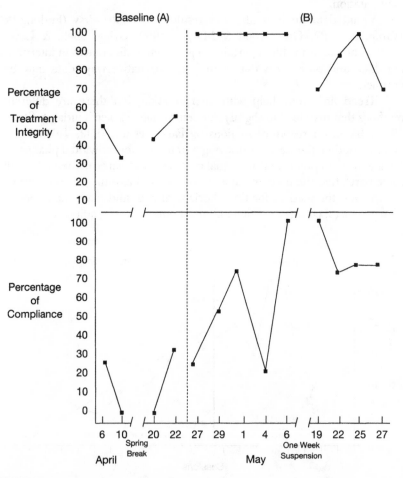

FIGURE 5.6. An example of coplotting outcome variables. From Barnett et al. (in press). Copyright 1999 by PRO-ED, Inc. Reprinted by permission.

5.6 combines these analyses by coplotting the data in order to help examine these relationships over time. One practical method to achieve additional confidence in the data is to coplot the results of a second observer; this could be carried out across the significant phases of the intervention (Kazdin, 1982b). We also have coplotted the ongoing results of social validity measurement in this way.

Figure 5.6 shows a data set for a child referred for noncompliance. Included are both treatment integrity data (top) and child data (bottom). In baseline observations, partial steps of an intervention were noted in narrative real-time observations (e.g., proximity, clear commands), but not always. The intervention consisted of developing a compliance training script. Elements of successful scripts may include sequences of steps (e.g., rule learning for the child to clarify expectations for behavior, practice with the behavior, starting with individually determined high probability requests such as "come here" said nicely, eye contact or proximity, giving choices, giving clear and developmentally appropriate requests). The top part of the figure continues, after a natural baseline, with estimates of the teacher's script use reported as a percentage of steps. The bottom part of the figure shows the child's data as a percentage of how often the child complied with requests. However, disciplinary actions should have been integrated into the intervention plans (note the 1 week suspension).

In summary, the essentials of having confidence in intervention outcomes include careful measurement of important personal, social, and contextual outcomes over substantial time periods (Wolf, 1978). Methods for coplotting data are more fully described in Ehrhardt et al. (1996).

Professional Practices and Time-Series Methods

Time-series methods are considered as fundamental to evaluating interventions, but there are difficulties and complexities in their use. First, *phases* are traditionally used in single-subject research to denote *consistent conditions*. However, outside of idealized research scenarios, conditions are only consistent to a degree. In practice, it is likely that conditions change in ways that are only partially revealed to the consultant. Changes in different ecologies can profoundly influence behavioral programs. The term "phase" in the present context reflects the consultant's understanding and working assumptions that are expressed as plans and professional behaviors. Phase changes also are related to the persistence of change agents and caregivers, their ability to cope with realities, and their creativity in responding to changing conditions.

A second potential point of concern is with the concept of internal validity, a requirement that is basic to outcome research. Internal validity pertains to evidence that the treatment—not external or extraneous factors—was responsible for the outcome. Threats to internal validity are well described by Kratochwill (1978); we briefly review several.

Multiple-treatment interference is a potential threat to internal validity if two or more interventions are introduced. Combinations of interventions make it difficult to determine which effects are attributable to a specific intervention. However, in practice, various intervention strategies are combined either deliberately or through parent and teacher embellishments (an issue of treatment integrity). While experimental design strategies that compare treatments may fit professional-practice circumstances, ideally, they need to be planned before starting the interventions. Most important, time-series methods can be used to evaluate an overall plan. Attributing success to individual facets of the plan may not be possible in many circumstances, but the evaluation of the overall plan is essential.

Another pertinent threat to internal validity involves reactive interventions (Kratochwill, 1978). These are similar to regression effects, where the professional intervenes in reaction to changes in the data. For example, if intervening in a crisis situation (B design), there is an increased probability that the situation will improve as a result of naturally occurring processes rather than (or in addition to) the planned intervention. Practical considerations should prevail and overrule the need to provide evidence for internal validity. Still, general time-series methods are appropriate for accountability in such circumstances.

Third, in many situations, the requirements of data collection are imposing. For example, it may not be feasible to obtain baseline data. In such cases, time-series methods can still be used to keep track of the trend of the behavior, and to adjust or replan interventions based on the data obtained (the B-only design). Also, the requirement of continuous data collection may be eased through the use of strategically planned time sampling, the use of probes, and the use of structured participant observations.

Fourth, it is necessary to assess outcomes in multiple ways, including behaviors that were not specifically treated and behaviors in alternative settings (sometimes termed "side effects"; Willems, 1977). This can be done by using a multibehavioral code and tracking caregivers' behavior, satisfaction with the intervention, and difficulties involved with maintaining behaviors. Outcomes may focus on *reducing* the necessity of some caregiver behaviors such as extensive monitoring or assistance.

Fifth, we would be remiss not to mention criticism of single-case designs (see Evans & Meyer, 1987, and the rebuttals by Test, Spooner, & Cooke, 1987; Meyer & Evans, 1993). Some of the traditions associated with design requirements and control features may not fit questions of practice. As other examples, rarely are parents or teachers concerned with carefully isolated behaviors. Furthermore, interventions achieved in highly controlled environments may not generalize to actual settings. As a final example, response covariation may be profitably studied through a multiple-baseline design, but this is the opposite of its traditional use.

In summary, time-series methods are an important means of determining changes that occur in behavior. To accommodate real-world exigencies, professionals can use "core elements" to evaluate the overall effectiveness of interventions (Hayes, 1981). The A-B design may be used for basic accountability. Most important, single-case designs imply that behavior is continuously assessed, as are the likely effects of well-defined and executed interventions.

LEGAL AND ETHICAL PRACTICE

Another significant way to evaluate intervention design and outcome is through close scrutiny of legal and ethical issues, and professional standards. There are tenuous links between theoretical perspectives related to changing children's behavior, research-based interventions, idealized measurement and intervention situations, and challenges and difficulties in applying what is known about intervention design to real-world practice. School district and building-level policies and practices are important in creating effective environments for professionals to provide services. Fundamental problems in many situations are the lack of resources, training, and support needed to fully implement and evaluate interventions in a manner consistent with exemplary practices. Also, researchers may not report critical features of interventions (Foxx, 1996) that practitioners are trying to carry out.

Psychological and educational services should be based on a coherent theoretical model, on appropriate research, and on a workable practitioner model. Given the absence of rules, formulas, and cookbook procedures, the best that can be offered are the foundations of assessment and intervention design, knowledge of effective interventions and practices that are applicable to young children and the roles of caregivers, problem-solving methods, and the creative, sensitive, and careful implementation and evaluation of professional plans. Professional practices often involve approximations to various ideals, but scientific methods can still be applied (Hayes, Follette, Dawes, & Grady, 1995).

Legal and Ethical Issues

There are numerous reviews of the legal and ethical implications of educational and psychological intervention decisions (Corrao & Melton,

1988; Martin, 1975; Rekers, 1984; Stolz & Associates, 1978). The field is quite complex and changing (e.g., Hart, 1991; Melton & Wilcox, 1989). The most significant changes are related to children's rights, use of research-based interventions, dignity as a guiding construct, reconfirmation of family (Hart, 1991; Hayes et al., 1995; Melton, 1991), and cautions about aversives. Certain legal foundations have been well established, including due process and equal protection. We review basic issues involved in designing and carrying out behavioral interventions.

Consent to Treatment

The major premise of consent to treatment is that clients are *informed* as to all relevant aspects of the intervention that are required for making decisions. In other words, informed consent "refers to the clients' right to decide whether they want to participate in a proposed program, after they have been told what is going to be involved" (Stolz & Associates, 1978, p. 30). There are three especially significant elements of informed consent.

1. *Competence.* "Competence refers to the individual's ability to make a well-reasoned decision, to understand the nature of the choice presented, and to give consent meaningfully" (Kazdin, 1984, p. 264).

2. *Knowledge.* "Knowledge . . . includes understanding the nature of treatment, the alternatives available, and the potential benefits and risks involved" (Kazdin, 1984, p. 264). One important aspect is that the pros and cons of intervening versus not intervening should be established as firmly as possible. In reality, this requires difficult predictions, or a "prognosis" (Rekers, 1984) based on research in developmental psychopathology and treatments regarding specific behaviors, classes of behaviors, or syndromes.

3. *Volition.* The client must agree to participate in treatment without duress. Voluntary consent means that the parent or guardian also has the right to withdraw consent without any condition or penalty. One potential danger is that the trappings of professional authority can be compelling; thus, the parent may feel considerable pressure to consent even though they may have questions or reservations about the intervention. At times, it may appear that consent for intervention is a condition for the child to remain in a childcare setting. The professional needs to be sensitive to these issues and should take proactive measures outlined in the subsequent section on intervention guidelines.

Determining consent is quite difficult in some cases. In practice, we have frequently advised parents to bring trusted family or community members to assist in the process. Within the context of Federal legislation, informed consent also means that requests are given in the parent or guardian's native language. Accommodating for adult literacy skills may be important. Communication should be jargon-free and easily understood.

Although parents are typically placed in a position to make intervention decisions for children, a growing body of literature has raised questions about a minor's so-called limited competence to consent, at least from elementary-age children upward. Many children can be involved in intervention planning to various degrees. Several authors have suggested a "Bill of Rights" for children in psychotherapy, including "The Right to Be Told the Truth," "The Right to Be Treated as a Person," "The Right to Be Taken Seriously," and "The Right to Participate in Decision Making" (Gelfand, Jenson, & Drew, 1982; Koocher, 1976; Ross, 1980). The findings of the American Psychological Association Commission on Behavior Modification suggest that obtaining consent from preschool children should be considered by the professional (Stolz & Associates, 1978). Children's rights also have been affirmed internationally (United Nations Convention on the Rights of the Child, 1991).

Sometimes, parents' and children's rights may conflict. Also, children's rights may take precedence over parents' rights in cases whereby parental behaviors present risks to children (Martin, 1975). This situation is discussed in a subsequent section.

Controversial Treatments

Many attacks on various forms of behavioral interventions have been made. Namely, these have involved aversive procedures such as punishment and time out, but have included other interventions such as token economies (e.g., Corrao & Melton, 1988; Repp & Singh, 1990). Corrao and Melton (1988) wrote:

> In legal terms, these [interventions] have been regarded as issues of mistreatment, abuse, and neglect. . . . Though they constrain the behavior therapist's discretion slightly, the resulting rules probably do so little more than common sense would in most cases, while serving to protect the health, safety, and welfare of minors in behavior modification treatment programs. (p. 391)

We include some interventions that have positive as well as negative consequences as components when data support their overall effectiveness. Many positive procedures discussed throughout the book may be used to potentially reduce the aversiveness of these interventions.

Another class of situations falls under experimental therapy (Barlow et al., 1984) when there are no known effective treatments. In these cases, informed consent and all of the other protections are necessary. However, given the requirements of informed consent under these circumstances, it will be impossible for information to be conveyed to parents or guardians concerning an intervention in any "complete" sense, because information is lacking about an intervention or novel applications of interventions. In such situations, the *uncertainty* needs to be communicated to parents or guardians.

Many widely disseminated interventions lack validity support. While this does not mean that they will be ineffective, it does mean that they cannot be used with great confidence, since the outcomes are unknown. Examples include various parent training programs. Such programs are proliferating due to the family emphasis of recent preschool legislation. Sapon-Shevin (1982) provided an extensive review of ethical issues surrounding parent training programs.

Protection for the Professional

While the client's rights have been clearly established, significantly, Griffith (1983) points out that many safeguards discussed here help protect the change agent as well.

> The issue of harm is as significant for the treating clinician as it is for the recipient client. An injured client, especially in situations where the treatment is questionable, has significant legal redress potential. If directed toward the clinician in the form of liability or malpractice litigation, the results are minimally professionally embarrassing, and quite possibly destructive in terms of liability. (pp. 328–329)

Guidelines for Intervention Programs

As protection for the child and change agent, and for those responsible for administering services, the consultant should adhere to general professional guidelines. Our review is based on guidelines developed by the Association for Advancement of Behavior Therapy (1977), the American Psychological Association (American Psychological Association, 1992; Stolz & Associates, 1978), the Association for Behavior Analysis (Van Houten et al., 1988), in addition to many other sources (National Association of School Psychologists, 1984a, 1984b). Martin (1975), Kazdin (1994) and Rekers (1984), have discussed these issues within a context of broader social values. Lovaas and Favell (1987) provided an analysis of protections for aversive interventions.

The fundamental principles are that selected intervention procedures are likely to be effective for the child and problem situation; that participants, parents, or guardians are fully aware and approve of the intervention, and that competent professionals are available to help carry out planned interventions. The end result logically may take the form of a contract whereby the conditions, goals, procedures, and roles are explicitly stated (Kazdin, 1984).

1. *Define and clarify who is the client.* The definition of the "client" may not be obvious in some circumstances. One important ethical and practical consideration is the possibility that the environment(s) and not children's behavior may need to be changed, or that both may need to be changed. For example, a child's activity level may be appropriate, but the parent's or teacher's developmental knowledge may lead to inappropriate expectations. In other cases, a child's behavior may be related to the caregiver's behavior or practices, and both the environment and the child's behavior may need to be addressed. As examples, a teacher may refer a child, but, based on the problem clarification, teacher behavior may be the focus of change efforts. Classroom management practices may need to be effective before individual behavior can be the focus of intervention. Likewise, parents may refer children, but depending on the problem behavior and intervention, most of the professional efforts may be toward modifying parental behavior. Family environments may be exacerbating problem behavior or may not support the most likely or promising intervention for a child's problem behavior.

More broadly, the client also may be defined as the institution or agency that employs the professional as a consultant. Institutions frequently have significant control over professional behavior. Ethical issues may arise when these relationships are not properly clarified. Thus, defining the *client* is important, because the client needs to be actively involved in intervention planning.

2. *Consider the ethics of target variable selection.* The result of consultation should be explicit written goals and methods to achieve those goals. An excellent device to test communication at key places is to have caregivers restate the goals and other significant features of the intervention program in their own words. One way to offer ethical "protections" and also to help decide on intervention targets and strategies is to clarify potentially different "systems of values and attitudes" that relate to a client's problems (Stolz & Associates, 1978, p. 22).

3. *Consider the ethics of intervention selection.* In practice, intervention design is guided by logical generalizations from research and idiographic problem solving. In essence, the client has a "right to an effective treatment"; the child should be receiving the most reasonable intervention available for the problem behavior (Gelfand & Hartmann, 1984, p. 20;

Van Houten et al., 1988). Thus, a major point of decision making involves the acceptability of interventions, the degree of empirical support for interventions, or the need for an experimental approach to intervention design. To help with the collaborative effort and to help prevent sources of bias, professional roles include assisting with the enumeration and evaluation of a range of intervention alternatives, including possible risks and benefits, and conducting a functional assessment. Related ethical considerations involve selecting the most natural, least intrusive, least restrictive, and least aversive intervention. However, these last four guidelines need to be balanced with considerations of potential effectiveness.

4. *Develop replicable procedures.* The specific treatment components and steps should be described in adequate detail. The reasons for this are at least twofold. First, it is an important element of informed consent. Second, it is basic to developing treatment integrity measures. This is why we emphasized the idea of script development in the last chapter.

5. *Obtain written and verbal permissions from parent, agency, teacher, (and perhaps child).* Even though agreed upon procedures are arrived at through parent and teacher consultation, they should also be obtained in writing. The intervention is described in a form of psychological report. Native language considerations also are important. Another significant aspect of consent is to clarify the individuals who have access to the information. The professional and agency are guided by established rules and procedures for such record keeping and review (Martin, 1975).

6. *Carefully select repeated measures to evaluate intended and potential unintended outcomes.* Multiple measures over appropriate time periods are necessary for evaluating interventions. Data should be analyzed and shared with parents or guardians. Possible harmful outcomes for others (classmates, teachers) need to be evaluated. While all interventions need to be evaluated in this regard, group contingencies and aversive procedures have been identified as being especially vulnerable with respect to unintended outcomes. Another example is that when using home–school notes or contingencies, a child's unmet criteria may result in unplanned aversive consequences for children of abusive parents (Kelley, 1990).

7. *Plan for intervention modifications, failures, follow-up, and transitions following intervention.* Plans should include an agreed upon time span for evaluating the intervention. Usually, this includes a brief trial period for the intervention based on predictions made from research (e.g., 3 days to 2 weeks, logically generalized from published studies). If similar interventions for other children have had relatively immediate effects, it is important to consult with parents during the first few days of an intervention. Expect that interventions need to be replanned or adjusted. Mutual agreement is necessary to replan an intervention or to refer the child, parent, or guardian to another professional or service agency for treatment based on

unsuccessful efforts. Planning for generalization is an explicit part of intervention design.

8. *Use professional, agency, and public review.* Accepted best practice dictates that professionals consult with others (supervisors, peers) regarding standards for practice and difficult or controversial situations. Memberships in relevant professional organizations are critical in this regard. Specific intervention decisions may affect the entire agency. Many agencies have functional teams and procedures to review service delivery to children, parents, and teachers. The goals of interventions, and the interventions themselves, should be open to such scrutiny and demystified.

9. *Ensure professional competence.* Two factors stand out. First, the behavior change agent should have experience or training in the procedures that will be used (Van Houten et al., 1988). Second, competent decisions need to be made on a case-by-case basis. This is why we developed the theme of technical adequacy of intervention design earlier in the chapter.

10. *When caregivers do not act in the best interest of the child.* Caregivers may be unable or unwilling to act in a manner consistent with the child's interests for a number of reasons related to competence, motivation, stressors, health, or psychopathology. At the same time, "[a] physical and social environment that is safe, humane, and responsive to individual needs is a necessary prerequisite for effective treatment" (Van Houten et al. 1988, p. 381). The professional cannot simply act as the agent of the parent (or school), but must determine how best to serve all those concerned in a situation. Gelfand and Hartmann (1984) wrote, "Therapists cannot respond automatically to requests to change a child's behavior but must independently assess their own ethical and legal responsibility in the matter" (p. 16). Such situations are typically ambiguous, and peer review, consultation with other professionals, and supervisory relationships under more experienced professionals are essential.

Some parents or guardians present dangers to children through lack of supervision or through specific acts of violence or forms of sexual or psychological abuse. In such cases, professionals must work within the context of accepted practices. In considering "best practices," guiding frameworks are legal requirements for reporting abuse and the empirically established validity support for intervention effectiveness.

11. *Interventions that require special considerations.* Interventions that fall under this category include the use of aversives, punishment, and group contingencies. The use of aversive techniques may be prevalent in the experiences of many children with severe learning and behavior problems, and their *ineffective use* (including reprimands, spanking, and time out) is an important point of parent and teacher consultation.

Specific permissions and agency review are recommended for all interventions. As discussed earlier, there is general support for the proposition that positive approaches should be used before aversives (e.g., Repp & Singh, 1990). Exceptions to this guideline were discussed by Axelrod (1990). The core issue is the use of the "least restrictive yet effective treatment" (Van Houten et al., 1988, p. 383). The situations for the use of punishment are tested by the question: "How urgent and important is it that a particular behavior cease?" (Axelrod, 1990, p. 63). Another important context is the analysis of positive features of the environment and whether there are potentially effective nonaversive procedures for changing behavior (LaVigna & Donnellan, 1986).

Punishment

The following steps, procedures, and considerations are typically employed for treatments considered as punishing or aversive (Green, 1990; Griffith, 1983; La Vigna & Donnellan, 1986; Lohrmann-O'Rourke & Zirkel, 1998; Lovaas & Favell, 1987; Matson & DiLorenzo, 1984; Repp & Singh, 1990).

1. Conduct risk appraisals and functional analyses to determine settings and variables that exacerbate or control the behavior, and consider nonaversive interventions whereby a new behavior that serves the same function is taught to replace the problem behavior (Foxx, 1996; Schrader & Gaylord-Ross, 1990).

2. The decision-making steps and criteria should be clearly specified for all in advance. The decision-making steps include establishing the need for intervention, the feasibility of carrying out an intervention within the present context or situation, the evaluation of prospective interventions, interdisciplinary team participation, and a written plan including goals and intervention components and steps specified in detail. High-quality data useful for decision making are essential (Lovaas & Favell, 1987).

3. "Insure the maximal amount of [positive] reinforcement possible in the environment" (Matson & DiLorenzo, 1984, p. 87). As Matson and DiLorenzo point out, time out, as an example, will not be effective unless the environment has attractive properties. Reduce, eliminate, or restructure frustrating or boring situations and long periods of inactivity related to the problem behavior (Foxx, 1996). Identify and define antecedent behaviors related to the problem behavior that may be helpful for caregivers in "interrupting the sequence of behaviors" and directing the child to more positive tasks (Matson & DiLorenzo, 1984, p. 91).

4. Restrictive use of time out may be commonly used by parents. Focal points of parent consultation include the search for less aversive means of control or discipline, parental monitoring of behavior and safety issues, and the evaluation of intervention effectiveness. The child should not be

able to hurt him- or herself, either intentionally or unintentionally. Thus, the room should be devoid of potentially harmful objects, and parents should remain in close proximity. In addition, potentially harmful objects in the child's possession may need to be removed. The procedures may be abused by being kept in effect too long, or by reducing the need to evaluate less aversive methods or positive intervention strategies (Axelrod, 1990).

5. If verbal prompts are used, as with time out, a "calm but firm voice" should be used (Matson & DiLorenzo, 1984, p. 88). Furthermore, the prompt should be a brief statement (e.g., "You are getting a time out now"; p. 89).

6. Medical or physical problems should be taken into account prior to the use of punishment or aversive procedures.

7. Agency regulations should be established and adhered to. Appropriate reviews help protect the client's rights in addition to those of the staff members carrying out the intervention. Institutional interdisciplinary panels should review aversive procedures with respect to the adequacy of plans, effectiveness of the procedures, quality control, and constitutional rights of the client(s). Institutional statements of policy are essential (Griffith, 1983). Peer review by knowledgeable professionals, especially those with responsibilities that are independent of the program in question, can help determine the appropriateness of the intervention (Griffith, 1983).

8. The "least restrictive, or drastic" but effective intervention should be considered for use (Griffith, 1983; Van Houten et al., 1988). Support for the effectiveness of the intervention for the behavior problem should be made available to those participating in the intervention decisions. If the intervention is not successful, changes in the intervention or therapist may be necessary.

9. Staff training and supervision is essential (Lovaas & Favell, 1987). The person responsible for the intervention should be appropriately qualified. Furthermore, since the use of aversives may focus caregivers' attention on inappropriate behaviors and noxious consequences, it is critical that caregiver skills in the development of functional and appropriate behavioral repertoires as alternatives to maladaptive behaviors receive primary emphasis. Lovaas and Favell (1987) wrote, "Thus, one should expect to see intensive and competent instructional and reinforcement procedures in place in any program in which aversive/restrictive procedures are also employed" (p. 317).

Group Contingencies

The use of group contingencies discussed in later chapters, merits additional considerations and safeguards. (Also, some of the concerns may apply to sibling interventions, discussed in Chapter 8.)

First, target children may become scapegoats if the intervention program is unsuccessful. Second, peer pressure may be considerable and result in coercion, and thus unintended and potentially harmful outcomes. It is especially important that all members of the group be able to perform at a sufficient level. Third, as peers gain control over behaviors, personal control and autonomy is diminished. Fourth, confidentiality may be breached when class members are able to identify individual performances. Fifth, intervention programs require informed consent and permissions from children who serve in roles as peer change agents.

As with other interventions, group contingencies require expanded observations in order to detect undesirable outcomes. Cooper et al. (1987) stated: "If the practitioner is unable to observe the behavior of individuals within the group periodically to determine whether the desired effect is produced, the group-oriented contingency should probably not be used" (p. 502).

Confidentiality

In designing and evaluating interventions, many communications are required between a wide range of persons in the schools. We recommend that, as an element of informed consent, the professionals who will be consulted and individuals who will participate in the intervention be made known to the parent or guardian.

Although there are some exceptions, basically parents or guardians have the right to control access to educational and psychological records and information. The exceptions to this generally involve other school-based professionals who have legitimate educational interest in the information or in situations of potential harm to the child or others. Still, it is important to clarify parental rights and share the process of record and information control with parents.

RIGHT TO EDUCATION AND TREATMENT[2]

Although we have not discussed early intervention within the context of special services defined by Federal Law (most recently, Public Law 105-17), important changes in recent legislation include (1) an emphasis on parental involvement during initial eligibility determination and reevaluation as well as other educational decision making, (2) the recommended use of pre-referral interventions and school-wide intervention programs to decrease categorical labeling and placement, and (3) support for educa-

---

[2]This section is adapted from Barnett, Bell, et al. (in press). Copyright 1999 by PRO-ED, Inc. Adapted by permission.

tional opportunities which provide access to the general curriculum to the maximum extent possible including participation in extracurricular activities with nondisabled peers. Fundamentally, recent amendments increase the emphasis given to the development, implementation, and evaluation of effective interventions. We have presented the intervention issues within the context of functional service delivery, and thus have deliberately avoided the categorical implications of the legislation. However, many of the general intervention principles and procedures that have been discussed have been applied to children described as having disabilities.

Furthermore, we have been unable to identify any convincing discussions of how to accomplish the identification of preschool children characterized by traditional, high-incidence disabling conditions, or "developmental delays," given the considerations associated with decision reliability and validity and standardized tests. Although experimental, given the controversies, we think that the basic principles of parent and teacher consultation and intervention design should guide the eligibility process.

For special services eligibility, from Public Law 105-17, preschool teams comprised of parents and professionals must determine: (1) a category of disability for a child based on one or more developmental delays in physical, cognitive, communication, social or emotional, or adaptive development (or a traditional category based on state and local agency discretion); (2) present levels of performance and educational needs; (3) special education and related services needed to support involvement and progress in the general education curriculum or appropriate preschool activities; and (4) modifications of special education and related services needed to meet annual Individualized Educational Programs (IEP) goals and to facilitate participation in typical child activities. Of primary importance in meeting the intent of Public Law 105-17, evaluation methods must be able to demonstrate that discrepancies exist from expected student performance *and* that data support the *need* for interventions or services.

Intervention-based assessment (IBA), a term currently used in an Ohio statewide pilot project, may be defined as the use of high-quality, low-inference data obtained by direct assessments in natural settings for the design and evaluation of interventions to meet referral concerns. Intervention-based multifactored evaluation (IBMFE) includes IBA procedures and adds disability evaluation components for special services. Decision-making teams are appropriately composed of professionals and parents to determine disability upon completion of a multifactored evaluation.

Operationalizing Logical, Natural, and Meaningful Discrepancies

Our recommendation is to use a collaborative problem-solving approach with parents and teachers in order to derive a meaningful ecological and setting context for analyzing developmental delays and making eligibility decisions through the analysis of discrepancies in performance. We define a "logical" discrepancy as a pattern (over time) of differences in behavior between a child and typical peers in specific settings, and the necessary intervention-related tactics necessary for inclusion. "Natural" means that the discrepancies are found in real-world interactions and are not contrived. "Meaningful" implies that individual differences matter greatly in the lives of children, parents, and teachers and focuses on features of the child or supporting context that are modifiable. In some instances, child variables themselves are not modifiable (e.g., chronic illness), but the focus remains on what *is* modifiable in the setting context to support the child's competence.

In IBMFE, discrepancies may be operationalized in at least two ways: by using peer micronorms and by examining differences in the instructional or related classroom strategies that are required to meet children's needs. Several of the measurement tactics we suggest require the collection of explicit peer micronorms (or local norms if peer micronorms are not feasible or appropriate) to clarify the manner in which a child's skills or behavior differ from those of typically developing peers in the same setting. Local norms are developed for a specific setting such as a district, school, or classroom.

In order to illustrate a discrepancy, peer performances may be monitored in an ongoing fashion or sampled, and coplotted along with data from the targeted child (Bell & Barnett, in press). Eligibility decision making is based both on (1) a discrepancy between educational performance in a critical or significant curriculum area of the referred child in comparison to expectancies for the performance of a typical child (Wolery et al., 1988, p. 287) *and* (2) a desired change in performance that is resistant to planned intervention efforts that are naturally sustainable within the educational service unit. The performance discrepancy and actual intervention data are used to clarify the special education services or supports needed for a teacher and child in order to meet the needs of the child in the present environment or to establish needed environmental modifications to do so. During the intervention period, documentation of failure of normal classroom modifications and the necessity of "special" effort is collected. Together, discrepancy and resistance analysis clarify the unique and special curriculum that *is* special education. Eligibility decision making related to instructional strategies and curricular content is based on empirical evidence of a significant discrepancy between regular classroom procedures and those actually required for a child.

At least three patterns or combinations of patterns derived from direct measurement of "intensity of the need for special support" are used for making decisions (Hardman, McDonnell, & Welch, 1997, p. 64): (1)

An intervention may be successful but requires extraordinary effort to be sustained; (2) an intervention may need to be in place extensively or throughout the school day for appropriate inclusion; (3) interventions carried out by a teacher may be unsuccessful, requiring replanning and special resources to be added to a situation.

We have identified seven IBMFE measurement tactics from intervention research and related literature that can be used to analyze aspects of the differences discussed (child and environmental differences) that may exist between a referred child and typical peers (Table 5.1). These tactics are elaborations of the well-established idea of analyzing discrepancies between a child's behavior and environmental expectancies as fundamental to educational programming (Evans & Meyer, 1985; Wolery et al., 1988). The tactics may be directly linked to intervention decisions and service delivery costs. The end result is the ongoing measurement of a problem or instructional situation to distinguish between those that are resistant to intervention efforts and those that can be logistically supported without special services. Eligibility for special services is determined by patterns of discrepancies (over time), demonstrated interventions (supports and services) required to address the discrepancies through technically adequate problem solving, and the data-based judgment of teams within the parameters discussed. They are illustrated in Figures 5.7 through 5.13 based on hypothetical cases representing our experiences with actual implementation. Note that many of the examples overlap. While demonstrating performance discrepancies, they simultaneously demonstrate the effects or need for more intense services.

Tactic 1: Caregiver Monitoring

Rationale

There are several major reasons for measuring the natural rates and effectiveness of teacher or parent monitoring: (1) Monitoring is a foundation for interventions that requires responsivity to children's behavior; (2) when the intervention demands are too great, indicated by high levels of required monitoring, the result may be fatigue and loss of caregiver motivation or the unintended consequence of learned helplessness on the part of a child; (3) special settings, in contrast to typical classrooms, are characterized by relatively greater teacher effort in supervising and monitoring behavior for individual children with special needs. Reducing the need for caregiver monitoring may lead to placement in more typical settings; (4) the type of monitoring may be inappropriate or ineffective (e.g., yelling, reprimands, repeat commands), or inconsistent, and may be contributing to the problem (e.g., Forehand & McMahon, 1981). Thus, important out-

TABLE 5.1. Measurement Tactics for IBMFE Eligibility Determination

1. Caregiver monitoring

The caregiver (e.g., parent, teacher, related service personnel) may spend a great deal of time watching the child because of potential concerns (e.g., safety, following routines). Caregiver monitoring may be measured as a rate (or state, if highly prevalent) and compared to peer micronorms.

2. Activity engagement

The child may spend less time participating in classroom routines or activities. Activity engagement may be measured as a state or event (rate of activity changes) depending on preliminary observations, and the data may be compared to peer micronorms.

3. Levels of assistance

The caregiver may spend increased amounts of time interacting with the child while facilitating learning, play, or adaptation to routines through assistance or prompts. Levels of assistance are measured through specific prompting strategies and may be compared to peer micronorms. The comparison may be unnecessary if peers require minimal or no assistance.

4. Rate of learning (trials to criterion)

The caregiver may interact with the child in a manner that requires more direct instructional time through the use of repeated structured trials (or practice). The number of learning trials for specific tasks may be compared to data from peer micronorms. Other similar measures include rate of acquisition, mastery, retention, maintenance, or generalization.

5. Behavioral fluency

There may be pronounced differences in the fluency (accuracy and rate) of the child's performance of specific skills or behaviors (e.g., specific language or play-entry skills). The fluency of performance may be compared to data from peer micronorms.

6. Modifying activities

Activities or instruction for the referred child may involve unique or more complex interventions in comparison to other children. The tactics are compared to typical activities or instruction.

7. Curricular adaptations

Domains, skill sequences, or instructional techniques may need to be modified (as in an IEP). Peer micronorms help establish the need for modifications in curricular content or presentation. Curricular adaptations are measured by the integrity of implementation and continuous progress monitoring.

comes may focus on *increasing, reducing, or improving* required caregiver monitoring of student behavior.

Operational Definition, Measurement, and Example

Saudargas and Lentz (1986) defined a teacher initiating a contact with a child as an event. Bramlett (1990) measured caregiver monitoring as a state scored when the teacher is in close proximity (6 feet) to the target child and is looking at the child or the child's activities. Bramlett also included prompts, but we have separated these for discussion purposes.

Figure 5.7 illustrates logical discrepancies in rates of caregiver contacts between the target child and typically developing peers within the same caregiving environment. Initial observations indicated baseline rates of caregiver monitoring for the target child to be five to seven times higher than the median peer rates over three observation sessions. Following implementation of an intervention targeting the child's play skills, the need for caregiver monitoring, while decreasing, continued to be four to five times that of typically developing peers. This discrepancy with regard

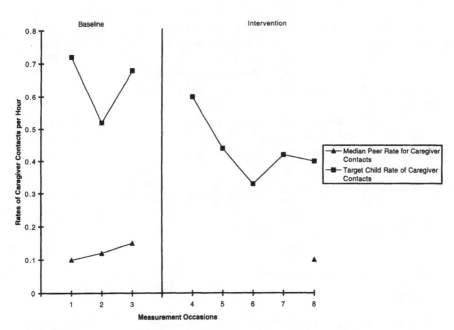

FIGURE 5.7. Rate of caregiver contacts and data from comparison peers. From Barnett et al. (in press). Copyright 1999 by PRO-ED, Inc. Reprinted with permission.

to monitoring could be among the considerations for demonstrating a need for services or supports.

Tactic 2: Activity Engagement

Rationale

Child engagement in meaningful activities in preschool classrooms is generally considered as an important indicator of the quality of the environment and of instructional effectiveness. Activity (task or play) engagement promotes learning, reduces the opportunity for disruptive behaviors, and generally contributes to the impact of the preschool experience. Although engagement is partially a function of child characteristics (e.g., interests), instructional strategies (e.g., incidental teaching, praise) and environmental variables (e.g., accessible and interesting play areas) also contribute to a child's engagement.

Operational Definition, Measurement, and Example

Activity engagement has been defined as the time a child spends interacting with the environment in a developmentally and contextually appropriate manner (McWilliam & Bailey, 1995). Play engagement and preacademic engagement may be measured as states using time sampling (Bramlet, 1990; see also Saudargas & Lentz, 1986). A target child's activity engagement is compared to that of typical peers in terms of patterns of duration and appropriateness of the engagement. A discrepancy is determined by comparing the target child's engagement in play or learning activities with those of typical peers in the same setting.

Figure 5.8 compares percentage of activity engagement for the target child and typical peers during baseline and intervention phases. While there were large discrepancies in percentage of activity engagement during baseline observations (e.g., 30% for the targeted child, 82% for the typical peers), the gap initially closed with the introduction of an intervention incorporating curricular adaptations and teacher facilitation strategies. However, subsequent observations found the activity engagement stabilizing at half the rate of the typical peers.

Tactic 3: Levels of Assistance

Rationale

Levels of assistance is a method of recording the support needed for participation in activities, and alternatively, the support that must be ultimately removed before the child can function independently (Wolery, 1989).

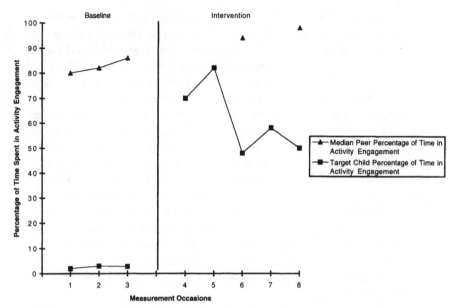

FIGURE 5.8. Percent of activity engagement and data from comparison peers. From Barnett et al. (in press). Copyright 1999 by PRO-ED, Inc. Reprinted with permission.

There are many ways to organize and measure levels of assistance, the most common being response-prompting strategies. There are three common features of prompting strategies: (1) They help teach skills or initiate performance; (2) prompts are removed as soon as possible; (3) and they are combined with differential reinforcement. Prompts must be matched to the individual activity or task and the child's learning characteristics.

Operational Definition, Measurement, and Example

Levels of assistance can be operationalized in terms of instructional prompts. We use as an example the system of least prompts, which involves the presentation of a target/task stimulus and the introduction of a series of the least to most intrusive prompts necessary for the production of a correct response. Prompts include verbal instructions, gestures such as pointing, models or graphic illustrations, and physical prompts, such as hand-over-hand assistance. The occurrence–nonoccurrence of behavior is recorded based on different levels of assistance provided to the child. A discrepancy is determined by identifying developmentally appropriate levels of assistance for peers in the same preschool setting and comparing that level of performance with prompts required for successful performance of a desired skill or behavior by the target child.

Figure 5.9 compares the levels of assistance defined by the type of prompt (group direction, individual verbal prompt, physical guidance by taking the child by the hand for a few steps) the target child and typical peers required in order to transition from lunch to group time. (The child must have the skills necessary to comply with the request, or the focus of the intervention would shift to teaching the specific routine.)

Classroom data (interviews and observations) indicated that the target child knew the transition routine but still required the teacher's physical prompt during the transition, whereas typical peers complied with the group direction. The intervention consisted of a least-to-most prompt hierarchy for the transition period (group direction [1], to individual verbal prompt [2], to physical guidance [3]). Data represent compliance to requests based on the type of prompt. After the intervention was introduced, the target child began to transition following an individual verbal prompt, while the typical peers transitioned following the group direction. However, other classroom activities also required intensive levels of assistance, and these data become useful in decisions about the necessity for support services.

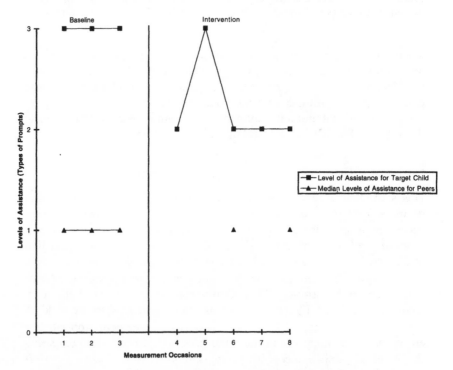

FIGURE 5.9. Levels of assistance and data from comparison peers. From Barnett et al. (in press). Copyright 1999 by PRO-ED, Inc. Reprinted with permission.

Tactic 4: Rate of Learning (Trials to Criterion)

Rationale

Recording the number of learning trials required for acquisition of a new skill is a direct measure of learning rate and the effort involved in teaching a child through a direct instruction. The need for repeated trials in comparison to peers may indicate attention to both the quality and quantity of the learning trials. This measure also is helpful for comparing time allocated for learning or alternative teaching techniques for the same skills.

Operational Definition, Measurement, and Example

"Trials to criteria is the report of the number of times response opportunities are presented before an individual achieves a preestablished level of accuracy or proficiency" (Cooper et al.,1987, p. 74). An example of measurement would be that a particular child needed 10 trials to perform a needed task at 100% accuracy. This would be compared to the number of learning trials from peer performances.

Figure 5.10 illustrates both the use of peer comparisons to establish expectancies for the rate of learning a set of discrete skills (counting) and resource-intensive intervention (direct instruction). For the baseline, educational games were played in a large group format in which children were incidentally taught to count objects. During the incidental teaching condition, typical peers took a median of eight trials to master counting

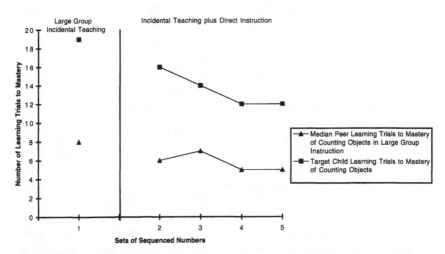

FIGURE 5.10. Trials to criterion for counting objects and data from comparison peers. From Barnett et al. (in press). Copyright 1999 by PRO-ED, Inc. Reprinted with permission.

three objects. Counting was considered mastered when peers counted objects on three consecutive days without teacher prompts or assistance. In comparison, the target child required 19 trials to reach the mastery criterion. Brief direct instruction (incorporating increased feedback and direct learning opportunities) was added to the classroom routine for the targeted child. Subsequently, there was a slight decrease in the number of instructional trials the targeted child required to reach mastery of counting increased sets of objects (5, 7, 10), but large discrepancies with peer performance still continued (7–10 additional trials). This is an example of documentation of the need for special instruction and additional resources while using peer micronorms to assess performance discrepancies. Likewise, it provides evidence that the child can learn and move toward curriculum mastery with special assistance.

Tactic 5: Behavioral Fluency

Rationale

A skill may be performed but not adeptly, thus indicating the need for fluency building. Lack of fluency is observed in performances that are too slow, or not natural or smooth (Wolery et al., 1988). Fluency in performance increases the potential for maintenance, transfer of skill to new situations, and positive affect related to mastery of a skill (Binder, 1996).

Operational Definition, Measurement, and Example

Fluency of response refers to accuracy *and* rate of response that describes relatively effortless, flowing, or automatic competent performance in a natural setting. Fluency may be measured by comparisons of the time required to complete some task by a targeted child in comparison to criterion performances of selected peers or social validity judgments through interviews (Wolery et al., 1988).

Figure 5.11 demonstrates the use of continuous peer comparisons for goal development and intervention effectiveness for behavioral fluency in a cleanup routine, as measured by minutes until completion. During baseline peer comparisons, the target child took 5 to 6 minutes longer to initiate and complete cleanup responsibilities and begin the transition to the next activity. Following the intervention consisting of a teacher prompt combined with a peer mediated "buddy system," minutes to completion steadily approached peer levels. However, from collaboration with the teacher and observations, other activities were identified that needed similar intensive intervention, and data were collected that would be useful in subsequent interventions or special services decisions.

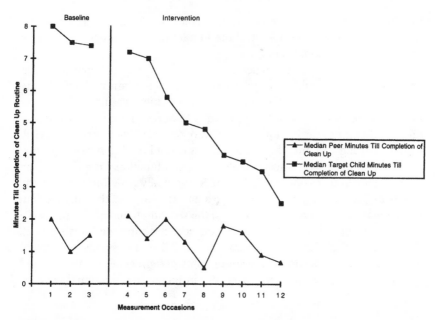

FIGURE 5.11. Completion of cleanup as a measure of fluency and data from comparison peers. From Barnett et al. (in press). Copyright 1999 by PRO-ED, Inc. Reprinted with permission.

Tactic 6: Modifying Activities

Rationale

Environmental intervention to support children with disabilities is one of the most important historical and philosophical ideas in inclusionary educational programming and IBA/IBMFE. It has impressive empirical support over many behaviors of concern (Dunlap & Kern, 1996) and is limited only by a team's creativity.

Operational Definition, Measurement, and Example

Including children with disabilities in typical settings may be based on making changes in activities, routines, or classroom management. These required changes or differences in activities may be used as natural discrepancies for special services consideration.

There are well-developed steps for defining interventions in inclusionary settings and their outcomes. Two critical steps are *identifying* and *quantifying* the events and behaviors comprising the intervention (adapted from Lelaurin & Wolery, 1992, p. 281). The end results are estimates of the amount of time and resources a teacher would spend planning and carrying out an intervention, and the impact of the planned changes on the overall instructional ecology.

Figure 5.12 illustrates logical discrepancies in instructional strategies necessary for successful child performance. In this example, the missing-item format (Tirapelle & Cipani, 1992) intervention was used to increase functional requesting of a target child. Measures of functional requests during other times throughout the day were recorded for potential generalization. During baseline, the target child was not heard to make any functional requests. Based on successfully increasing functional requests during lunch, other instructional periods were sequentially added to increase the number of trials using the technique in a natural way (e.g., the missing-item format was carried out during lunch in the second phase, lunch and toothbrushing in the third phase, and art was added during the fourth phase). This hypothetical data set also illustrates the use of a single-case design (changing criteria) beyond the accountability designs generally used.

Intervention efforts were successful in increasing functional request-

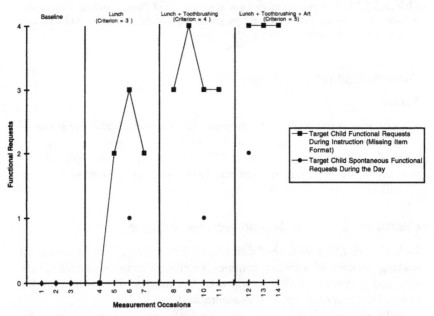

FIGURE 5.12. Introduction of a functional requesting routine (missing-item format) during instructional periods and measurement of spontaneous functional requests. Criterion indicates the total number of instructional trials with missing-items format during the day. From Barnett et al. (in press). Copyright 1999 by PRO-ED, Inc. Reprinted with permission.

ing by the target child during instructional sessions and nonintervention periods. In this case, a discrepancy is indicated by the need to modify activities, and, related, the nature of the teacher's sustained effort. Future goals also would involve language competence.

Tactic 7: Curricular Adaptations

Rationale

One of the most useful approaches for making educational decisions involves the systematic and ongoing assessment of children within the contexts of a well-constructed curriculum, instructional techniques, and environmental conditions necessary for competent performance (LeBlanc, Etzel, & Domash, 1978). Curriculum-based assessment circumvents many problems because developmental sequences are tied to ongoing measurement related to instructional efforts and skill progression rather than a "profile" of skills at one point in time, and the results are used in planning for intervention decisions.

Operational Definition, Measurement, and Example

To enable decisions about interventions, a curriculum must have (1) a wide range of functional, developmentally sequenced tasks; (2) ongoing measurement of progress; and (3) a variety of teaching and learning strategies. Children who remain at a particular level of a skills sequence, or who are unable to complete a task, determined by the above tactics, may require a change in instructional strategies in order to progress to the next step (Wolery et al., 1988).

The developmental domains may be assessed by ongoing observations of the child's performance in preacademic, social, and other developmental areas through curriculum-referenced measurement if the curriculum includes the developmental sequences. If not, sequences of developmental skills from a specialized curriculum, along with progress monitoring, may be added for children. Judgments about developmental delay may be made through peer micronorms, taking into account the appropriateness of instructional strategies that are being used.

The most basic measurement strategy is monitoring of a child's progress through a sequenced curriculum. Progress is reported as objectives that are mastered.

Figure 5.13 compares the number of curricular objectives mastered for the target child and randomly selected typical peers. From October to January, the target child consistently mastered approximately five curricular objectives. The peers steadily increased the number of objectives mas-

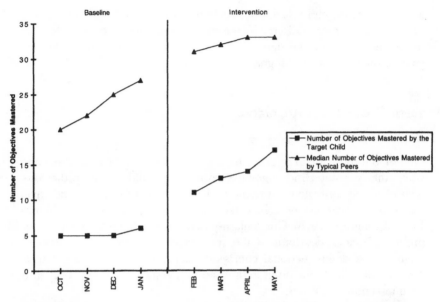

FIGURE 5.13. Number of objectives mastered by the target child and data from comparison peers. From Barnett et al. (in press). Copyright 1999 by PRO-ED, Inc. Reprinted with permission.

tered from 20 to 27 during this same time period. An intervention was implemented in order to help the target child increase the number of objectives mastered. The intervention was successful in increasing the number of curricular objectives mastered to 17 by the end of the school year. The peer data continued to steadily increase to 33 objectives mastered. The discrepancies demonstrate the need for sustained, individualized instructional efforts, and the possible adaptation of a specialized curriculum.

SUMMARY AND CONCLUSIONS

We approached designing and evaluating interventions in four ways. First, measurement theory was applied to behavioral assessments. Second, we connected those concepts to the problem-solving model. Accountability for intervention outcomes was addressed through the use of single-case experimental designs. Third, ethical and legal intervention decision frameworks and practices were reviewed. Fourth, an experimental approach for making eligibility decisions by using intervention-related measurement tactics also was introduced. Foundations for navigating through all of these discussions were ecobehavioral collaborative consultation, and sequential and iterative decision making.

CHAPTER 6

◆◆◆

Developing New Behaviors and Modifying Existing Behaviors

◆

One of the most significant foundations for professional practice is the analysis of research-based interventions. In Chapters 6 and 7, we review interventions that have research support and that have been used in a wide range of settings. In later chapters, we present examples of intervention applications that have been oriented to home and school.

NATURALISTIC LEARNING EXPERIENCES[1]

Perhaps the most important foundation of early intervention, and the most difficult to rectify when not present, is the availability of a responsive, guiding, caring, and nurturing adult. Safe physical environments that are conducive to development also are necessary. Thus, the learning and mediational environments of families (Hart & Risley, 1995; Laosa & Sigel, 1982) and classrooms (Bredekamp & Copple, 1997; Rogers-Warren, 1982) are a point of broad-based intervention for many children. Mediation refers to the manner in which adults (or peers) select, focus, organize, and give meaning to experiences for children. Adult–child and child–child interactions that occur naturally across a variety of situations and environments provide rich opportunities for facilitating children's cognitive, language, and social development. For parents, interacting with a child in a naturally educative manner during daily events—dressing, meals, television viewing, reading, play, shopping, or household tasks—holds many opportunities for teaching basic concepts, problem solving, and related language skills within the con-

---

[1]John D. Hall contributed to writing this section.

text of an important relationship. For teachers, classroom and instructional design include the development of play and learning areas that help promote curiosity, task engagement, and appropriate peer interaction, and routines that minimize disruptions, promote self-regulated behavior, and contribute to learning objectives. Opportunities for direct and incidental teaching occur during planned instruction and on serendipitous occasions.

The cumulative power of brief encounters may be underestimated by parents and teachers (as well as by other change agents and consultants). Cognitive, language, and preacademic skills development occur incidentally through play and countless daily events. Modeling necessary skills and encouraging social maturity and coping occurs within real-life contexts of problem solving and resolving conflicts. Learning takes place within an interpersonal context characterized by the caregiver's responsivity and warmth. Adult–child interactions should avoid unnecessary restriction, and physical and verbal punishment.

Play experiences are particularly important. Hobbs wrote, "A child should know joy" (1966, p. 1113). Play behaviors can be explored through interviews and observations. Interventions may include (1) structuring or monitoring play experiences that incorporate cognitive, language, affective, social, and motor learning; (2) facilitating or modifying adult–child and child–peer interactions; and (3) enabling appropriate periods of solitary play. In subsequent discussions, we elaborate on specific interventions that involve play.

In summary, the most significant elements of intervention design depend on responsive and capable adults, and on safe and interesting environments that support a wide range of learning objectives that include peers, materials, and functional activities. Initial intervention efforts should be directed toward assisting adults who are available to children and who are capable of fulfilling these roles. Many children are being raised in precarious environments. For this reason, throughout this text, we have stressed naturalistic principles in intervention design, because they are intended to fit real-world exigencies, and they enhance intervention acceptability and generalizability. Other reviews of naturalistic teaching techniques are provided by Wolery, Ault, and Doyle (1992).

Naturally Occurring Strategies

The degree to which an intervention is deemed natural is dependent on the beliefs and practices of the individual caregiver. Wolery and Wilburs (1994) further described interventions as falling along a continuum from those more likely to result in child-initiated interactions with the environment (e.g., structuring the environment) to those that are caregiver-initiated and more likely to result in a specific response or behavior (e.g., prompting). Professionals involved in the design of early intervention efforts consider basic procedures rather than more complicated ones, at least initially. We present strategies that are potentially powerful but can easily be overlooked or misused. These strategies are used by effective caregivers to teach, eliminate, shape, and maintain many types of behaviors. We also include common, naturally occurring aversive strategies, since they easily may be misapplied or abused, and thus also may contribute to maladaptive behavior. Therefore, these strategies often deserve systematic attention in interviews and observations as a starting place for intervention design.

Quality Interactions

Perhaps it is not too challenging to bring to mind impressions of quality interactions as they are features, hopefully, of our everyday lives. Many have been well established as educational principles and through intervention-related research.

Bredekamp and Copple (1997) describe the role of the early childhood educator as one who provides novel and challenging experiences that sustain individual children's effort and engagement through focused attention. Hart and Risley (1995) found the following features of parent interactions to be a powerful predictor of children's language development: "They just talked; they tried to be nice [even when enforcing rules]; they told children about things; they gave children choices; and they listened" (adapted from p. 149). Similar strategies have been a highly effective first step during intervention for children with challenging behavior. Parents use attention to show interest in their child, to communicate approval, and to reinforce their child's appropriate behavior. These are important parental behaviors and should be in place before addressing disruptive behaviors (Forehand & McMahon, 1981).

Providing Significant and Interesting Experiences

Play is the vehicle through which children learn to understand their world, interact with others, develop adaptive and functional skills, and begin the process of self-regulation (Bredekamp & Copple, 1997). Fostering child engagement in a variety of play activities is one indicator of the quality of the environment and of instructional effectiveness (McWilliam, 1991; McWilliam, Trivette, & Dunst, 1985). Engagement is a function of child characteristics, instructional strategies and environmental variables (McWilliam & Bailey, 1995). Kaiser (1993) wrote, "Child engagement functionally defines the aspects of the physical and social environment that influence the child's language learning and use" (p. 71). Children frequently self-engage with persons and materials in their environments, but engagement also is prompted by others and by the presence of objects or the occurrence of events. Child engagement, including the idea of trying out and practicing emerging skills, may be considered a keystone behavior influenced by features of the environment. We build on these ideas, referred to in various places as environmental enrichment, during many intervention descriptions.

Opportunities to Respond

One of the most powerful interventions involves giving children more frequent chances for learning and for practice. Most of the examples are for older children, but the general principles apply. Greenwood, Delquadri, and Hall (1984) provide the following definition of opportunity to respond: "The interaction between (a) teacher formulated instructional antecedent stimuli (the materials presented, prompts, questions asked, signals to respond, etc.), and (b) their success in establishing the academic responding desired or implied by the materials" (p. 64).

The term includes such factors as practice, time on-task, at-task behavior, and specific child responses, but attention is directed to the *antecedents* of instruction. Greenwood, Delquadri, and Hall give examples of antecedents:

> scheduling and . . . implementation of instructional time on a systematic basis for specific academic subjects; providing level-appropriate materials that facilitate directly the desired academic responses; organization of the classroom physical structure so that it is conducive to academic responding; and teacher interaction patterns with students as individuals or as groups, that support academic responding at high levels. (1984, p. 64)

Another important distinction implied in these characteristics is that children are actively rather than passively responding, feedback is given, and performance is monitored.

Overall, research has demonstrated a strong relationship between the "quality and frequency of academic interactions" and academic gains (Greenwood et al., 1984, p. 86). The major focus is on identifying instructional methods and materials that promote frequent, diverse, and systematically planned preacademic behavior. Applications are discussed in Chapter 10.

Modeling

We make reference to modeling throughout the chapters on interventions. Indeed, "most human behavior is learned by observation through modeling" (Bandura, 1986, p. 47). Through observing the behavior of others, children learn rules for behavior that later serve as guides for action. In addition, values, attitudes, patterns of cognition, cognitive competencies, and the consequences for behaviors also are learned by observing others.

In addition to teaching new behaviors, observational learning may have the effect of strengthening, weakening, or facilitating learned behavior. Basic to these processes is observing the consequences of behavioral acts for others. For example, it is safe to say that many, if not all, children in a preschool classroom have in their repertoires behaviors that are inappropriate to the school or other settings (hitting, spitting, swearing). When one child behaves inappropriately and receives negative consequences, all of the other children may become more "restrained" in similar behaviors. However, if the consequences for inappropriate behaviors are inconsistent or not effective, more children may exhibit the behavior. Wolery et al. (1988) discuss vicarious reinforcement of others' behavior as a basic strategy for behavioral change. Children who are behaving in the desired manner are reinforced while the target child observes. As another example, if children with high status in the classroom often share and other children observe that, sharing is likely to increase. Other possible outcomes are that modeling may enhance the value of the object or setting that was the focal point of the modeled behavior. Bandura (1986) concluded that the effects of modeling depend on the information that is actually conveyed:

> The direction and strength of the impact of such information on personal restraint largely depends on three factors: on observers' judgments of their ability to execute the modeled behavior, on their perception of the modeled actions as producing rewarding or punishing consequences, and on their inferences that similar or unlike consequences would result if they themselves were to engage in analogous activities. (p. 49)

Emotions are "coeffects" of learning and performing (Bandura, 1986). Emotions are an inextricable part of social interactions, and emotional reactions to events are pervasively modeled. Gottman (1986) argued that "emotional development organizes social development" (p. 85). Because of these properties, modeling also may be useful for dealing with fears.

Observational learning involves four major processes (Bandura, 1986).

1. *Attentional processes* focus analysis on what is observed. Features of the modeled activities and the cognitive processes of the observer determine what events will be observed, how they are perceived and interpreted, and how they affect subsequent behaviors.

2. *Retentional processes* incorporate the ways brief experiences are encoded or remembered. "Retention involves an active process of transforming and restructuring information about events" (Bandura, 1985, p. 90).
3. *Production processes* involve the ability to carry out acts based on a cognitive or symbolic organization of the response and a plan for the activity. Actual performance is compared to the conceptual plan. Points of analysis include the physiological or developmental limitations of the person and factors related to prior learning.
4. *Motivational processes* have to do with whether a new behavior is learned and whether a learned behavior is performed. The reinforcement may be external, based on environmental contingencies and on the consequences of behavior. Reinforcement also may be self-generated or vicarious.

All four processes are important for understanding the effects of observational learning. Furthermore, positive changes in behavior can occur through any combination of the four: (1) by improvements in selective observation (attentional processes); (2) by improvements in memory encoding; (3) by enhancement of the child's ability to perform based on sensory, motor, and cognitive processes; and (4) by improvements in the anticipation of the consequences of acts. It may be important to assess what relevant people (child, caregivers, and consultant) *believe* about their contributions to the processes of change, which helps define *self-efficacy*.

The practical applications of modeling are unlimited. Interventions that involve observational learning may be applied to individual children, groups of children, parents, and teachers. Furthermore, opportunities for learning through modeling may be planned or unplanned (Striefel, 1998). One of the major points of assessment is the evaluation of the models and modeled behavior that are available to children. Specific examples of interventions using modeling are given in this and in subsequent chapters.

Differential or Systematic Attention

Differential attention consists of approval. It is defined as social reinforcement given to a child contingent on the display of desired behavior. Hall and Hall (1998a) described it as "noticing when someone is doing something desired and then giving him or her attention by commenting, looking at, touching or expressing approval" (p. 6). The effectiveness of differential attention has been well established in research studies, and it serves as one of the best examples of a systematically replicated intervention. On the other hand, Hall and Hall (1998a) wrote: "Unfortunately, many persons squander their attention and approval in an unsystematic or haphazard way—worse yet, some give nearly all their attention to unwanted behavior" (p. 3). *Misplaced* differential attention can serve to reinforce inappropriate behaviors.

Systematic attention is only effective when attention is reinforcing; that is, when it increases the probability of occurrence of a desired response or appropriate child behavior. If attention is not reinforcing, or is having a weak effect, then it first must be paired with an effective reinforcer. Basic steps for providing systematic attention are described here (adapted from Hall & Hall, 1998a, except as noted).

1. Define the behavior to be changed. Systematic attention and approval are designed to increase behaviors to be strengthened. Paine and colleagues (1983) described an "if–then" good praise rule: "*If* the student is doing something you want to encourage— something you want the student to do again or do more often in the future (and if you are sure that is what the student is doing)— then (and only then) you should praise the student for it" (p. 46).
2. Use basic observation procedures in measuring the behaviors to be changed.
3. Set a goal for the target behavior.
4. Select appropriate types of attention and approval. Use a variety of different reinforcing verbalizations immediately following the desired response. Use *specific* and descriptive praise ("I like the way you helped Sally put the blocks away"). Note that praise may be easily misused or overused, or used perfunctorily. It should be convincing: genuine, warm, and sincere. Consider whether to use public or private praise, or both. Systematic attention or approval also may be used in conjunction with backup reinforcement, other interventions, and treatment packages. The most notable are compliance training and classroom management procedures discussed in later chapters. Another example is the use of positive attention in shaping programs if the child lacks the prerequisite skills or behaviors.
5. Determine when and how often. A basic principle of systematic attention is that it should occur while the targeted behavior is occurring or immediately after. Also, praise should not be used in a way that disrupts ongoing activities.

Choices

Choice making adds quality to interactions (Hart & Risley, 1995) and structured choice making fits the criteria of being a natural and research-based strategy to help manage or modify behavior. It is incorporated into intervention design in many ways: for reinforcement appraisal and goal setting (Guevremont, Osnes, & Stokes, 1988), and as a foundation of strategies, developed in later chapters, such as functional communication training (Durand, Berotti, & Weiner, 1993) and contingent observation. Procedurally, it may mean that children have choices over objects or activities, such as when to take a break or get a drink. A thorough illustration of choice making with young children having multiple and severe problems is provided by Peck et al. (1996).

High-Probability Requests

A brief, rapid sequence of usually three (to five) high-probability requests, defined as those likely to be complied with based on observations (80% compliance has been used in research), may be used to increase appropriate responding to a low-probability request (i.e., 50% compliance) when the low-probability request is given soon after the high-probability requests (i.e., 5 seconds). As an example, at school, a child may have left a play area without cleaning up. A sequence of requests might be "Come here and give me a hug" and "Point to your picture," followed by "Put your name on your picture" and then, "Put the markers and glue away on the shelf." This sequence may be more likely to lead to compliance than "Put the markers and glue away on the shelf" alone. Practical interest stems from Mace and colleagues' (1988) research based on behavioral momentum (Nevin, 1996), but numerous studies have appeared showing effectiveness with many potential referral questions such as compliance and social behaviors. Davis and Reichle (1996) found that varying sequences of high-probability requests helps maintain compliance with requests. They also found that the intervention procedures could be carried out with young peers delivering the requests.

Errorless Teaching

In learning new skills, it is important to maximize the amount of early success. In errorless teaching (sometimes referred to as errorless learning), early teaching tasks are simplified through prompts that are gradually faded. More difficult tasks are introduced slowly. Errorless teaching stresses the control of antecedent teaching procedures to enable the child to perform with no (or few) errors. There are two basic types of procedures. One involves a system of teacher prompts to help children perform. A second (and more elaborate) procedure uses systematic stimulus modifications whereby the task is initially made easy and progressively becomes more difficult by fading prompts. In later chapters, we give examples for parenting (Chapter 9) and teaching (Chapter 11).

Praise

A powerful strategy for management of classroom behavioral challenges is the use of brief, specific, contingent and sincere verbal reinforcement commonly referred to as praise. We have referred to praise in numerous places. Some early childhood educators have cautioned against the use of nonspecific and evaluative praise, indicating that such efforts may (1) lead to negative emotions (e.g., the child experiences fear and anxiety about the quality of his or her efforts or products), (2) foster reliance on external approval and adult dependency, and (3) encourage rote responses rather than creativity and individual problem-solving (Hitz & Driscoll, 1988). Others emphasize the importance of incorporating frequent praise throughout the day in order to develop a positive atmosphere in the early childhood classroom (McCloskey, 1996).

Descriptive praise is a form of specific feedback regarding the appropriateness and desirability of the child's behavior in a designated classroom activity (Brophy, 1981). Bredekamp and Copple (1997) suggest the developmental appropriateness of the use of verbal encouragement and reinforcement as effective strategies "to sustain an individual child's effort or engagement in purposeful activities" (p. 19). This topic is developed more fully later in this chapter in the section on the use of reinforcement.

The next strategies are commonly used or abused by caregivers to reduce problem behavior. It may be profitable to appraise their misuse for many referrals related to children's misconduct.

Reprimands

Reprimands are perhaps the most common overt strategy for behavior control. They can be used in combination with many other interventions. However, when used ineffectively, they can intensify maladaptive behaviors. Many of the children referred to us for problem behaviors are growing up in environments dominated by aversives. Perhaps most important, reprimands should be used in the context of positive attention. Specific training for caregivers in the use of reprimands is often needed. Van Houten (1980) identified the following guidelines for the use of reprimands.

1. Specify the inappropriate behavior, state why the behavior is inappropriate, and provide an example of an appropriate behavior.
2. Use a firm tone.
3. Use appropriate nonverbal expressions of disapproval.
4. Deliver the reprimand within close proximity.
5. Avoid ignoring inappropriate behavior.

6. Use a more intrusive intervention with a dangerous behavior.
7. Use social reinforcement for appropriate behaviors.
8. If necessary, follow reprimands with other acceptable behavioral strategies.
9. Maintain emotional control.
10. Outcomes should reveal decreasing use of reprimands while maintaining or improving behavior.

Ignoring

Planned ignoring is "noticing when someone is trying to get your attention by engaging in an undesirable behavior and ignoring that behavior in a preplanned manner" (Hall & Hall, 1998b, p. 3). It may be viewed as a form of time out in which "usual attention, physical contact, and any verbal interactions are removed for a short duration contingent upon the occurrence of the unwanted behavior" (Sulzer-Azaroff & Mayer, 1991, p. 457).

Many behaviors are difficult if not impossible to ignore. Planned ignoring will not be effective for modifying inappropriate behaviors if positive attention of the caregiver is not serving as a reinforcer (or if the caregiver's circumstances interfere with the plan). In other words, the child must be responsive to positive attention in order for ignoring to work as an intervention. Even if the caregiver is appropriately ignoring the behavior, the attention of others (peers, adults) may sustain the behavior. Also, ignoring is an aversive procedure. Thus, children may become upset and undesirable behaviors may increase when the procedures are first used.

The term "extinction" is closely related. This means no longer reinforcing a behavior that was previously reinforced. All sources of reinforcement that are maintaining the behavior need to be removed for the length of time extinction is in effect. Several characteristics of extinction are well established by extensive research (Lerman & Iwata, 1996) and we summarize some of them. Its effect in reducing behavior is gradual rather than immediate. At first, the target behaviors may increase in rate and intensity (referred to as an extinction burst; found in 24% of cases analyzed by Lerman & Iwata, 1996). As the target response decreases, the behavior may be "extinguished," only to reappear at the beginning of a new session or at a later point in time. This is termed "spontaneous recovery." The original responses may appear if a new extraneous stimulus or event occurs. Also, other behaviors, such as aggression, emotional behavior, or escape, may increase (termed "indirect effects"). The predicted consequences are important for teachers and parents. Although extinction has been used successfully for a wide range of problem behaviors such as crying, whining, and tantrums, in fact, both planned ignoring and extinction may be difficult interventions for many caregivers to apply.

DEVELOPING LANGUAGE SKILLS

Many referrals in preschool populations have to do with language problems. Language skills are linked to cognitive and social competencies, and they are often the target of formal interventions. Numerous sources extensively discuss various language interventions. We have too much respect for the complexities and specialization necessary to do more than give an overview of language intervention consistent with naturalistic intervention design: research on milieu language intervention (Warren, 1992) and functional communication training (Carr & Durand, 1985; Reichle & Wacker, 1993). Note also that definitional concerns about "natural" have been raised (Hepting & Goldstein, 1996).

Naturalistic Language Training Techniques

Naturalistic strategies focus attention on the roles and skills that caregivers need in order to help children acquire, generalize, and maintain new behaviors. The rationale is straightforward; caregivers, primarily mothers, are natural language teachers for infants and young children, and language learning is a critical part of the preschool curriculum. The most important initial aspect is adaptive caregiver–child communication that may be described as contingent verbal responsiveness (MacPhee, Ramey, & Yeates, 1984). Feedback or modeling given in a way that does not undermine the integrity of social interactions may be a critical component (Camarata, 1993). Subsequently, pragmatic language is critical for developing social competence in peer interactions.

Language Development

Learning "events" include experiences intentionally provided and those that result from incidental opportunities. Teaching can be a part of ongoing daily routines. Based on a review by Hart (1985, p. 67; see also Hart & Risley, 1995), the following characteristics of environments contribute to language development:

1. *Stimulation*: the richness and variety of objects, and experiences provided. Hart wrote,

   For language acquisition to progress, it is essential that nonsocial stimuli such as materials and activities evoke verbal behavior: that a child want to talk not just to people, but about *things*. The more things in the environment that the child is interested in talking about, the greater is the pressure to acquire language as a means of communicating perceived properties, actions, and relationships. (1985, p. 85)

2. *Adult–child ratio*: the one-to-one nature of early interactions.
3. *Topic*: child selection of the topic for interaction.
4. *Routines*: the standardized framework of early interactions.
5. *Models*: the language the child hears.
6. *Initiation*: repetition of models by child or adult.
7. *Prompts*: method of evoking language from the child.
8. *Function*: the consequences of language use for the child.

Warren and Kaiser (1986) summarized common premises of naturalistic language interventions: (1) Language and communications skills are taught in natural environments; (2) a conversational context is used for acquisition and skill development; (3) dispersed trials are used; (4) learning follows the child's "attentional lead"; and (5) functional reinforcers are revealed by the child's "requests and attention" (p. 291). Halle, Alpert, and Anderson (1984) and Warren and Gazdag (1990) review applications for young children with more severe disabilities.

Pragmatic Language

The emphasis of pragmatic language is on the real-life context of language performance. "Establishing the *function* of the communicative act is as necessary to language development as the acquisition of conventional form (syntax) and content (semantics)" (MacDonald, 1985, p. 95). Social competence is an important context of pragmatic language performance (Prutting, 1982). For these reasons, parent, teacher, and peer roles and social contexts are critical for improving or facilitating language development. The analysis of pragmatics has two main thrusts (adapted from Alpert & Rogers-Warren, 1985, pp. 133–134): (1) determining how prelinguistic and linguistic behaviors function in communication—as in requests, protests, answers, vocatives, declaratives, and so on; and (2) evaluating social skills that tend to promote effective communication such as taking turns, maintaining the topic of conversation, relating new information to old, avoiding saying what the listener already is likely to be aware of, and using the apparent interest level of the listener as a cue for modifying one's verbal behavior.

In the next sections, we discuss basic naturalistic strategies to facilitate language acquisition: mand–model, the use of brief time delays, incidental teaching, and missing-item format. All are based on naturally occurring strategies used by caregivers and have experimental support.

Mand–Model

A mand is a request, question, demand, or instruction to respond (Skinner, 1957). The mand–model strategy is a systematization of a type of natural interaction between mothers and young children (typically at 12 to 15 months) described by Bruner (1978) and Snow (1977). At the most basic level, the mother directs the child's attention, as by saying, "Look." After the child attends, the mother asks a "Wh . . . question" such as "What's that?" After the child vocalizes, the mother provides a model or label. Developmentally, labels first are object words or proper nouns (Bruner, 1978). In natural settings where language is readily acquired by children, the interaction is repeated often. While the mother's behavior may remain relatively unchanged, Bruner (1978) reported changes in child initiations of the behavior and the frequency of responses by the child to the mother's initiations.

Rogers-Warren and Warren (1980, p. 367) outline the sequence of steps for the mand–model strategy as follows:

1. Teachers direct children's attention by providing a variety of attractive materials with which children want to play.
2. When a child approaches material (such that joint teacher–child attention is focused on that material as topic), the teacher asks, "Tell me what this is," or "Tell me what you want." (Open-ended questions that require responses beyond "Yes" or "No" are used.)
3. If the child does not respond, or gives a minimal response, the teacher provides a model for the child to imitate. The teacher may also prompt within this step, as for example, by elaborating the request to "Give me a whole sentence," and then providing a model if the child does not respond appropriately.
4. The teacher praises the child for responding appropriately to the mand, or for imitating, and gives the child the material.

The mand–model technique has many potential applications across settings because of the brevity of the caregiver–child interactions. It also may have positive effects on general language behavior. Furthermore, the technique may be used naturally and systematically.

Brief Time Delay

Another normal process is that parents expect and wait for more mature forms of behavior (Hart, 1985). The use of a brief delay (5 to 15 seconds) during natural routines when children need assistance, or otherwise need to initiate communication, has been found to help with the development of language (Halle, Baer, & Spradlin, 1981). Delay is an adaptation of incidental teaching (Warren & Kaiser, 1986). The delay is used as a nonverbal cue or stimulus to respond.

Halle et al. (1981) give an example: The caregiver holds a glass of juice, faces the child, and waits for the child's vocal initiation. Delay can be used with any natural or functional opportunities that occur on a regular basis, such as gross motor play (putting hands on the object to be moved and waiting before moving the object, or stopping a moving object) or when the child needs help with a shoelace or button, or with bathroom requests. Delay also may be used to fade from the mand–model strategy (Hart, 1985).

Steps in using the delay procedure include (1) The caregiver is within 3 feet of the child and is oriented toward the child, may kneel or sit at the child's eye level; (2) the child is attending to the caregiver and assumes an expectant look; (3) the caregiver does not vocalize to the child but may use visual prompts; (4) a 5-second delay is instituted; (5) the child's verbalizations must be appropriate for the context of the request; (6) if the child does not make a response or the response is incorrect, the adult models the behavior.

Incidental Teaching

Incidental teaching takes advantage of naturally arising interactions between adults and children in unstructured situations. Through brief interactions, adults transmit new information or enable the children to practice communication skills. Experimentally, the procedure was used to increase compound sentences in spontaneous speech for children with mild language problems whose language use was sufficient to provide adequate learning opportunities (Hart & Risley, 1975, 1980).

Incidental teaching is described as "loose" training that follows the child's attention. The topic is chosen by the child; the adult focuses attention on what the child says and encourages elaboration. Incidental teaching is one of the best examples of a language intervention that combines conversational and behavioral elements.

Nine steps or conditions are included in the procedure (Hart & Risley, 1982):

1. The setting must have attractive and appropriate materials and activities.
2. The caregiver's attention must be important to the child.
3. The caregiver waits for the child to begin a conversation.
4. When the child vocalizes, the caregiver looks at the child, smiles, and focuses on the child's conversation.
5. If the caregiver is unsure of the child's language, the caregiver clarifies the topic.

6. The caregiver asks the child a question that allows the child to elaborate.
7. The caregiver prompts the child as necessary throughout the conversation.
8. The caregiver models a correct response as needed, and asks the child to practice the modeled response.
9. The caregiver confirms the child's correct response, models the language, and gives the appropriate adult response.

Several examples follow (Barnett, Silverstein, & Miller, 1988):

Example 1:

JILL: *(Points to doll.)*

CAREGIVER: She's a pretty doll. What is her name?

JILL: Baby.

CAREGIVER: Well, Baby has on a bright red dress today.

Example 2:

JILL: Help.

CAREGIVER: What do you need help with, Jill?

JILL: Help with coat.

CAREGIVER: You need help putting on your coat.

Example 3:

JILL: *(Reaching for cup at mealtime.)*

CAREGIVER: What do you want, Jill?

JILL: Cup.

CAREGIVER: Good, Jill. You asked for your cup with juice.

Warren and Kaiser (1986) provide a comprehensive review of incidental teaching. They underscore its potential in educational and family settings. Other potential applications include social behavior (Brown, McEvoy, & Bishop, 1991), and peer tutoring (McGee, Almeida, Sulzer-Azaroff, & Feldman, 1992).

Missing-Item Format

The missing-item format (Tirapelle & Cipani, 1992), used to increase functional requests, involves choosing a classroom routine (e.g., teeth brushing, eating cereal), providing all of the materials necessary for the activity except one, and in a game-like fashion, withholding (or as alternatives covering, removing, or giving the child the wrong item) the one needed item. The child is instructed to begin the activity, and the caregiver waits for the child's response (for 5 seconds), or encourages the child's response if necessary. For example, a child can be presented with cereal, milk, sugar, a bowl, and a fork, or the spoon can be covered.

Functional Communication Training

Communication skills are frequently targeted as functional behaviors for children. Carr and Durand (1985) proposed a "communication hypothesis" where behavior problems function as "nonverbal communicative acts" to obtain socially mediated reinforcement (p. 124). The intervention component may be referred to as differential reinforcement of communication. This intervention is elaborated in the next chapter.

Summary of Early Language Intervention

We have stressed language intervention in terms of the roles of primary caregivers rather than by specialists. This is not intended to minimize the contributions of specialized disciplines, but, rather, to emphasize the importance of language for personal and social development, the pragmatic and functional nature of early language acquisition, naturalistic learning strategies, and an ecobehavioral emphasis for assessment and intervention design. While not necessarily causal, if language problems persist into school age, they are likely to be associated with a broad range of academic and social problems. Furthermore, the strategies involving the roles of parents and teachers are directly related to issues concerning skill generalization—a topic for which research is lacking.

Incidental learning experiences are important because they have the potential for flexible adaptation to a wide range of settings and change agents. Incidental teaching is successful because it incorporates both behavioral principles such as shaping, prompting, and contingent reinforcement (discussed in subsequent sections) and factors gleaned from basic developmental research. Recent research trends suggest the importance of integrating language interventions into the child's usual routines and interactions.

OTHER BASIC INTERVENTION STRATEGIES

We began the chapter with everyday or naturalistic techniques that may be used by parents and teachers in many situations. Many of the techniques that have been introduced can be built on to achieve more powerful interventions. Next, we expand our discussion of intervention foundations for children that are hard to teach, parent, or befriend.

Reinforcement

A reinforcer is a contingent event that follows a response and increases the "future probability of responses in the same *class*" (Skinner, 1953, p. 87). The concept of response class is important because typically interrelated behaviors are the unit of analysis, not isolated responses. For example, aversive behaviors of children such as whining, tantrums, and crying often are treated as a response class due to their functional interrelatedness (see Chapter 4 on keystone behaviors).

Reinforcement may be either positive or negative. In both cases, however, behavior is strengthened. The reinforcement increases the probability of the occurrence of behaviors belonging to a response class.

Positive reinforcers "add something" to the situation (Skinner, 1953). Positive reinforcement is most widely applied and is a cornerstone of intervention design with young children. One of the best examples, positive attention, was introduced earlier in the chapter. We will return to positive reinforcement in a later section on differential reinforcement.

Negative reinforcement increases the probability of a response class of behaviors through "removing something . . . from the situation" (Skinner, 1953, p. 73). After the child makes the desired response, the caregiver takes away the aversive stimulus. Thus, the use of negative reinforcement requires "a prior worsening of the environment" (Cooper et al., 1987, p. 261). The potentially undesirable outcomes of negative reinforcement may be reduced by combining it with positive procedures. Negative reinforcement may be a factor in learning disruptive behaviors, such as tantrums, to avoid or escape difficult or unpleasant tasks. Negative reinforcement also may be used therapeutically (Iwata, 1987; Peck et al., 1996).

Punishment is different from negative reinforcement. Furthermore, technically it is *not* the opposite of reward (Skinner, 1953). Punishment involves introducing (rather than removing) an aversive consequence or removing a positive reinforcer (Skinner, 1953). When contingently applied to a response, punishment decreases the rate of the response. Punishment also applies to the contingent *withholding* of positive reinforcement, such as in the time-out intervention. These definitions do not always fit lay interpretations of the term "punishment."

Current views of rewards, punishment, and the use of aversives vary widely. Use of rewards is sometimes dichotomized as *intrinsic* or *extrinsic*. The use of extrinsic reinforcement has led to widespread concern over undesirable outcomes related to motivation and creativity. However, these detrimental effects have *not* been reliably found in research (Eisenberger & Cameron, 1996). Use of aversives or punishment typically is considered as a last-resort and controversial intervention. Wolery and Gast (1990) make the point that aversives may be placed on a continuum, and much of the debate has centered on extremes. What is needed is to establish the conditions for use of specific and effective interventions, whether positive, aversive or nonaversive, mild or extreme. The focus is on a decision model that systematically is used to protect a client's right to an effective intervention; to ensure appropriate planning, implementation, and review; and overall, to establish the reasonableness of professional actions (Wolery & Gast, 1990). At the same time, many alternatives to punishment have been developed.

While punishment is common in parental discipline, numerous ethical and legal concerns apply when it is used by professionals. One of the first steps for the professional is often to examine the aversiveness of techniques that caregivers already use for discipline and control, such as unintentional or ineffective negative scanning, reprimands, and punishment. (We resume the discussion of aversives in Chapter 7; procedural safeguards, guidelines, and resources for the use of aversive interventions were presented in Chapter 5.)

Types of Reinforcement

When social attention is not sufficient, it is necessary to consider other types of reinforcement. *Primary* or *unconditioned* reinforcers have biological importance; the most widely used example is food. *Secondary*, learned, or *conditioned* reinforcers become reinforcing only after they become paired with primary reinforcers (or other secondary reinforcers).

Several groups of reinforcers have been used with young children. *Tangible* reinforcers are objects, such as toys, stickers, balloons, and pennies for a bank. *Activity* reinforcers are events or privileges that may be used to increase behaviors and include trips to the park, the zoo, or any special outing; playing with special friends; listening to music or stories; feeding the class pet; playing games; or piggyback rides. These may be superior to edibles and toys for many children (Hall & Hall, 1998c). Making choices about activities may be reinforcing. Novel events also may be rewarding, for example, an activity or "surprise box" containing slips of paper with various activity reinforcers (draw a picture, get a drink, and so on). If the contingency is met, the child pulls out a slip and completes the brief activity (Sulzer-Azaroff & Mayer, 1991). *Social reinforcers* include physical contact such as hugs, attention, proximity (e.g., standing or sitting near someone), or verbal statements (e.g., recognition or approval) (Hall & Hall,

1998c). Helping others may fit this category and be effective as a reinforcer. Praise by caregivers such as "Yes," "Great," "That's right," or "I like the way you . . . ," can be effective with young children. Reinforcers can include smiles, eye contact, and handshakes. *Feedback* from self-recordings or charts showing improvements in behaviors may be reinforcing for many children. *Tokens* serve as *generalized reinforcers*; these tangibles can be exchanged for other backup reinforcers. Group reinforcement and tokens are discussed in Chapter 7. *Automatic reinforcers* may be functional when behavior is not maintained by social or environmental reinforcement, as in forms of solitary play, some self-injurious behaviors, self-stimulation (Vollmer, 1994), and aggression (Thompson, Fisher, Piazza, & Kuhn, 1998).

Selecting Reinforcers

A reinforcer is defined by its effect on the behavior of an individual child. Thus, change agents must decide what to try as a reinforcer. Basic strategies involve asking the child, teacher, and parent, and observing the child for data on such factors as play preferences or different responses to consequences. As a general guideline, the selection of reinforcers should start with those that are "most natural or indigenous to a situation" (Sulzer-Azaroff & Mayer, 1991, p. 179). This would include judgments of acceptability by parents and teachers. If artificial reinforcers are selected, natural reinforcers ultimately should be introduced. Several strategies are discussed that are based on observations.

The *Premack Principle* (Premack, 1959), or Grandma's Law, is a powerful strategy whereby access to high-frequency behaviors (playing with a favorite toy) is made contingent on low-frequency behaviors (completing a preacademic task). Further analysis of the Premack Principle has led to a contrasting general principle. The *response deprivation hypothesis* (Timberlake & Allison, 1974) states: "If access to one of a pair of events is restricted below free operant levels (baseline), an organism will work to regain access to that activity" (Redmon & Farris, 1987, p. 327). In other words, a low-probability behavior can function as a reinforcer for a high-probability behavior if there are restrictions placed on responses as assessed at baseline levels (Konarski, Johnson, Crowell, & Whitman, 1981). The practical implications are enormous: "Almost any behavior in which the individual engages is a potentially effective reinforcer, provided access to that response can be restricted" (Sulzer-Azaroff & Mayer, 1991, p. 160).

Another strategy involves *reinforcer sampling* (Ayllon & Azrin, 1968) in which the child is given a brief exposure to the potential reinforcer. If a child does not have experience with an object, it may have only minimal appeal (Sulzer-Azaroff & Mayer, 1991). The child can be given several samples of reinforcers and the child's preference can be observed directly. Modeling of another child using the reinforcer also may be helpful (Ayllon & Azrin, 1968). Once the child begins to enjoy the activity or event, it may become a reinforcer.

Given the array of decisions, one can see that the task of selecting reinforcers may be quite complex. Outside of the use of direct observation, it may also be subjective. However, the use of direct observation will restrict the classes of potential reinforcers to those that are currently available. Typically, the process is not carried out systematically. Furthermore, reinforcement preferences may vary by day and by sessions. Satiation may also be a problem for some reinforcers.

In summary, the ongoing assessment of child-preferred reinforcers or activities is strongly linked to intervention outcomes and typically is carried out through interviews of caregivers and observation. However, it is a topic that will likely benefit from the development of structured procedures.

Reinforcement Assessment Packages

Mason, McGee, Farmer-Dougan, and Risley (1989) studied a procedure in which children selected their own reinforcers on an ongoing basis. The basic strategy followed earlier work by Pace, Ivancic, Edwards, Iwata, and Page (1985), who assessed reinforcement preferences by sampling from stimulus items selected for accessibility and ease of presentation. The items also represented different sensory qualities (mirror, juice, hug, clap, swing). To determine potential reinforcers, approach behavior and compliance to instructions were observed. This package capitalizes on variety and novelty.

In the study by Mason and colleagues (1989, p. 173), the reinforcer assessment package involved the following categories along with two stimuli, each from one of eight groups:

1. Olfactory: potpourri, coffee beans
2. Gustatory: juice, animal crackers, or cookies
3. Visual: flashing light, mirror
4. Tactile: vibrating wind-up toy, fan
5. Thermal: ice, heating pad
6. Vestibular: rocking, spinning
7. Auditory: touch-tone telephone beep, music
8. Social: clapping, hugs

Reinforcement was individualized. About half the child-preferred reinforcers identified in the comprehensive assessment were used in teaching. The range of reinforcements across children and conditions was two to five. The researchers described the comprehensive procedure used at the beginning and end of the study, and the daily minisession assessment.

Comprehensive Procedures

Each item was alternated randomly among stimuli for 10 trials. If a child failed to approach (that is, reach for or correctly label) an item within 5 seconds of its display, the experimenter prompted the child by providing a model of the response (the experimenter picked up and manipulated the item), and then re-presented the trial after a 5-second delay. Preferred items were those that children approached on 80% of the initial trials.

Daily Procedures

The presession mini-assessment consisted of one presentation of each of the items designated as preferred in the initial comprehensive assessment. The experimenter simultaneously displayed two preferred stimuli. The order and position of items varied across presentations, and two stimuli from the same sensory category were never presented as pairs. The child was told once to "pick one." The experimenter continued to display the two items until a selection or active rejection was made. (Adapted from Mason et al., 1989, pp. 173–174).

The results of the study with 3 preschool children having behaviors described as autistic showed positive effects (on maladaptive behaviors, correct responses on a teaching task, out-of-seat behavior) and positive side effects. One side effect was the broadening of reinforcement interests over the period of the study. Whereas the process of obtaining reinforcer information from teachers was about 5 minutes, the average experimental procedure based on children's selection of reinforcers ranged from 30 seconds to 1 minute.

Northup, George, Jones, Broussard, and Vollmer (1996) investigated choice-making and reinforcement assessment. They found that adding verbal or pictorial choice procedures may aid in detecting preferences, and that choice making may be superior to asking children to name preferences.

Schedules of Reinforcement

Reinforcement may be given on a continuous basis whereby every occurrence of the targeted behavior is reinforced, or it may be administered intermittently. *Noncontingent reinforcement* is the scheduled delivery of a preferred reinforcer *independent* of either positive or negative behaviors (its intervention use is discussed in Chapter 7).

During the initial stages of interventions, continuous reinforcement is used primarily to strengthen behavior. Intermittent reinforcement is used later to maintain behaviors. The term "thinning the schedule" refers to the process of changing from continuous to intermittent reinforcement. Lovaas (1981) described the thinning procedure:

> How "thin" you can make the reward schedule depends on many variables, and differs between children and tasks. Thin the schedule and look for *schedule strain*; if his behavior falls apart or begins to fluctuate widely, "thicken" the schedule, that is, reward him more often. Once you have recovered his behavior, start thinning again. (p. 13)

Advantages of intermittent reinforcement include resistance to extinction for desired behavior, maintenance of relatively high rates of responding, control for satiation, and cost-effectiveness. "Intermittent reinforcement is usually necessary for the progression to naturally occurring reinforcement" (Cooper et al., 1987, p. 277).

The effects of intermittent schedules of reinforcement have been extensively studied in laboratory experiments. The four basic schedules of intermittent reinforcement and characteristics are summarized in Table 6.1. Schedules of reinforcement can be much more complex than this. Lattal and Neef (1996) have expanded discussions of schedules of reinforcement.

Matching Law

For many interventions, one of the most important and often challenging tasks is to assess for competing contingencies of reinforcement. Matching Law (or Herrnstein's Law of Effect) expresses the rate of a target response as a function of *reinforcement context*. Examined in research for over three decades, this is a naturalistic view of reinforcement, because it takes into account other concurrent reinforcers present in environments.

The practical importance of Herrnstein's formulation is that "a given rate of contingent reinforcement may produce a high or low response rate depending on the context of reinforcement in which it occurs" (McDowell, 1982, p. 773). Regarding treatment implications, problem behavior may be reduced by extinction, by increasing reinforcement for appropriate response alternatives, or by "increasing the rate of free or noncontingent reinforcement" (p. 777). To increase desirable behavior, the reinforcement rate can be increased for the target behavior, the reinforcement rate for a concurrent inappropriate response can be decreased, or free or noncontingent reinforcement can be decreased. Tryon (1983) pointed out the benefits of selecting modification strategies to reduce reinforcement rates.

TABLE 6.1.   Schedules of Intermittent Reinforcement

Ratio schedules: Reinforcement is contingent on a specified number of responses.

● *Fixed ratio (FR)*: A set number of responses is performed before reinforcement. After the FR schedule has been in effect, there may be a postreinforcement pause or cessation in performance if the interval is relatively large, followed by typically high rates of responding. During extinction, performance may be characterized by bursts of responding, followed by increasingly longer periods of nonresponding until it reaches its prereinforcement level.

● *Variable ratio (VR)*: The number of responses required to earn a reinforcement for each trial is variable. The average number of responses across trials is used to describe the ratio. Steady rates, high rates of responding, and greater resistance to extinction are characteristic of VR schedules.

Interval schedules: Reinforcement is based on the passage of time.

● *Fixed interval (FI)*: The subject is reinforced following the performance of the targeted response after a set period of time. A scalloped performance effect is characteristic of FI schedules, whereby the subject responds at a low (or zero) rate following reinforcement, and performs at an increasing rate prior to the end of the interval. Under extinction, similarly, performance is interspersed with periods of nonresponding. Generally, extinction performance is less persistent compared to performance under other schedules.

● *Variable interval (VI)*: The subject is reinforced for performing the desired behavior following a time period that varies around an average interval. Like VR schedules, VI schedules typically generate stable levels of responding, with rates of responses depending on the size of the intervals, and they are resistant to extinction.

More formally, the equation asserts that behavior increases (hyperbolically) as a function of contingent reinforcement of the target response, but also as a function of extraneous concurrent reinforcement. Extraneous reinforcement may include reinforcement for a response other than the target behavior, noncontingent reinforcement, or spontaneous reinforcement (McDowell, 1982). The equation is expressed as

$$R = k(r/[r + re])$$

where R is the rate of target response, k (a constant) is the maximum possible rate of response, r is the rate of reinforcement contingent on the target response, and re is the rate of reinforcement for all other behaviors (Herrnstein, 1970). Martens, Halperin, Rummel, and Kilpatrick (1990) successfully demonstrated Matching Law for teacher-contingent attention and the on-task behavior of a 6-year-old boy. Teacher attention for off-task behavior influenced the rate of target responding by changing the relative amount of contingent attention for the target response.

Establishing Operations

From earlier discussions, one of the major points is that reinforcement has overall idiosyncratic and sometimes momentary effects on behavior based on reinforcement history and context. Changes in the environment can alter the momentary effectiveness of reinforcers as well as rates of behavior that have been previously reinforced by a specific contingent event or object. The term "establishing operations" (Michael, 1982) is used to describe how alterations in conditions (i.e., hunger, activity, social reinforcement, task difficulty) may establish the reinforcing value of stimuli (food, activity reinforcers, time out from social reinforcement, escape from a difficult task) and the likelihood of behavior occurring as a function of a reinforcer. An establishing stimulus describes the antecedent event that sets up the relationship (or need for food, activity, and so on). Establishing operations to increase reinforcement value can build on common events and natural levels of deprivation (Vollmer & Iwata, 1991).

Neutralizing Routines

"A neutralizing routine is . . . an establishing operation that reduces the value of reinforcers that are associated with problem behaviors" (Horner, Day, & Day, 1997, p. 601). The benefit of a neutralizing routine occurs when it can be introduced prior to the activity that serves as a stimulus for problem behavior. The idea is to reduce the reinforcing value of the consequences associated with the problem behavior. Neutralizing routines are based on a functional analysis of behavior, but we offer examples of how they may be used. A common example for young children is to let sleep-deprived children nap before activities that are associated with misbehavior. A second example has to do with favored routines. If expected and highly preferred activities need to be delayed (i.e., gym), this may occasion problem behavior for some children for the activity that is substituted. A neutralizing routine would be the introduction of a familiar preferred activity prior to the activity that is substituted. For children that require a great amount of teacher attention, a third example may be to develop positive *entry into the classroom routines*, such as a review of rules and practice, along with positive teacher attention.

Stimulus Control

Stimulus control—meaning that behaviors are performed in response to specific cues or stimulus conditions—is fundamental to the environmental analysis of behavior (Skinner, 1953) and to behavior modification programs (Kazdin, 1994). An event that functions as a signal that behavior will be reinforced is termed a "discriminative stimulus." "A discriminative stimulus sets the *occasion* for the behavior: it increases the probability that a previously reinforced behavior will occur . . . [and] eventually becomes a reinforcer itself" (Kazdin, 1994, p. 43). Thus, these antecedent events help control behavior. The control of the antecedent events over behavior is termed "stimulus control." The importance of stimulus control is that responsibility for learning rests with the person arranging the "conceptual environment" (Etzel, LeBlanc, Schilmoeller, & Stella, 1981). There are many examples of simple and effective stimulus control procedures for young children. Modeling and a brief time delay, discussed earlier as ways to promote language development, are two examples. Other examples in later chapters include improving parental commands for compliance, and the use of classroom rules and prompts. Stimulus control is used to teach concept formation and in differential reinforcement and errorless learning. The effects of stimulus control may be used to explain why behavior of children may vary considerably in different settings. Stimulus control also is used in self-control intervention procedures (Kazdin, 1994). Stimulus *generalization* occurs when a response transfers or generalizes from one stimulus condition to other similar conditions.

In the next four sections, other applications of stimulus control are discussed. Stimulus control procedures also need to be *faded*. Examples of fading procedures are given in the discussion of prompts.

The Use of Prompts

"Prompts are events that help initiate a response" (Kazdin, 1994, p. 45). There are three common features of prompting strategies (Wolery, 1994; see Wolery et al., 1992, for a full discussion): They help teach skills; they are removed as soon as possible; and they are combined with differential reinforcement.

Common prompts include verbal directions, modeling, and physical guidance. Gestures are often used as prompts or in combination with verbal prompts. Pictures or photographs also may be used as prompts in a wide variety of situations to depict rules, goals, steps in completing tasks, or models for performance.

Prompts may be ordered on a continuum of intrusiveness. Physical guidance is the most intrusive of the prompting procedures. However, without physical prompts, some children are unable to perform the behavior. *Partial* physical prompts require that caregivers touch the children but not control their movements. *Full* physical prompts involve moving children through the desired behaviors. Wolery et al. (1988, pp. 226–227) suggest the following guidelines for prompts:

1. Select the least intrusive, effective prompt.
2. Combine prompts if necessary.
3. Select natural prompts and those related to the behavior.
4. Provide prompts only after students are attending.
5. Provide prompts in a supportive, instructive manner before the student responds.
6. Fade prompts as soon as possible.
7. Plan fading procedures before using prompts.

Ultimately, the prompts are "faded," gradually diminished until the responses occur without them. There are several methods to accomplish fading. Cooper et al. (1987) described *least-to-most* as an appropriate fading procedure for most applications involving skills development. "Least-to-most" fading involves giving the child the opportunity to perform a response with the least amount of assistance needed on each successive trial. A brief delay (i.e., 5 seconds) is required between stimulus presentation that begins the task and the opportunity to respond. If the child does not respond within the time frame, a prompt of "least assistance" is provided by the caregiver. If, after the delay, the child has still not correctly responded, an additional prompt and guidance, such as a gesture, are given. Partial or full physical guidance can be provided when the child does not respond to less assistance.

Time delay is another method to fade prompts. Other fading strategies include the following (Wolery, Ault, & Doyle, 1992; Wolery, Bailey, & Sugai, 1988):

1. *Most-to-least prompting procedure.* In contrast to the least-to-most, most-to-least prompts involve progressively less intrusive prompts or decreasing levels of assistance as children demonstrate performance at the specified criterion.
2. *Antecedent prompt and test procedure.* This involves presenting children with "prompted trials" and giving them practice with the prompts removed.
3. *Antecedent prompt and fade.* Prompts are given on initial trials, but are faded (rather than removed) systematically by reducing the intensity or frequency of the prompt.
4. *Graduated guidance.* This procedure involves beginning each trial with sufficient assistance (or prompt), so that the child is able to perform the desired behavior, but withdrawing the prompt immediately when he or she does so. Prompts are provided as needed. *Shadowing* means that the caregiver's hands follow the child's movement in carrying out the behavior but do not touch the child. It enables immediate prompting as necessary.

Shaping and Chaining

In *shaping*, a complex behavior is achieved by teaching and reinforcing steps or *successive approximations* to the final behavior. Panyan wrote, "Shaping fosters the gradual development of a new behavior by repeatedly reinforcing minor improvements or steps toward that behavior. Instead of waiting for a new behavior to occur in its final form, we reinforce every resemblance of that new behavior" (1980, p. 1). From Panyan, first, the initial and goal behavior are defined in specific terms, and the condition under which the behavior is to occur is described. Second, a behavior that the child performs well and that approximates the desired behavior is identified. Third, the current behavior is reinforced when it resembles the desired behavior and reinforcers are withheld for behaviors that are not steps to the desired target behavior. This step is repeated with closer approximations to the desired behaviors. Fourth, as approximations occur with regularity, the requirement for reinforcement is increased and new approximations are consistently reinforced. Reinforcement is discontinued for behaviors that are not in the direction of the desired behavior. Finally, the criterion for reinforcement continues to be increased until the target behavior is fully demonstrated and occurs consistently.

Behaviors can be shaped in five ways (Panyan, 1980). First, the time that a child is engaged in an activity can be *lengthened*. An example is allowing a child engaged in appropriate solitary play to continue; shaping is used to increase existing behavior. Second, the time that it takes for a child to engage in a behavior following a stimulus or cue (e.g., replying to a request or dressing) can be *shortened*. Third, the *frequency* of a behavior can be increased. An example is increasing the rate of spontaneous language in play situations by a child with limited social interactions. Fourth, the *form* of the original response may be changed. Typical examples involve shaping sounds into recognizable language or teaching social skills. Fifth, shaping can be used to modify the *intensity* of a response. An example is shaping the force a child uses in coloring or drawing, or the loudness of a social greeting. Other techniques such as modeling and physical guidance may be combined with shaping.

A "*chaining procedure* is the reinforcement of a specified sequence of relatively simpler behaviors already in the repertoire of the individual to form a more complex behavior" (Sulzer-Azaroff & Mayer, 1991, p. 338). Whereas in shaping the steps only are useful because they lead to the desired response, in chaining the desired goal is typically the sequence of the separate behaviors (Kazdin, 1994). The individual responses are usually within the child's repertoire. The stimulus conditions and responses are components of the chain. The stimulus linking the components together serves two functions: as reinforcer and as discriminative stimulus for the next response.

There are three major varieties of chaining (Cooper et al., 1987). *Forward chaining* involves teaching the behaviors identified in a task analysis in temporal order. The first step is reinforced when the initial behavior in the task analysis is achieved. After that, each successive step is reinforced, contingent on adequate performance of prior steps to a specified criterion. The steps for *backward chaining* require that all behaviors in the task analysis, with the exception of the last behavior in the chain, be completed by the caregiver. Reinforcement is contingent upon the child performing the final behavior in the chain at a predetermined level. Next, reinforcement is delivered when the child performs both the last and next-to-last behaviors in the chain. Once this criterion is met, the child is reinforced when the last three behaviors are performed at the predetermined level. The sequence continues until the child has mastered all of the steps in the chain. Lovaas (1981) suggested that backward chaining is useful for skills such as undressing; since undressing is easier to learn than dressing, it may be taught first. Also, backward chaining builds on the reinforcement provided by the completion of the entire chain (Sulzer-Azaroff & Mayer, 1991). *Total task presentation* also begins with a task analysis. The difference is that the child receives training in each step for every session. Assistance is given as needed for each step, and steps for the entire chain are trained until the child is able to perform to a preset criterion. Skills that may benefit from chaining include dressing, feeding, and chores. Which procedure to use is an empirical question that depends on specific situations.

Preattending Skills

For many children, *preattending* skills may be an important focal point of assessment and intervention. Preattending is a preliminary step in learning; it involves looking at the materials, listening, and sitting quietly during instruction. With adept learners, preattending behaviors occur with minimal adult prompting in a learning task.

Attention to tasks can be improved by first teaching specific preattending behaviors through shaping. For example, in teaching a child the preattending behavior of sitting quietly, the adult first verbally models the behavior ("Watch how I can sit quietly in my chair." For some children, other prompts may be added: " . . . without talking to others or getting up."). The teacher physically models the behavior by sitting next to the child for a brief period (approximately 5 seconds). Next, the adult verbally prompts the child to exhibit the behavior ("Now show me how you can sit quietly."). Upon successful completion of the behavior, the child may receive a reinforcer such as praise. After each session, the time criterion for the reinforcer can gradually be increased. If the child is not imitating the model, different strategies need to be used.

The components for teaching preattending skills are summarized as follows:

1. *Modeling.* The caregiver verbally models the behavior for the child. For example, in teaching the child to look at a page of a book, the teacher would say, "Watch how I look at the page of this book without looking anywhere else."
2. *Physical prompting.* The caregiver models the behavior for the child. Continuing the example, the teacher would look at the book for approximately 5 seconds while the child watched.
3. *Verbal prompting.* The caregiver prompts the child to engage in the looking behavior ("Show me how you can look at the page of this book just like I did without looking anywhere else"). The interval should be kept brief, 5 seconds or less.
4. *Reinforcement.* Sometimes children's attention to tasks can be improved simply by providing reinforcement for attending. When the child successfully completes the looking behavior, the caregiver should praise the child. Other reinforcers may be added as needed.
5. *Following sessions.* During following sessions, model and prompt as necessary, while gradually increasing the time interval for looking (6 seconds, 8 seconds, 10 seconds). Also, shift reinforcement from preattending responses to task completions.

SUMMARY AND CONCLUSIONS

This chapter introduced basic interventions for learning new behaviors or modifying existing behaviors. Naturalistic strategies—differential attention, opportunities to respond, and modeling—are fundamental techniques for acquiring or modifying behaviors and for learning rules that guide subsequent behaviors. An expanded discussion of language skills emphasized the role of caregivers and the importance of language to other developmental tasks.

In addition, other basic principles and strategies for behavior change were presented, including reinforcement and stimulus control. The use of prompts, shaping, and chaining procedures are foundations for many interventions discussed in later chapters.

♦♦♦

Managing Severe Problem Behaviors

♦

Problematic child behaviors may lead to serious disruptions in home, school, and community settings in ways that have potentially broader implications for development and quality of life. Problem behaviors may be viewed as either excesses or deficits in behaviors desired or expected in specific settings. However, concern with these children's behaviors alone cannot serve as a guide for intervention design. It is necessary to focus on the environment in the form of intervention plans that lead to desired changes in behaviors. This chapter suggests effective intervention strategies to consider when designing intervention plans for severe problem behavior.

As these strategies necessitate individualized and sometimes complex departures from routine parent or teacher activities, it is recommended that: (1) these strategies be considered for severe and intractable behavior problems which do not respond to more naturalistic intervention strategies, and (2) frequent progress monitoring guide implementation of fading procedures as soon as the problem behaviors are under control.

DIFFERENTIAL REINFORCEMENT

Differential reinforcement simply means that certain responses or classes of behaviors are reinforced while others are not. This strategy is especially effective for building skills or for altering patterns of behaviors. Differential attention (Chapter 6) is an application of differential reinforcement. Some of the best and earliest examples in the intervention literature used parent and teacher attention as reinforcers.

This section presents techniques used to reduce maladaptive behaviors. They are referred to as "positive reductive procedures" for decreasing inappropriate behavior (Deitz & Repp, 1983, p. 35). Since the procedures involve changes in reinforcement, a functional analysis to identify and alter environmental variables as a basis for modifying or maintaining behaviors is an important prerequisite (Chapter 5). There is a confusing array of differential reinforcement strategies; some terms are widely used, while others have been selected to communicate key features of intervention plans.

Differential Reinforcement of Alternative Behavior (DRA)

In this technique, a more acceptable behavior is substituted for the maladaptive behavior, and occurrences of the acceptable behavior are selectively reinforced. The alternative behavior should appropriately occur during the time when a child would otherwise be exhibiting the undesirable behavior. As examples, a child cannot be attending and be off-task or isolated and engaged in peer play at the same time. Increasing engagement in activities or appropriate play would be alternative behaviors. DRA procedures have great possibilities for reducing classroom disruptions (Lentz, 1988). In addition, DRA is a positive procedure, without known negative side effects.

The alternative behavior must be selected with care. LaVigna and Donnellan (1986) proposed the 100% rule: The target behavior and the alternative response taken together should cover all possibilities for behavior. "By definition, the learner can either engage in the target behavior or in the alternative response with no third option available" (p. 44). Also, the alternative behavior must be in the child's repertoire. If it is not evident in preintervention baseline data, other procedures such as modeling, instruction, and prompts must be added to the intervention package.

Differential Reinforcement of Incompatible Behavior (DRI)

DRI is a subclass of DRA. Reinforcement is presented if the child performs a desirable behavior that cannot be performed simultaneously with the problem behavior. The rationale is that since both behaviors cannot be performed simultaneously, by increasing an acceptable but incompatible behavior, the unacceptable behavior must diminish. The behaviors selected as incompatible should be "natural opposites" (Donnellan & LaVigna, 1990). Table 7.1 suggests guidelines common to both DRA and DRI.

Differential Reinforcement of Functional Behavior (DRF)

This term, described by Rolider and Van Houten (1990), is also logically related to DRA. Based on a functional analysis of behavior, a new behav-

TABLE 7.1.   Guidelines for the Use of DRA and DRI

1. Appropriate alternative or incompatible behaviors should be in the child's repertoire of skills, and should be observed with regularity. Furthermore, the skills should lead to acquiring additional skills, and should be likely to be maintained by the child's natural environment.

2. The alternative behaviors should be "as physically different from the target behaviors as possible, in addition to being incompatible" (LaVigna & Donnellan, 1986, p. 52). Thus, alternative and target behaviors cannot be performed simultaneously.

3. Guidelines for the selection and administration of reinforcers should be carefully considered. The reinforcement should be contingently, consistently, and immediately administered. The reinforcers need to be stronger than those maintaining the maladaptive behavior, or, if possible, the maladaptive behavior should be subjected to extinction.

4. A continuous schedule of reinforcement should be used initially, and then should be gradually thinned.

5. DRA and DRI can be effectively combined with other techniques (e.g., DRO, DRL).

ior that serves the same function as the maladaptive behavior is selectively reinforced. Functional behaviors are taught because they are likely to enable children to access reinforcement that is naturally available in the environment or to help them learn appropriate ways to deal with difficult tasks. DRF stresses teaching new and adaptive behaviors to replace maladaptive behaviors. It is important to make certain that the new behaviors are more effective than the current behaviors in earning the desired reinforcers: "The new response should access the relevant reinforcer with a shorter delay, greater consistency, and less effort" (Carr, Robinson, & Palumbo, 1990, p. 367).

Differential Reinforcement of Communication (DRC)

Children's disturbing behaviors may serve a communicative function for parents and teachers when children seek to avoid or escape situational demands. Differential reinforcement of communication is a subset of differential reinforcement of alternative and functional behavior. Communication is used as a metaphor conceptualizing challenging behavior (e.g., self-injurious behavior, aggressive behavior, tantrums) for intervention purposes (Durand, 1990, p. 22; Reichle & Wacker, 1993). Examples are teaching a child to ask for help (such as signaling the need to use the toilet), to receive attention appropriately ("I'm finished"), or to appropriately "escape" stressful or demanding situations ("I need a break").

Since complete training manuals are available (Carr et al., 1994; Durand, 1990), we emphasize the basics that build on earlier discussions. First, the reinforcers maintaining the challenging behavior must be identified through a functional analysis. Second, these reinforcers are made contingent on appropriate child communicative responses that serve the same function as the challenging behaviors, and are withheld for the occurrence of challenging behavior.

Durand (1990) suggests the following steps for functional communication training (DRC):

1. Describe in detail each behavior of concern, taking care to focus on observable and measurable aspects of the problem situation.

2. Determine whether the behavior merits intervention (i.e., dangerous, of long duration, disruptive, interferes with learning, of great concern to caregivers).

3. Using a functional record review, structured caregiver interviews and direct observational methods, assess the function of the targeted behavior (i.e., escape, assistance, attention, sensory stimulation) and the variables maintaining its occurrence.

4. Using a variety of methods (e.g., surveys, pretesting and direct observation) identify reinforcers which are naturally available within the child's environment (e.g., activities, objects, edibles, classroom materials).

5. Choose a developmentally appropriate form of communication based on the child's skills, abilities, and materials present in the current environment (e.g., pointing, signing, verbal responses, symbols).

6. Teach the child a functionally equivalent response within the chosen communicative modality.

7. Provide reinforcement contingent upon occurrence of the functionally equivalent response.

Differential Reinforcement of Other Behavior (DRO)

In using DRO, the caregiver provides reinforcement for all responses *except* the target behavior. Reinforcement is given when the child does not perform the target behavior for certain time intervals. Carr, Robinson, and Palumbo (1990) reconceptualized DRO by its stimulus properties. They pointed out that DRO provides systematic discriminative stimuli for appropriate behaviors, thereby reducing problem behaviors.

For children with more than one problem behavior, those behaviors prioritized for change may be introduced sequentially or, preferably, target behaviors may be defined by response classes where several behaviors are included in the criteria for acceptable performance (if not, undesirable responses may be reinforced). Also, the child must have functional and appropriate behaviors in his or her repertoire. Most typically, DRO has been applied to self-injurious, aggressive, and disruptive behaviors (Poling & Ryan, 1982). Parent-administered programs for thumb-sucking and for inappropriate car behavior are described in Chapter 8.

There are several possible alternatives in designing a DRO program. For example, "whole" DRO involves a specified time period in which the child must not emit the targeted behavior in order to receive reinforcement. In momentary DRO (Barton, Brulle, & Repp, 1986), reinforcement is provided if the child is not performing the behavior at the moment of observation ("spot checking"). Whole-interval DRO is likely to be more effective in initial modification, whereas momentary DRO may be helpful in maintaining behavior change.

Generally, the interval is reset if the target behavior occurs. For example, if a child misbehaves 3 minutes into a 5-minute interval, the timer is reset for another 5 minutes. Another practical variation is to set the interval at a specified length and only provide reinforcement if the behavior was not emitted during the interval. Intervals also may be variable in length, and may be increased based on the child's performance (termed an "escalating schedule").

Like other differential reinforcement procedures, DRO may require substantial vigilance and effort. However, only the target behaviors (in contrast to the alternative behaviors) and the time interval need to be carefully monitored. DRO may be combined with other interventions. For example, Rolider and Van Houten (1984) found that the appropriate use of disapproval and correction increased the effectiveness of DRO. DRO is generally viewed as an alternative to punishment (LaVigna & Donnellan, 1986), whereas Rolider and Van Houten (1990) describe it as a punishment procedure. Suggestions for improving DRO include making the conditions more discriminable (e.g., visual or auditory timer) and using verbal mediators to describe the conditions when possible to help develop rule-governed behavior (e.g., no hitting) (Rolider & Van Houten, 1990). General procedures for DRO are outlined in Table 7.2.

Differential Reinforcement of Low Rates of Behavior (DRL)

DRL is a procedure to *reduce* rather than eliminate behavior. It may be used as a first step in eliminating undesirable behavior when behavior rates are very high. To use DRL, a criterion is specified for the targeted response and the child is reinforced if the rate of behavior is less than the criterion for a specified time period. DRL is appropriate when it may not be desirable to reduce the behavior to a zero level. For example, a child who makes numerous comments during group discussions may be allowed only a set number (established through the use of peer micronorms or teacher consultation).

TABLE 7.2.   Guidelines for Using DRO

1. Establish an appropriate time interval for reinforcement. One guideline is to set the initial time interval less than the mean interresponse time (IRT) found during baseline observations (Deitz & Repp, 1983) or one-half the baseline IRT (LaVigna & Donnellan, 1986).

2. Reinforce the child at the end of the interval if the target behavior, or other inappropriate behavior, was not performed during the interval.

3. Establish procedures to increase the length of the DRO interval by small increments after behavior is effectively controlled. Three recommended ways to increase the interval include the following: (a) Intervals can be increased by a constant amount of time; (b) intervals can be increased by a proportionate amount of time (e.g., 10%); and (c) the interval length can be based on the child's performance (e.g., the mean IRT interval from the preceding session can be used to set the new DRO interval) (Poling & Ryan, 1982; see LaVigna & Donnellan, 1986, for other recommendations). It may be helpful to inform the child about the change in interval length (Poling & Ryan, 1982).

4. Since DRO is not a constructive procedure, it should be combined with DRA (Sulzer-Azaroff & Mayer, 1991) or other strategies for positive programming in order to increase adaptive and appropriate behaviors.

5. DRO can be effectively combined with other reductive procedures.

Note. Except where noted, the procedures as described have been adapted from Cooper, Heron, and Heward (1987). Copyright 1987 by Simon & Schuster and Prentice Hall, Inc. Adapted by permission.

DRL may be specified by the number of responses allowed within a time period or by how much time passes between responses. Once the behavior is under control, the criterion for the number of responses can be changed to lower the average rate of responding. New criteria for performance may be introduced after the behavior has reached a "steady state" (LaVigna & Dollellan, 1986).

The opposite of a DRL is DRH, differential reinforcement of high rates of behavior (contextually appropriate). An example of its use would be with children having low rates of social interaction or communication.

As with all differential reinforcement procedures, there are several alternative strategies (Deitz, 1977). In *full-session DRL*, reinforcement is administered if responses during the session are equal to or below a specified criterion. Full-session DRL involves the fewest demands on practitioners. The practitioner simply has to count the number of targeted behaviors exhibited during the session and reinforce or withhold reinforcement (Deitz, 1977).

Interval DRL requires dividing the session into equal, smaller intervals of time. Reinforcement is administered at the end of each interval if the child's responses were equal to or below the set criterion. Longer intervals can be subsequently reinforced, thereby reducing the rate of behavior. In *spaced-responding DRL*, a response is reinforced that is separated by another response by a preset minimum amount of time (interresponse time, or IRT). After behavioral control has been obtained, the length of the IRT is increased. General procedures are presented in Table 7.3.

Differential Reinforcement of Diminishing Rates (DRD)

DRD is reinforcement contingent on a *reduction* in response rate (Sulzer-Azaroff & Mayer, 1991). This may be a helpful procedure for disruptive behaviors when a change from 15 acts to 14 is reinforced, but the next criterion would be 13 or fewer disruptive acts. Similarly, a parent self-monitoring program in which 32 yells reduced to 31 may occasion self-reinforcement on a particular day, with the next criterion being 30 or fewer, and so on.

The opposite of DRD is the differential reinforcement of increasing rates of behavior. An example of differentially reinforcing *increasing rates* would be having teachers self-monitor and increase the ratio of positive/negative statements made to children.

As these examples show, self-monitoring or other feedback systems may be combined with differential reinforcement procedures. While effective across many applications, some cautions are in order regarding differential reinforcement procedures. Appropriate alternative behaviors must

---

TABLE 7.3.   Guidelines for Using DRL

1. Baseline data are used to set the initial DRL criterion. When using full-session DRL, the criterion should be set at or slightly lower than the response rate found in baseline conditions. Similar considerations are used when selecting the IRT for interval or spaced-responding DRL.

2. The DRL criterion is gradually and systematically decreased. Prior sessions are used to make decisions concerning new criteria.

   a. For full-session DRL, a criterion equal to or less than the average number of responses per session may be used as a guideline.

   b. For interval DRL, the length of the interval can be increased if the criterion is one response per interval, or the number of responses per interval may be lowered. If the criteria is not met (i.e., the child behaves inappropriately in excess of the criteria), the interval is reset.

   c. With spaced-responding DRL, the IRT is used to reestablish the criterion and is set equal to or less than the IRT in recent sessions.

3. A decision rule needs to be established for changing the DRL criterion. Example: Change the criterion when the criterion is not exceeded in three consecutive sessions.

Note. Adapted from Deitz (1977), Deitz and Repp (1983), and D. E. Deitz (personal communication, August 29, 1991). Copyright 1983 by PRO-ED, Inc. Reprinted by permission.

be within the child's performance capabilities. Also, DRD, DRO, and DRL focus on negative and not constructive behavior, although other procedures such as DRA or modeling may be added.

Noncontingent Reinforcement (NCR)

Noncontingent reinforcement is a behavioral reductive procedure developed to help resolve the potential problems associated with differential reinforcement (continuous monitoring of behavior, potential side effects due to extinction, and possible low rates of reinforcement because of high rates of inappropriate behavior). It has been used to reduce self-injurious behaviors and aggression.

Studies show that when a functional reinforcer (one that is linked to behavioral maintenance) is administered noncontingently, a target response will be reduced. While Marcus and Vollmer (1996) propose that extinction is the most likely mechanism, in that the relationship between reinforcement and behavior is altered, NCR also is predicted to be effective based on Matching Law.

NCR consists of the following components (Marcus & Vollmer, 1996, pp. 43–44): (1) a functional analysis to determine potential reinforcers; (2) NCR, during which a fixed-time schedule determines when the individual will receive access to preferred reinforcers during the session, independent of occurrences of aberrant or adaptive behaviors; (3) extinction, during which the experimenter provides no programmed consequences contingent on the aberrant target behaviors; and (4) fading, in which the schedule of noncontingent reinforcement is gradually decreased from a dense (continuous) to a lean schedule (e.g., one delivery per 5 minutes).

Possible side effects may include unintentional reinforcement of the undesired behavior and extinction bursts. A procedure may be added to reduce these potential effects by omitting reinforcement if the targeted response (i.e., aggression) occurs during a preset interval (i.e., 10 seconds) prior to the scheduled time for reinforcement (Vollmer, Ringdahl, Roane, & Marcus, 1997). This added procedure may be described as a momentary DRO.

AVERSIVE PROCEDURES AND PUNISHMENT

The use of aversive procedures has prompted many considerations of legal and ethical issues that were discussed earlier. In many ways, aversives also should be viewed as a strategy that is naturalistically used, or misused, by caregivers (Axelrod, 1990) and often merits analysis in referrals for misbehavior for at least two reasons. First, many children are growing up in very aversive environments, and second, the punishment administered to children may be reinforcing to caregivers.

In this section, we discuss interventions traditionally considered as aversive: time out, response cost, and overcorrection. Other aversive strategies were presented earlier, such as the use of planned ignoring, extinction, and reprimands. DRO and DRL also may be considered as aversive procedures because reinforcement is reduced contingent on inappropriate behavior (Rolider & Van Houten, 1990). Also, both focus on undesirable behaviors and "negative scanning" for occurrences.

Some think that punishment never should be used (Donnellan & La Vigna, 1990); others argue that for certain behaviors involving risk, harm, or disastrous consequences of intervention failure, interventions involving punishment may be considered from the outset (Axelrod, 1990). Except in unusual circumstances, interventions that involve harsh and restrictive punishment should be considered only after positive procedures have been adequately tried and failed, and only if legal, ethical, and procedural safeguards have been followed. Thus, at the minimum, the use of punishment or aversives merits the following considerations: the likelihood of risk or harm to the child or others, the results of functional analysis, and the likelihood of intervention effectiveness. If punishment is used, appropriate alternative behaviors should be reinforced.

Time Out (from Positive Reinforcement)

Time out is considered to be a punishment procedure; it involves a child being denied access to the opportunity to earn positive reinforcement for brief periods of time contingent on a targeted maladaptive behavior. Nelson and Rutherford (1983) noted that time out "involves a combination of extinction, punishment, positive reinforcement, and negative reinforcement" because it includes multiple contingencies for different possible behaviors (p. 56). Planned ignoring can be considered as a form of time out when attention is the major reinforcer.

To be effective, the "time in" environment must be reinforcing. Thus, the first step in using time out is to assess the *time-in* environment—a step basic to ecobehavioral analysis in general. Schrader and Gaylord-Ross (1990) described environmental enrichment in the following way:

> Enrichment refers to the provision of a wide range of activities and materials that create a stimulating and reinforcing environment. . . . An enriched environment . . . provides availability of and reinforcement for interacting with materials and activities, opportunity and reinforcement for the use of language and other forms of communication, a high interest curriculum, novelty in available stimuli, frequent rein-

forcement for adaptive behaviors, opportunities for structured and incidental social interaction, an adequate amount of personal space, choices within a predictable schedule, and the opportunity for community participation. (pp. 408–409)

Time out can be easily overused and misused. Reasons for this are (1) an insufficiently reinforcing "time-in" environment, (2) reinforcement the caregiver receives for placing children in time out, (3) inappropriate use of time out (for mild problems, or for problems that are out of control), and (4) unenforceable time outs (Nelson & Rutherford, 1983). Time out is subject to significant criticism and legal concerns (Lohrman-O'Rourke & Zirkel, 1998) when used to exclude or seclude children.

Because of the many challenges to time out and other aversives, the professional must be especially cautious about *introducing* aversive interventions into intervention plans. Often it will be important to work toward making intervention designs more positive. Regardless, consultation regarding time-out procedures may be beneficial. It may be the intervention of choice by parents, or a mild time out may be used as an end point in sequenced intervention plans.

Procedures for teaching the use of time out have been well described (McGimsey, Greene, & Lutzker, 1995). Flanagan, Adams, and Forehand (1979) suggested that modeling (such as through the use of videotape) may be the best procedure to help parents competently perform time out. The effectiveness of the training should be assessed by observing the parent's use of the technique. Parents will benefit by systematically planning time-out procedures.

Considerations for planning time out are identified in Table 7.4. Time out can be conducted in many ways, perhaps best represented on a "continuum of aversive procedures" (Nelson & Rutherford, 1983). Some evidence suggests that one brief warning may decrease the number of time-out occasions (Roberts, 1982). Time-out durations for most preschool applications should be relatively brief but are also dependent on the child's history with the procedures. Short durations of time out (2 minutes) may be useful if they have not been preceded by longer intervals (Harris, 1985), but still, this would be a function of the attractiveness of time in. A reason for concern over long or frequent time outs is that they reduce learning time. Backup procedures or contingencies also are a necessary part of plans for time out.

Frequently, time-out interventions include a step whereby the interval is extended if the child behaves inappropriately. This is called contingent delay. For example, if the child is crying, whining, or yelling at the end of the time-out interval, the time-out duration is extended until a brief contingency is met for appropriate behavior (say 15 seconds). The rationale is

TABLE 7.4. **Considerations in Planning and Using Time Out**

1. Enriching time in.
2. Type and location of time out (i.e., removing reinforcing conditions or removing child from reinforcing conditions).
3. Selecting the duration of time out.
4. Using a warning prior to time out.
5. Selecting and using verbal explanations in conjunction with time out. If used they should be brief, and perhaps only used during the first occasion.
6. Presence or absence of a signal to indicate the beginning and end of time out, and/or that time out period is in effect.
7. Using verbal instructions (vs. physical assistance).
8. Scheduling of time out (e.g., time out for each occurrence of misbehavior vs. warnings).
9. Selecting criteria and procedures to release children from time out.
10. Selecting back up contingencies.
11. Presence or location of adult during time out.
12. Training staff and monitoring implementation.
13. Collecting and analyzing data: the use of time out should be decreasing based on improved behavior.

Note. Adapted from Harris (1985), Matson and DiLorenzo (1984), and Wolery, Bailey, and Sugai (1988). Copyright 1985 by the Council for Exceptional Children. Copyright 1984 by Springer Publishing, Inc. Copyright 1988 by Allyn & Bacon. Reprinted by permission.

that if the child is released from time out while misbehaving, the misbehavior may inadvertently be reinforced. However, the efficiency and effectiveness of the contingent delay procedure have been questioned (Mace, Page, Ivancic, & O'Brien, 1986). Potential problems with the contingent delay include unnecessarily longer time outs, time out for relatively minor offenses, and practical factors related to a more complicated intervention. Mace and colleagues (1986) compared time out with and without the contingent delay and found both to be effective across 3 children.

A key decision is to plan for noncompliance with time out. In some early treatment programs for parents, spanking was used as a consequence for noncompliance with the procedure. Studies suggest that room time out may be useful for this purpose (Roberts, 1988). Potential noncompliance with a procedure like time out is one reason for considering sequenced interventions introduced in Chapter 4.

An Example of Time Out

Firestone (1976) evaluated the use of time out with a 4-year-old boy in a nursery school. The child had a substantial history of aggressive behaviors and was expelled from a nursery school at age 3. In addition to verbally and physically aggressive behavior, other behaviors were observed in order to determine the side effects of the intervention: (1) cooperation (such as being compliant, sharing), (2) interactions with teachers (such as asking questions, helping with chores), (3) isolation (such as playing alone), and (4) activity level.

For every physically aggressive act, the child was placed in a chair in the corner of the classroom for 2 minutes. The rationale for time out was shared with the child the first time.

Physical and verbal aggressiveness decreased significantly. In addition, the intervention demonstrated beneficial side effects. Isolate behavior decreased, while cooperative play increased. Interactions with teachers were reduced, but were variable. Activity level increased slightly over the baseline condition but was variable, and the data did not suggest a trend. The most notable findings were the reductions in physical aggressiveness and increased positive interactions with peers.

Other more drastic forms of time out, such as isolation or seclusion, are not discussed here as they typically are not recommended for preschool practices. However, these forms of time out are often practiced by parents (sending a child to his or her room). Many other forms of time out have been used in home and educational settings. Parental strategies and the use of time out in treatment packages are discussed in Chapter 9.

Contingent Observation

For problem behaviors, a strategy easily adapted to many play routines is contingent observation. Contingent observation involves incidental teaching, choice making, and "mild" time out from active participation in an activity. The description of the procedures is from Porterfield, Herbert-Jackson, and Risley (1976).

First, the inappropriate and appropriate behaviors need to be described to the child ("Don't take the ball from other children" "Ask for the toys you want"). The child is guided to the periphery of the activity and sits on the floor without toys or play equipment. The child is told to watch the way the other children play ("Sit and watch how the other children ask for the toys they want to play with"). When the child has been watching for less than 1 minute, the child is asked if he or she is ready to join in play activity and use appropriate behavior. The child indicates his or her readiness for play by nodding or verbalizing, and the child returns to the group. If the child does not respond to the question or gives a negative reply, the child is told to sit and watch the children play until he or she is able to ask for the ball appropriately. The child is then required to sit for another 30 seconds to 1 minute and then is asked again if he or she is ready to join in the play. When the child returns to play, reinforcement (i.e., positive attention) is provided for appropriate behavior ("Great, you asked for the ball"). Should the child continue to cry or have tantrums and disrupt the play of other children, or if the child refuses to sit and observe quietly, he or she is removed from the immediate setting, is given a reason for leaving and criterion for returning, and goes to a "quiet place" (e.g., a brief time out), away from the "sit and watch" location close to other children. When calm or sitting appropriately, the child is returned to the sit-and-watch location following the child's positive response indicating that he or she is "ready to sit quietly and watch" (p. 59), and ready to rejoin play. Contingent observation provides an example of a sequenced intervention and consequence hierarchy building on choice making (Chapter 4).

Response Cost

Response cost is used to decrease inappropriate behaviors. It is the removal or loss of a positive reinforcer held by the child (or one that would normally be available) if a target behavior is performed, with a result of a decrease in occurrences of the behavior. Alternatively, it sometimes involves a fine or penalty for every occurrence of the targeted behavior. Most often, response cost has been applied to earned points, tokens, chips, stars, check marks, money, or similar reinforcers, but it can also apply to privileges. It has been effectively used with token economies. Also, it has been used to describe contingent unpleasant routines, such as assisting with cleanup after soiling accidents (Reimers, 1996).

Response cost, in one form or another, is pervasively used by parents or teachers—sometimes ineffectively, such as removing toys or other positive experiences in ways that do not decrease misbehavior but limit positive experiences and learning. For this reason, we examine considerations for its use. Prerequisite skills are necessary and may have to be taught. Ineffective response cost may undermine a treatment program. Also, because it is an aversive procedure, unwanted side effects such as aggressive behaviors, avoidance, or emotional outbursts may occur.

Response cost is likely to be an acceptable procedure to many caregivers. Advantages are that response cost may result in effective decreases in inappropriate behavior, and it is convenient to use in group or classroom settings. In comparison to time out, the child is not removed from ongoing activities.

There are different ways of implementing response cost. First, response cost can be used along with a system of reinforcement; the child earns points or tokens for appropriate responses and loses points for inappropriate behaviors. Second, participants may be fined, and reinforcing events such as free play are taken away. In a third strategy, referred to as a "bonus response cost" (Sulzer-Azaroff & Mayer, 1991, p. 442), additional reinforcers that are not typically available to the child are made accessible. An example would be additional time in the gym or play with an attractive toy. The bonus time, but not the usually scheduled time, would be lost in specified amounts for inappropriate behavior. The advantages are the potential use of backup reinforcers and less critical legal and ethical concerns, since positive experiences available to all children are not removed. Fourth, group contingencies may be involved. These are discussed in a later section.

Guidelines for response cost have been suggested by several writers (Kazdin, 1977b, 1982a; Pazulinec, Meyerrose, & Sajwaj, 1983; Thibadeau, 1998; Walker, 1983).

1. Clearly define the behaviors or rules and carefully determine the amounts of the fine. The target behaviors should be significant inappropriate behaviors and not minor transgressions. The amount of fines or penalties may need to be determined empirically.

2. The effective use of positive attention for appropriate behaviors may be critical. For this reason, response cost frequently should be combined with other positive differential reinforcement procedures, because it alone does not teach adaptive behaviors, and it causes behavioral change agents to focus unduly on inappropriate behavior.

3. Children need to have clear descriptions of both how to earn positive reinforcement and the behaviors that result in response cost. Carefully evaluate the natural reinforcers that are available, or the "bonus" reinforcers that can be made available. Consider gradual reductions in behavior, and different penalties for more or less serious rule violations.

4. Depending on the response cost system, children may need to have experience with the reinforcers, and need to be able to earn or build up a sufficient amount to establish a "reserve." Baseline data should be used to help determine the amount of reinforcement that may be set aside for possible losses.

5. Role play with the system may be helpful, and prior training in prerequisite skills may be necessary (such as how to enter play groups to prevent playground fighting).

6. The "economics" of response cost need to be considered carefully to prevent situations where children fall into debt and give up, or amass large amounts of the tokens or rewards, with the result that fines may be of insufficient concern. The fine should be sufficiently substantial to affect behavior but not so large as to result in bankruptcy. Increasing the amount of fine will decrease behavior only to a point, after which large fines are not likely to decrease behavior significantly. A child should not be allowed to accumulate fines. If at zero, other consequence can be applied until the child can earn points or a new session begins.

7. Administer the fine as soon as possible following each targeted inappropriate behavior. The fine should not be administered in a harsh, punitive, or personal way. Records should be kept for each inappropriate behavior and resulting response cost.

8. Plan for collecting response-cost fines and plan backup interventions for children who refuse to give up tokens. Home–school contingencies may be added.

9. Evaluate the program for unplanned outcomes.

Overcorrection

Overcorrection involves two procedures that may be used separately or in combination. In *restitution*, the child is required to restore the environment to an improved condition, contingent on the performance of a target behavior: (1) A request is made to stop responding, the activity is interrupted, and feedback is provided about the behavior to be corrected; (2) a requirement is made to do work and provide assistance, and prompts are given as necessary; (3) the work is performed repetitively; and (4) the child is then returned to the ongoing activity (Matson & DiLorenzo, 1984). In *positive practice*, appropriate behaviors are practiced in situations that have been associated with misbehavior, contingent upon performance of the targeted maladaptive behavior. The child is requested to perform a suitable and incompatible behavior repetitively and is then returned to the ongoing activity.

Conceptually, overcorrection may be viewed as punishment—a time out from reinforcement, during which the child is required to perform a positive task (or work) logically tied to the misbehavior (Matson & DiLorenzo, 1984). It also is viewed as a complex treatment package and can be combined with other interventions such as DRO. In contrast, simple correction means that the child only "corrects" the result of his or her behavior. *Negative practice* requires the child to engage in the undesired behaviors repetitively for a specified time period under supervision and contingent on the targeted maladaptive behavior.

The intervention originated with toilet training for adults with mental retardation (Azrin & Foxx, 1974). Restitution and positive-practice overcorrection have helped with severe problems such as toileting problems of children, stereotypical behavior (self-stimulation), self-injury, aggression, and disruptive behaviors for individuals with severe disabilities (e.g., autism, mental retardation). The procedures can be applied to a wide range of maladaptive behaviors of typically developing children as well, "such as throwing food on the floor and leaving toys and clothes strewn all over the house" (Spiegler, 1983, p. 156). However, negative reactions to the procedures may be extreme (Foxx, 1996).

Overcorrection may have a number of components that vary within specific treatment programs. Important conditions are that (1) the additional task must be similar or related to the original task or behavior; (2) the overcorrection should occur immediately after the misbehavior if the child is calm; (3) the duration of the overcorrection should be longer than the original problem situation; (4) the child must be engaged actively in the positive practice overcorrection task; and (5) appropriate alternative behaviors should be reinforced when not applying overcorrection.

Shapiro (1979) applied restitution and positive-practice overcorrection to reduce paper shredding and book tearing by a 5-year-old girl described as nonverbal with moderate retardation. Restitution (2 minutes) consisted of instructions to pick up all torn paper and then clean the area (place toys in the toy box). Physical prompting was given when necessary. Positive practice (5 minutes) consisted of looking through books with the experimenter without tearing them. The behaviors were successfully eliminated, and the results were sustained for 18 months after the program ended.

Overcorrection is potentially acceptable to parents, teachers, and other change agents across a variety of target behaviors. The procedures can follow an analysis of naturally occurring caregiver responses to misbehaviors and incorporate ways to teach socially appropriate behaviors and provide natural consequences for specific maladaptive behaviors. However, it is important to follow established procedures whenever possible. Also, since overcorrection is viewed as a punishment or aversive technique, special precautions are necessary. The caregivers should be prepared to handle a child who becomes upset or refuses to perform the required behaviors.

Overcorrection can be abused by angry or unskilled caregivers; thus, it may require close supervision. It can be punishing to caregivers due to children's aversive reactions and may be very difficult to use correctly and consistently by some caregivers or in certain situations. Medical consent may be required in addition to the safeguards outlined in Chapter 5. However, durations for overcorrection applications may be quite brief (30 seconds to 3 minutes), and partial corrections may still be effective. An important application of overcorrection is dry bed training described in Chapter 8. Studies using overcorrection and negative practice for firesetting behavior are mentioned in Chapter 9.

SELF-MEDIATED INTERVENTION TECHNIQUES

Self-Regulation

Self-regulation is considered to be a keystone behavior that is pivotal in behavior change efforts, and the development of responsibility and self-regulation serves as a primary objective of early childhood education (Bredekamp & Copple, 1997). Self-regulatory processes involve self-observation or monitoring, judgmental processes concerning one's performance, and self-reactions. Kanfer and Karoly (1982) suggest that self-regulation or management "signifies the *gradual* assumption of control by the individual over cueing, directing, rewarding, and correcting his or her own behavior" (p. 576). Methods of external control (by parents, teachers, peers) are used to teach self-management skills. Furthermore, in practice, interventions that are usually "externally controlled" may benefit from combining self-control procedures, usually in the form of verbal mediation by caregivers.

There are many reasons to further the development of self-regulation. First, much behavior is missed by parents, teachers, and other potential observers. Second, observers, behavioral change agents, or settings may become "cues" for the target behavior, so that the child performs the behavior depending on the setting or presence of another person. Self-regulation is an inherent mechanism for generalization. Third, practical benefits of successful interventions include giving caregivers additional time for other responsibilities. Successful self-regulation reduces the vigilance required in monitoring children's behavior that results in fatigue and loss of caregiver motivation. Fourth, the goal of intervention is often that of self-control, defined as a set of generalizable skills such as coping responses or rules of conduct in identifiable problem situations. A projected end goal of self-regulation interventions would be the ability to follow group rules, resolve conflicts, and solve problems that arise in a variety of situations (Bredekamp & Copple, 1997).

Self-monitoring may have treatment effects, termed "reactivity." Thus, self-monitoring may be an important intervention in itself. With young children, we have used self-monitoring with such behaviors as thumb-sucking and tantrums, and have included it as a component in other interventions to the greatest extent possible. Other techniques of self-control for young children involve applications of stimulus control, self-instruction and self-statements, self-reinforcement, and alternative response training (Kazdin, 1994).

Teaching Self-Regulation

The general strategies for teaching self-regulation are outlined here; specific home and school applications are discussed in later chapters.

1. The child must be able to observe his or her own behavior. These skills may be taught prior to an intervention. The component strategies of self-monitoring were reviewed in Chapter 3.

2. Rule learning is essential. Rules involve behaviors that are appropriate for various tasks and situations, and awareness of the consequences of behaviors.
3. The child must have the necessary skills to perform the behaviors.
4. The child is taught to evaluate his or her own behavior and compare it to standards for the behavior.
5. The child is taught to self-record and self-reward.
6. Self-regulation may be used in combination with other interventions (DRO) and other reinforcers. Public goal setting (Hayes et al., 1985) may be an important aspect of self-regulation training.

Poth and Barnett (1983) combined self-regulation with other intervention components to reduce occurrences of a 3-year-old boy's tic-like behavior. The child had an extensive history of abuse and neglect. Parent and teacher consultation, plus a review of his educational and psychological history, revealed multiple concerns, including delayed fine and gross motor development, reduced attention span, and difficulties with speech and social skills. Of special concern were his tic-like behaviors, described as "shuddering episodes" in which his upper body and arms became tensed and rigid, and he displayed palsylike movements in his hands for 2 or 3 seconds.

The intervention plan was implemented first in the resource room, followed by intervention in the classroom. In the first phase, self-observation and self-regulation techniques were used, following the general steps discussed in Chapter 4. The child was taught to discriminate tensed from relaxed positions and behaviors, and was reinforced for engaging and completing activities in which the shuddering behaviors were not exhibited. The procedural steps were as follows:

1. "Charlie, this is relaxed" (Slowly rotate head, shake arms loosely, bend at the waist, hands near the floor. Slowly return to upright position. Extend arms forward in a slow and relaxed manner. Repeat "This is relaxed.")
2. "Charlie, show me relaxed; let's relax together." (Repeat relaxing the body as described in Step 1, talking softly through each movement.)
3. "Charlie, this is *not* relaxed. (Demonstrate rigid arms, legs, tensing the body, then repeat "This is not relaxed".)
4. "Charlie, show me *not* relaxed. Let's do *not* relaxed together." (Repeat tensing the body as described in Step 3.)
5. Repeat Step 2, then Step 4, and Step 2.

After the relaxation practice, it was explained to the child that if he remained relaxed during the planned activity, he would receive a star for his special card. In the classroom phase, the child received stars or stickers on a special card for completion of classroom activities while staying relaxed. A silent signal was used as a reminder to be relaxed. Like many interventions, specific techniques were combined. The intervention also used elements of DRO by reinforcing periods of time when the tic-like behavior was not evident. The results were described in Chapter 5 in the example of a multiple baseline across settings.

Self-instruction training involves teaching self-statements related to problem solving. Meichenbaum and Goodman (1971) developed the core procedure: (1) The adult models the behavior while talking aloud; (2) the child performs the behavior while the adult instructs out loud; (3) the child performs the behavior and talks aloud to him- or herself; (4) the child performs the behavior while whispering; and (5) the child performs the behavior while covertly verbalizing. Modeled verbalizations usually consist of (1) questions about the task, (2) answers to the questions, (3) self-guiding instructions, and (4) self-reinforcement (Bryant & Budd, 1982). However, there have been failures to replicate the procedure (Billings & Wasik, 1985).

Correspondence Training

In correspondence training, "reinforcement is made contingent on both promising to engage in a target response and then actually doing so, or on truthfully reporting past actions" (Baer, Williams, Osnes, & Stokes, 1985, p. 479). The rationale for *correspondence training* is quite simple. It involves developing the relationship between children's verbal accounts of behavior and their actual behavior, between saying and doing. It can be viewed as training in promise keeping (Baer, Osnes, & Stokes, 1983).

Language is a logical target for self-regulation efforts, for several reasons (Stokes & Osnes, 1986): (1) Relatively speaking, it may be a well-developed skill with a pattern that leads to some control over behavior; (2) it can be used readily across different environments; and (3) it may be used conveniently and requires little effort. A potential advantage is that it may facilitate behavioral programs across inconvenient situations and inaccessible settings (Baer et al., 1983). Although the focus of correspondence training is on verbalizations used to mediate behaviors, the procedures have been used with language-delayed or socially withdrawn children (Osnes, Guevremont, & Stokes, 1986).

First, careful consideration must be given to the child's ability to perform the task and to criteria for reinforcement. Baseline information is used to set initial criteria, and level changes are introduced by changing the criteria in planned increments. Final goals are set by peer comparisons through the use of micronorms.

For example, before a play period, the caregiver asks the child, "What are you going to do in play today?" If the child responds with "I'm going to talk to the kids a lot," he or she is sent to play. The criterion for "talking a lot" is set with baseline performance in mind. If the child does not spontaneously respond, the caregiver should prompt the child until the child verbally responds that he or she is ready to play. The play setting should have a minimum of four children. After the play period, the child is taken aside and given feedback about the play session. If the child talked a lot, he or she should be given praise, affection, and a reinforcer. Osnes et al. (1986) used a "Happy Sack" to provide reinforcement, a bag containing 10 slips of paper with attention or activity consequences that require less that 3 minutes to carry out. The child is then directed to return to play. In the case where the child does not meet the criterion (i.e., talk a lot), the caregiver says something like, "If you talk more next time, then you get to pick from the Happy Sack. You can go back to play."

Baer et al., (1983) demonstrated that it was possible to train correspondence between verbal and nonverbal behaviors across settings. Also, correspondence training may help with maintenance and generalization to facilitate entry into natural communities of reinforcement by increasing the likelihood of reinforcement and positive attention from adults and peers (Stokes & Osnes, 1986). Through correspondence training, children achieve a "successful history" between verbalizations and actions: what they say they will do, and how they actually behave (Stokes & Osnes, 1986).

Despite the demonstrated effectiveness of correspondence training, it is important to note that the facets of the intervention still merit study. A component analysis with typical preschoolers found that reinforcement of compliance ("Today you must do a letter or number worksheet when you get up from your nap in order to get your prize") was just as effective as reinforcement of correspondence (Weninger & Baer, 1990). Thus, the child's verbalization of the target behavior in correspondence training may not play an independent or important role (for further discussion, see Baer, Detrich, & Weninger, 1988; Deacon & Konarski, 1987). The results suggest the importance of prompts, reinforcement of appropriate behavior, and rule-governed behavior. Despite the ambiguities, for some children, learning rule-governing language and reinforcing its use may be quite beneficial.

GROUP AND PEER INTERVENTIONS

There are significant reasons for considering the roles of other children in interventions for target children. Interventions for those who have various skills deficits or interfering behaviors related to social competence must take place in a social context. In fact, social behaviors constitute one of the most significant goals of early intervention or prevention programs. Strayhorn and Strain (1986, adapted from p. 288) conclude that three broadband competencies are essential, all of which require a social context for learning:

1. The ability to be kind, cooperative, and appropriately compliant, as opposed to having a prevailing habit of being hostile and defiant.
2. The ability to show interest in people and things, to be appropriately outgoing, to socialize actively, as opposed to being withdrawn, fearful, and shy.
3. The ability to use language well, to have command of a wide range of vocabulary and syntax such that ideas may be both comprehended and expressed with facility.

In addition, there are practical reasons for including groups of children and peers as change agents. They provide powerful sources of reinforcement for learning and maintaining behaviors. Peers can model, reinforce, extinguish, and monitor broad classes of social behaviors. Peers may have more opportunities to observe specific social behaviors than adults. Similarly, the use of peers may greatly expand the situations where behaviors may be targeted for change, and evidence suggests that untrained supportive behaviors may emerge in the forms of encouragement, tutoring, and prompts (Kohler et al., 1995). Peer-related interventions encompass situations or behaviors where it would be impractical or impossible to intervene, and they may be both powerful and time efficient for teachers. Examples related to classroom ecologies are discussed in later chapters.

Alternatively, adult-mediated strategies for producing and sustaining changes in social behavior may result in limited outcomes. In some cases, adult intervention may increase the frequency of brief, appropriate social behaviors to the detriment of *sustained* social interactions with peers.

While many studies focus on specific skills and relatively brief play bouts, a desired result for children is to increase the likelihood of friendships. Friendships involve mutually established, stable and skillful play interactions, and positive affective ties. While children with disabilities make friends (Field, 1984), many of the interventions for improving social competence may not directly lead to friendship patterns. However, there still may be benefits for children in learning effective social skills and increasing positive interactions even when friendships are not the outcome.

Despite the potential benefits, the research related to how individual or peer-group behavior of preschool children may be used either to reduce target behaviors or increase developmental skills is encouraging but incomplete. Questions remain, especially about the durability of changes. The use of group contingencies also raises special ethical and legal questions, which were reviewed in Chapter 5. Foremost is the possibility of unplanned negative effects for individual children.

In this section, we introduce general intervention strategies involving groups of children and peer-mediated programs.

Group-Oriented Programs

Group-based programs vary widely in procedures and outcomes. General guidelines for using group-based programs include the following (Axelrod, 1998; Hayes, 1976; Kazdin, 1994; Litow & Pumroy, 1975):

1. Set measurable objectives for behavior change. Make certain that all children can perform the desired skills or implement a preliminary intervention as necessary to develop appropriate skills. As an example, Kohler et al. (1995) introduced social skills training with targeted children and peers before introducing group contingencies. Objectives may include those linked to individual performance (such as aggressive acts, talking out), or those used for the entire group. Appropriate target behaviors include those that are under peer control, and those where it may be difficult to pinpoint individual behaviors (classroom noise levels).

2. Plan a group-based program designed to meet specific long-term goals and establish methods for feedback about performance. Goals may be derived from peer micronorms.

3. Set an achievable criterion for performance. Baseline measures can be used to help set this criterion. Target children and group members must be able to meet criterion levels. There may be advantages for contingencies based on the performances of individual children (or subgroups) resulting in positive consequences for the class, or consequences contingent on every child in the class meeting the set criterion (Gresham & Gresham, 1982; Litow & Pumroy, 1975).

4. Establish measures for unwanted side effects. Monitor the behavior and performance of both the target child and other children in the group. Targeted children may experience extreme pressure from peers as a result of inadequate performance or to achieve the group contingency. On the other hand, a target child or subgroup may control the classroom by refusing to achieve the criterion, thereby creating a situation in which no class members receive reinforcement.

5. Select powerful reinforcers. One helpful strategy is the use of a reinforcement menu. Bonus reinforcement, beyond that which would normally be available to the children, can be made contingent on individual

or group performances. Consider ways to reduce the possibility of adverse consequences if a criterion is not met by the group.

6. As necessary, combine individual programs with group-based programs. Many individual behavioral programs, for example, DRO, can be integrated effectively into intervention plans. When a child meets a set criterion for individual objectives, such as receiving individual reinforcement for appropriate behavior, the entire class can receive a reward.

7. Record keeping may be facilitated in ways that engage children and reduce possible negative reactions. Teachers may design highways or railroad tracks on tagboard, with "towns" representing intermediate goals at planned intervals. The spaces on the highways or between the railroad ties can be used to indicate steps, and children can participate in "moving" the class to goals. If a child is successful in 6 (or 5, etc.) out of 10 DRO intervals, the class may move six "steps" to a group reward.

In summary, group-based programs have many potential advantages, and they may be combined with individual intervention programs. However, they also require special safeguards, discussed in Chapter 5.

Peer-Mediated Interventions

Rather than sharing the consequences of behavior, as previously described, peers (or siblings) may be directly involved as behavior change agents. Peer-mediated intervention strategies have been widely researched.

A basic design includes a peer confederate (or group) that is close in age to the target child and receives specific training in participating in an intervention. Many variables have been studied, such as the functioning level of the confederate child and various target behaviors. The adult role typically involves training, monitoring the intervention, and prompting behaviors, but not directly intervening. For older children, peer tutoring has been widely researched. For younger children, most research efforts have been directed toward improving the social behavior of withdrawn children and including children with disabilities into group or classroom settings.

Odom and Strain (1984) outlined three different "topologies" for peer-mediated interventions. First, *proximity* interventions entail placing socially competent children with target children and instructing them to "(1) play with the target children, (2) get the children to play with them, or (3) teach the target children to play" (p. 545). The distinguishing feature is that the socially competent children are not specifically trained for their intervention role, and behavior change is dependent on "a natural transmission of social skills" (p. 545).

The second type of peer-mediated strategy is referred to as *prompt and reinforce* (Odom & Strain, 1984). "[A] prompt is an instruction (e.g., 'Come play') to engage in some social activity, and reinforcement is an event that comes after the interaction (e.g., 'I like to play with you') and maintains or increases the frequency of the desired type of behavior" (p. 546).

The third type of procedure is termed a *peer-initiation intervention*. Peers are instructed to make "social initiations" including "asking a child to play, giving a toy to a child, providing physical assistance, or suggesting a play idea" (Odom & Strain, 1984, p. 547).

In each case, research suggests at least some success with the strategies, but, overall, proximity alone seems to be less effective than the other approaches. However, direct comparisons between the various methods are limited.

We describe general guidelines for implementing peer-initiation strategies (Chandler, Lubeck, & Fowler, 1992; English, Goldstein, Shafer, & Kaczmarek, 1997; Kerr & Nelson, 1998; Odom & Strain, 1984; Strain & Odom, 1986). In addition, peer-mediated interventions can be combined with group contingencies (Kohler et al., 1995).

Carefully Select Targets for Change and Specific Peer Initiations

Consider social skills training for the target child and peers (English et al., 1997). Targets for change include a variety of play strategies, including making eye contact, sharing, suggesting specific play topics, responding to a target child's play initiations, and offering assistance (Chandler et al., 1992). These have been condensed into "Stay with your friend. *Play* with your friend. Talk to your friend" (English et al., 1997, p. 223). Strain and Odom (1986) suggest "teachable" units based on naturalistic research. Recommendations include play organizers ("Let's play___"), sharing, assistance, and affection.

Carefully Select Peer Confederates

Frameworks for decisions include consistent school attendance and naturally frequent and appropriate peer interactions. Critical decision points also include likely compliance with training instructions and skill in imitating modeled behavior included in the intervention components. Furthermore, the confederate should be able to maintain on-task behaviors related to the intervention; Kerr and Nelson (1998) suggest 10 minutes. Also, specific play competence may be helpful depending on the game or activity.

Plan to Reduce the Effects of Fatigue

Many variables may contribute to declining rates of social interaction over time, including characteristics of the peer confederate and the target child (such as difficulty in maintaining positive social interactions). A variety of reinforcements have been used to maintain the behavior of the peer confederates. Teacher prompts may be a significant part of the intervention. Also, several confederates may be trained and alternated in play.

Plan and Monitor the Intervention Closely

Successful social interventions employ combinations of techniques or "packages." Three frequently successful techniques are prompting, positive reinforcement, and feedback (Chandler et al., 1992). Kerr and Nelson (1998) also suggest the possible use of *cue cards* that assist the peer trainer in conducting the intervention. For example, each cue card might depict a preferred toy or activity of the target child. There may be positive or negative side effects for the confederate that need to be monitored and evaluated. Overall, the effects of the intervention on peer confederates have not been found to be negative, whereas, on some occasions, the effects have been positive (Strain, Hoyson, & Jamieson, 1985; Strain & Odom, 1986).

Systematically Train Peer Initiations

Training involves teaching the peer confederates specific social initiations. The training suggested by Strain and Odom (1986, p. 546) incorporates the following features: (1) discussion of the importance of the intervention or a review; (2) description of the target social behavior that is the focus of the daily lesson; (3) modeling and role playing of the behavior, including the role of a nonresponsive child; (4) practice; and (5) verbal feedback. Figure 7.1 depicts a sample script. Consider having several peers rotate the mediator role (although this may detrimentally affect more stable relationships without long-term assignments), giving peers choices in participation and spacing brief (1 minute) refresher training periods (English et al., 1997). In addition, English et al. showed peers videotapes of various atypical communication attempts made by target children to gain attention and make requests (gestures, unintelligible vocalizations).

Make Necessary Changes in the Physical Environment to Enable and Facilitate Interactions

Ecological factors include the availability of play materials and activities, and the planning of play areas so that children will be encouraged to in-

Session 1: Introduction to System—Share Initiation—Persistence

Teacher: "Today you are going to learn how to be a good teacher. Sometimes your friends in your class do not know how to play with other children. You are going to learn how to teach them to play. What are you going to do?"

Child response: "Teach them to play."

Teacher: "One way you can get your friend to play with you is to share. How do you get your friend to play with you?"

Child response: "Share."

Teacher: "Right! You share. When you share you look at your friend and say, 'Here,' and put a toy in his hand. What do you do?" (Repeat this exercise until the child can repeat these three steps.)

Child response: "Look at friend and say, 'Here,' and put the toy in his hand."

Adult model with role player: "Now, watch me. I am going to share with ___. Tell me if I do it right." (Demonstrate sharing.) "Did I share with ___? What did I do?"

Child response: "Yea! ___ looked at ___, said, 'here ___' and put a toy in his hand."

Adult: "Right. I looked at ___ and said, 'here ___' and put a toy in his hand. Now watch me. See if I share with ___." (Move to the next activity in the classroom. This time provide a negative example of sharing by leaving out the "put in hand" component. Put the toy beside the role player.) "Did I share?" (Correct if necessary and repeat this example if child got it wrong.) "Why not?"

Child response: "No. You did not put the toy in ___'s hand."

Adult: "That's right. I did not put the toy in ___'s hand. I have to look at ___ and say, 'here ___' and put the toy in his hand." (Give the child two more positive and two more negative examples of sharing. When they answer incorrectly about sharing, repeat the example. Vary the negative examples by leaving out different components: looking, saying 'here,' putting in hand.)

Child practice with adults: "Now ___, I want you to get ___ to share with you. What do you do when you share?"

Child response: "Look at ___ and say, 'here ___' and put a toy in his hand."

Adult: "Now, go get ___ to play with you." (For these practice examples, the role-playing adult should be responsive to the child's sharing.) (To the other confederates:) "Did ___ share with ___? What did she/he do?"

Child response: "Yes/No. Looked at ___ and said, 'here ___' and put a toy in his hand."

Adult: (Move to the next activity.) "Now, ___ I want you to share with ___"

Introduce Persistence

Teacher: "Sometimes when I play with ___, he/she does not want to play back. I have to keep on trying. What do I have to do?"

Child response: "Keep on trying."

Teacher: "Right, I have to keep on trying. Watch me. I am going to share with ___. Now I want you to see if I keep on trying." (Role player will be initially unresponsive.) (Teacher should be persistent until child finally responds.) "Did I get ___ to play with me?" *Child:* "Yes." "Did he want to play?" *Child:* "No." "What did I do?" *Child:* "Keep on trying." "Right. I kept on trying. Watch. See if I can get ___ to play with me this time." (Again, the role player should be unresponsive at first. Repeat above questions and correct if necessary. Repeat the example until the child responds correctly.)

FIGURE 7.1. Sample script for peer-initiated training. From Strain and Odom (1986). Copyright 1986 by The Council for Exceptional Children. Reprinted by permission.

teract, play cooperatively, and share. Strain and Odom (1986) suggest that dolls, house materials, blocks, wagons, and kiddie cars help facilitate social interactions. Furthermore, some children may benefit from instruction in toy play. Sociodramatic activities also help promote social interactions (Peters, 1995).

Conduct Frequent Intervention Sessions

Strain and Odom suggest daily sessions. Strategies to encourage persistence also may need to be programmed, especially for the first few days of the intervention (Kerr & Nelson, 1998). Consider spacing the learning trials throughout the day (free play, snack time) rather then during a special time (English et al., 1997). Here we describe the daily event sequences for peer-initiated interventions adapted from Strain and Odom (1986, pp. 546, 548).

The group of children is first brought to the intervention setting (the target child and at least one confederate). The activities are introduced to the children, and the caregiver models ways in which play materials can be used. The children are directed to a play activity, except for the confederate child, who is taken aside and reminded about the steps in the intervention activity. The confederate child then is directed to engage the target child in play.

The confederate is observed carefully. If no spontaneous initiation occurs within 15 seconds, the caregiver verbally prompts the confederate to engage the target child. The first prompt should be explicit (e.g., "Remember, you need to get _____ to play"). If the confederate is unable to come up with an idea for approaching the target child, a prompt that tells the confederate exactly what to do may be necessary (e.g., "Tell _____ to help with the puzzle"). The confederate should receive several prompts (spaced 15–20 seconds apart) if play is not initiated. A verbal reinforcer should be given to the confederate for effective prompting if a contingency system is not in place. The target child should be reinforced for being a good play partner. Both children are then directed to the next activity.

Caregiver support for the confederate must be withdrawn gradually and systematically. For example, once the confederate is initiating to the target child within 15 seconds on 75% of the opportunities, the length of time before giving the verbal prompt may be increased to 30 seconds, and after 3 days the interval may be increased to 45 seconds. If the initiations do not decline, the interval can be further lengthened to 2 minutes, and finally 3 minutes. For teachers, two prompts to the confederate per session are an acceptable criterion. Each time the interval is increased, the behaviors must remain stable for a 3-day period. If noticeable reductions in behavior occur, the caregiver moves back to the previous prompting interval length.

Plan for Generalization and Maintenance

This topic is extensively reviewed by Chandler et al. (1992), Fox and McEvoy (1993), and in Chapter 4. Four promising strategies may be selecting functional target behaviors, using indiscriminable contingencies, teaching self-mediation skills, and ensuring fluency as a criterion. One important factor is the availability of "socially responsive peers" (Odom & Strain, 1984, p. 554). In addition, entire groups may receive social skills training to promote generalization of treatment effects. The behaviors and activities required in various settings, the planned roles of adults, and the timing and sequence of the intervention components are other important variables.

Long-term treatment effects have not received much attention from researchers (Chandler et al., 1992). One important caveat before deciding on a peer-mediated intervention is the warning by Odom and Strain (1984) that the "maintenance problem must be solved" before peer-mediated interventions can demonstrate clinical significance. For this reason, interventions may need to be carried out in each setting where the targeted behavior is observed. Peer interventions should be considered experimental. However, the same issues may also be applied to many other interventions, not only social skills interventions.

USING TOKENS

Token economies combine many procedures that have proven effective. In a token economy, children earn tokens based on a set criterion for performance. The tokens are exchanged for backup reinforcers at a later time.

Token economies were widely applied in the 1970s, and many reviews are available. However, research on token economies has waned since that time. This has been attributed by some (e.g., McLaughlin & Williams, 1988) to the demonstrated effectiveness of tokens, resulting in less need for research. An alternative explanation is the availability of other acceptable procedures that accomplish the same goals but require less effort, especially in monitoring and recording, and are more natural. In other words, token systems may not be necessary for instituting change. Examples of effective and less intrusive procedures include the use of performance feedback systems for classrooms (Van Houten, 1984) or daily report cards (Kelley, 1990).

However, token economies are versatile and may be adapted to many situations. One important advantage with young as well as older children is that tokens help bridge the delay between the response and reinforcement. Another benefit is that they may be backed up by a variety of reinforcers and thus may help avoid satiation or help with children that have reinforcement preferences that are difficult to predict.

The following procedures and guidelines have been used to set up token economies. Kazdin (1982a) specifically treats problem areas associated with token economies as well as possible strategies for dealing with the problems.

1. Define the targeted behaviors and rules. Definitions of the response(s) to be reinforced (or tokens lost; see the discussion of response cost) need to be specified. Preacademic skills and social behaviors may be addressed by token systems.
2. Select a token that is safe, durable, and standardized. The token itself may be attractive but not overly valued. The token should be easily administered. Earlier, examples of tokens were given in the section on selecting reinforcers.
3. Select reinforcers to serve as backups for the tokens to be exchanged. Activity reinforcers have been widely used. Do not rely on a single reinforcer for an individual. Children may help select backup reinforcers. Token delivery should be paired with praise or approval.
4. Specify the contingencies, exchange system, and the exchange ratio (or token value) whereby the number of tokens are "cashed in" for the backup reinforcers. At first, it may be important to reinforce a minimal performance "to allow for exposure to some sources of reinforcement" (Kazdin, 1977b, p. 50; see reinforcement sampling, Chapter 6).
5. Plan and establish a way to dispense tokens. Important elements of economic theory are discussed by Kazdin (1977b). Guard against satiation by controlling the contingencies for the reinforcement.
6. Plan to implement the token economy. The training of staff is an essential part of effective token economies. Assign individual responsibilities for specific occasions. Treatment integrity is a significant consideration.
7. Develop a record-keeping system to monitor the children's performance. Other records can include exchange preferences and reliability in carrying out the procedures. They also serve to reinforce those carrying out the intervention.
8. Plan a way to fade the token economy. Basically, in order to fade the use of tokens, their use should become reduced over time and

be replaced by natural procedures. Kazdin (1977b) discussed a number of procedures for fading. One critical approach is to select target behaviors that are adaptive and likely to continue to be reinforced after the intervention ends (Ayllon & Azrin, 1968). Having children earn their way off the token program is one way to fade tokens (Kazdin & Mascitelli, 1980). Another practical strategy is to build in a delay between earning and exchanging tokens. Issues related to generalization and maintenance are pertinent. Fading should have the desired outcome of increasing self-regulated behavior.

In summary, the literature surrounding the use of token economies is extensive. It has been applied across many populations and settings (including home, school, and community), and with many behavior change agents. Tokens may be effectively employed with group contingencies. One of the potential criticisms is whether the target behaviors help with adaptation to specific institutional settings or to broader treatment goals (Kazdin, 1977b). A further criticism that arose in the 1970s centered on the potential deleterious effects of extrinsic reinforcement. However, these negative effects have not been documented in the research literature on the use of tokens. Perhaps the most important criticism is the relative effectiveness, efficiency, and normalcy vis-à-vis other intervention alternatives. Many other potential concerns, such as the full evaluation of treatment effects, can be applied to most other forms of intervention. Staff and administrative demands may be considerable.

Alternatively, the defining characteristic of the token economy is simply "the delivery of tangible conditioned reinforcers contingent upon specific behaviors" (Kazdin, 1977b, p. 283). Thus, even in its simple form, token use may be versatile and effective. Specific family and school-based applications are discussed in later chapters.

SUMMARY AND CONCLUSIONS

Interventions commonly used for problem behaviors were presented. Problem behaviors may represent excesses or deficits related to expectations for desired performance, and a way to communicate. Differential reinforcement represents a family of procedures to increase positive or adaptive behaviors while reducing maladaptive behaviors. Other basic interventions that have been widely used with young children include time out, response cost, and overcorrection. Effort may be spent analyzing existing use of aversives and making intervention designs more positive. Building on earlier discussions related to self-observation as a keystone behavior, basic strategies for teaching and enhancing self-regulation in young children were reviewed. We closed the chapter with discussions of group and peer-mediated strategies, and the use of tokens.

The interventions described here and in Chapters 6 have been used to derive many of the interventions in the following chapters, where we present specific examples of how these and other interventions have been applied in the home and school.

CHAPTER 8

◆◆◆

Changing Roles within Family Systems

◆

Parents assume many roles in designing and carrying out interventions for young children. For school-based interventions, parents participate as problem solvers and decision makers. When the locus of the intervention is at home, parents also become observers and teachers or change agents. Many interventions successfully combine home and school elements. Parental contributions to problem solving, decision making, observation, and intervention were discussed in earlier chapters.

In addition, social networks and work-related responsibilities, apart from child responsibilities, often are critical considerations when working with parents. For these reasons, we have emphasized strategies to enhance parent–child relationships and naturalistic interventions based on parental and family realities and goals.

Discussion of professional roles and qualifications related to family assessment and intervention are outside the scope of this book. This chapter is written within the general context of a parent-consultation model using assessment methods described in earlier chapters.

FAMILY SYSTEMS ISSUES

The overall significance of family systems for assessment and intervention design can be stated succinctly: "The child is an inseparable part of a small social system of an ecological unit made up of the child, his family, his school, his neighborhood, and community" (Hobbs, 1966, p. 1108).

We begin with one assumption—that the relationship between child and caregiver is the primary factor in establishing a *general* model for early intervention. However, many factors may interfere with the relationship between parent and child. Family realities affect intervention decisions and may have direct and indirect effects associated with children's risk status and adjustment or learning difficulties. For these reasons, our focus is on family *systems* rather than solely on parent–child relationships. Although there are many other frameworks for early intervention, we place the child and the realities of families at the focal point of our analysis.

Family Realities

The assessment of family realities is an important first step in intervention design with young children. Family realities that may impact upon child behavior and childrearing practices include social, economic, and personal stress, illness, and disruptive life events. The daily care of a child who places unusual demands on parents also contributes greatly to stress.

Family situations often fall short of various ideals. However, many alternative strategies for rearing children and different social arrangements will lead to the development of children's competence. Children also vary greatly with respect to their vulnerabilities (Rutter, 1987).

Families, like other environments, present both "risks and opportunities" (Garbarino, 1982, p. 3). While risk status for young children may be increased in response to family stressors, early stressors have the potential for both beneficial and harmful consequences. "There may be *sensitization* to the effects of later stressors," thus compounding risk factors, "but also there are *steeling* effects involved in overcoming stress and adversity" (Rutter, 1981, p. 347). The effects of stressors may be buffered by at least one caregiver who provides a relationship characterized by warm, reciprocal, and supportive interactions; a continuity of experiences; and the active promotion of competence (Werner, 1986).

It is also important to recognize that there is not one "global" environmental effect for children, even for those being raised in the same family. Aspects of the environment uniquely influence individual development and may operate at discontinuous points in time (Plomin, 1987).

Mental health professionals frequently work with families in crisis, and, unfortunately, parents that most need help may be quite hard to reach. At the same time, demographics suggest increased numbers of single-parent families, use of day care by mothers joining the workforce, and considerable divergence from traditional practices in the structure of families. Therefore, because of their potential effects on parent–child relationships and early experiences, parental stress and coping may be important targets in assessment and intervention design.

Relatedly, risk status for young children is associated with the quality of the learning and mediational contexts provided by families where opportunities likely to encourage growth and competence are provided. As discussed in earlier chapters, qualities of the family system and interactions transform commonplace events into learning experiences. Methods of teaching, control, punishment, and underlying parental belief systems influence learning and behavior outcomes.

Parents as Teachers and Change Agents

The assessment of the parental role requires careful consideration. There is general agreement on parental "teaching" and family environment variables (Caldwell & Bradley, 1979; Hart & Risley, 1995): (1) emotional and verbal responsivity of the caregiver(s), (2) avoidance of restriction and punishment, (3) organization of the physical and temporal environment, (4) availability of play materials, (5) degree of maternal involvement, and (6) opportunities for variety in daily stimulation.

There have been many studies of parents' roles in early intervention (Guralnick, 1997). Shearer and Shearer (1972, 1976) developed several prototypic features of models based on the parental teaching role. The program included curriculum-based assessment, behavioral principles, parental input into curriculum planning and implementation, and a "home teacher" that demonstrated tasks and observed and gave feedback to the parent teaching the child. In addition, parents were taught the basics of recording behavior.

Greist and associates (1982) found that a *parent enhancement* program, including discussion and training in individual adult and family functioning, improved treatment outcomes, especially generalization. The program encompassed parental perceptions and expectations about child behavior, parental mood and adjustment, marital relationship, and extrafamilial interactions and relationships. The multifaceted training included direct instruction, discussion, modeling, role playing, and homework.

A simpler example of an intervention directed toward children at educational risk is establishing a routine for parents reading to children (Taverne & Sheridan, 1995; see also Dale, Crain-Thoreson, Notari-Syverson, & Cole, 1996). The key parts of the parental role in *interactive book reading* were (1) examining a storybook and pointing out its main parts, (2) labeling and discussing picture content, (3) reading aloud, and (4) pausing to question the child's understanding of the material (p. 46).

Although much attention has been focused on the parental role, many factors mediate the effectiveness of parent–child interventions. While parental involvement in early intervention often leads to successful outcomes, it is not a panacea, nor are the effective designs and outcomes of parent-based interventions well known. Sometimes parents will not be able to fulfill responsibilities because of a range of complicating factors, such as illness or economic stressors.

Maternal (or Caregiver) Responsiveness

Many view maternal responsiveness as a key behavior that underscores children's early competence in developmental skills. Parental factors such as depression, or child factors related to temperament, challenging behaviors, or other variables, may at least partially determine qualities of interactions related to responsiveness. Martin (1989) outlined the following *person and relationship variables* underlying responsiveness.

1. Interpersonal sensitivity: to be aware "of the interpersonal dimension of experience" and attuned "to characteristics of and variations in the interpersonal field" (p. 7).
2. Empathic awareness: to experience "another person's emotional reality as his or her own" (p. 8). Affective and cognitive components may be included.
3. Predictability: to provide "a stable, safe context for self-expression" (p. 8). Without predictable behaviors, the child may "experience the relationship as unsafe, unstable, and unresponsive" (p. 8). Excessive predictability may "result in relationships that are flat and arid" (p. 8).
4. Nonintrusiveness: to not intervene when the situation does not require intervention. An example of intrusive behavior is overprotectiveness.
5. Emotional availability: to be "affectively involved in a relationship and available for authentic exchange of feelings" (p. 8).
6. Engagement or involvement: to freely exchange values and ideas while considering the "needs and wishes" of the other person (p. 9).
7. Contingent reactivity: to respond to the behaviors of the child in appropriate ways regarding "content, timing, and intensity" (p. 9).
8. Interpersonal relations: to embrace "both personal and interpersonal components of mutually responsive mother–child relationships" (p. 11).
9. Interpersonal system: to consider responsiveness as a "domain" consisting of multiple variables "embedded within an interpersonal system" (p. 12).

Most specific studies have dealt with language (Hart & Risley, 1995; Kaiser, Hemmeter, Ostroksky, Fischer, Yoder, & Keefer, 1996; cf. Wahler & Meginnis, 1997). Kaiser et al. (1996, p. 19) outlined specific techniques adapted from Weiss (1981): (1) empathic nonverbal interaction strategies described by the acronym SOUL (silence, observation, understanding, listening), pauses, and nonverbal mirroring; (2) semantically contingent feedback strategies (descriptive talk by the intervention agent, expansion, requests for clarification of the child's communication attempts); and (3) linguistic modeling at the child's target level.

In summary, a first step in intervention design for early learning and behavior problems is to consider the relationship between parent and child in the context of daily events. The potential outcomes associated with this step may impact the range and quality of personal, social, and educational experiences that are provided in the home and community, or, if necessary, may help address parental needs in order to accomplish this goal. Despite the difficulties, the focus of early intervention decisions often may be directed toward improving the realities of family circumstances, since other factors in the caregiver's experience may be precluding the adequate expression of the parental role. However, there are many times when it may not be possible to alter family circumstances. In these cases, goals are associated with coping with realities. In the next sections, several factors related to planning family interventions are examined.

It should also be noted that the measurement of parent–child interactions is challenging (Mahoney, Spiker, & Boyce, 1996). Family needs and parent–child relationships need to be studied idiographically and in context (see our recommendations in Chapters 2–4).

Parental Beliefs

Parental beliefs directly and indirectly influence experiences that are provided to children and childrearing practices. Furthermore, they are likely to play a significant role in the decision process, including goals, efforts, and persistence related to change, and the acceptability of various intervention alternatives. However, beliefs are difficult to assess. Individuals may be unaware, unwilling, or unable to communicate beliefs that affect behaviors. Willingness to reveal belief systems to professionals is likely to be a function of rapport and trust. Home observations and interviews reveal parental beliefs only to a degree because (1) observations usually are too limited; (2) outcomes associated with beliefs may be subtle and cumulative, related to the basic organization of the home and family; and (3) they may be linked to influential factors outside the parent–child relationship (Sigel, McGillicuddy-DeLisi, & Goodnow, 1992).

Although parents may receive technical assistance in the course of an intervention, it should be provided in a way that is likely to encourage self-efficacy in the form of independent problem solving and relationship building through naturalistic means. Interventions can have the unintended effects of *reducing* self-sufficiency and confidence.

Dunst and his associates (i.e., Dunst & Trivette, 1987; Dunst, Trivette, & Deal, 1988; Trivette, Dunst, & Hamby, 1996) have focused on the ways that help can be provided by professionals. They argue that professionals should strive for relationships with families that enable and empower the family, so that parents may meet their own needs with increased self-sufficiency. A major factor is professionals' help-giving practices that actively engage parents in participating in decision making.

HOME AND SCHOOL INTERVENTIONS

Collaboration between home and school is a central theme of early intervention efforts. Collaboration may be expressed in many ways. First, parents may have a significant role in developing and conducting preschool programs. One of the legacies of Head Start is the focus on meaningful parental participation in programmatic decision making. Second, parent volunteers may be utilized for specific classroom interventions. Third, a critical area of professional practice involves conducting center-based interventions for parents. For example, preschools may offer programs on parenting skills desired by parents. Fourth, certain problem areas may benefit from collaboratively developed home–school plans for assessment and intervention.

In this section, we discuss strategies of developing home–school interventions and present examples. The basic procedures involve establishing ongoing parent–teacher communications and mutually agreeing on planned activities, target behaviors, and interventions. The behavior of concern—and the reinforcement—may occur at school or at home, or both.

The potential benefits are many (Kelley, 1990): (1) Such programs help promote parent involvement and reduce "blaming"; (2) they can be time- and cost-efficient; (3) they may be nonintrusive in the classroom; (4) for some children, the range of rewards in the home may be greater than in the school (although the opposite may be true); (5) there may be general beneficial outcomes for parent–child relationships in addition to those targeted; (6) the delay of reinforcement may enhance generalization efforts; and (7) home-based reinforcement may deal effectively with ethical concerns related to school-based behavior modification programs. While home–school interventions may be applied to a wide range of target behaviors, they will not be effective in all situations, especially with severely dysfunctional families.

The following steps are suggested for effective home–school notes (Atkeson & Forehand, 1979; Kelley, 1990).

1. *Use parental and teacher consultation strategies to evaluate realistic and acceptable roles.* For initially unwilling or resistive parents (or teachers), the roles may be minimal but still meaningful. In comparison with parent training programs or other classroom interventions, the involvement by a caregiver may be drastically reduced.

2. *Define target variables and decide on ongoing measurement strategies.* The general strategies discussed in earlier chapters apply. Frequently, we use parent and teacher consultation to design simple participant-observation strategies involving frequency counts (such as the number of fights). An important decision is whether to apply the measurement procedure (and intervention) for the whole day, for a portion of the day, or for a specific activity such as bus behavior or free play. Direct observations or probes may be useful when specific activities are targeted (such as behavior in group free play).

3. *Decide on a home–school communication system.* The most likely strategy involves a home–school *note.* The system should be tied to the target behavior and intervention, and behaviors and conditions should be described in ways that are appropriate for daily use. The note should be easy to use. Parents are frequently the recipients of bad news. Home–school notes that address accomplishments rather than misbehavior will be welcome. An important decision involves whether the note will include very specific information or a global description of the behavior. Factors related to this question include the complexity of the target behavior and the degree of possible involvement and acceptability by parents and teachers. Messages can be delivered daily or weekly, or only contingently (when the child meets a specified criterion). Phone contacts also may be useful with some parents. Lahey and associates (1977) reported the effective use of daily "report cards" for disruptive kindergarten behaviors.

For children with behavior problems, we have frequently used differential reinforcement of other behavior (DRO), or modifications of DRO, for home–school programs structured by classroom routines and planned activities (entering routines, large groups, transitions, snack, and so on). In these cases, the child may take home the record of intervals showing the occasions when reinforcement was earned in school and the occasions that will be reinforced by the parent. Many developmentally appropriate and attractive means may be used for home–school communications. For example, a ticket format may be used: Each section of the ticket is "punched" or marked when a planned activity is completed successfully.

Young children may be able to self-record behaviors, with assistance and structure. A prearranged private or silent signal can be given to the child when the targeted behavior is observed, and the child can be taught to mark a paper. The tallies, such as small circles colored in on a paper, can be recorded by the teacher or parent, and can serve as the basis for social and or tangible rewards. Strategies for self-observation and regulation may be considered as adjunctive procedures initially but may have important long-term benefits.

4. *Develop plans into scripts for teachers and parents concerning ways to carry out the daily communication.* Plan the specifics of how to introduce, monitor, and send the home–school communication, and the way parents receive it and provide consequences. One of the possible dangers involves the natural variability of behaviors in intervention phases and subsequent parental and teacher reactions. This likely variability and the possibility of "bad days" need to be discussed. Plans may range from simple, brief nonpunitive discussions about the behavior to the use of tokens, where each reinforced activity contributes to daily and weekly goals. Potential disruptions in family life and dysfunctional parent–child relationships need careful consideration. Parent and teacher training in the intervention is critically important in determining successful outcomes and should not be neglected. Behavioral contracts may be used to specify the roles and contingencies.

5. *Evaluate the intervention periodically and plan for ultimately fading it.* Given the many procedural variations that have an impact on overall intervention effectiveness, evaluation is essential. The home–school report is one important measure; it may be supplemented by direct observation probes conducted in the home or school. In other words, key elements of assessment and intervention design apply.

INTERVENTIONS TO EXPAND
LEARNING OPPORTUNITIES

One of the major parental roles is expanding learning opportunities in the home and community. Events such as shopping, dining, and sibling interactions hold potential for social, cognitive, and language skills development.

Shopping with Children

Clark and colleagues (1977) wrote, "While shopping offers many opportunities for constructive and educational family interactions, parents rarely seem to use them!" (p. 606). At the opposite extreme are coercive demands, punishment, and, frequently, embarrassment for family members.

"Indeed, many family shopping trips occasion a high level of inappropri-ate child behavior and an equally high rate of apparently ineffective parental coercion" (p. 606). Studies that focus on shopping behavior of parents and young children are described in this section.

Barnard, Christophersen, and Wolf (1977) assessed the effectiveness of two traditional interventions on shopping behaviors: token reinforce-ment and response cost. Three mothers, who had received prior training in behavior management, and their 3 young boys participated in the study. The study was conducted in a supermarket. Mothers were encouraged to shop in their usual manner except that children were not permitted to ride in the carts. We describe their study in some detail.

There were two key measurement and intervention targets. First, parent *proximity* (being "within reach" of the child) is viewed as a prerequi-site for effective parent–child verbal interactions and instructions in the supermarket setting. Second, *product disturbance*, defined as the child picking up, moving, pushing or disturbing merchandise without permission, also was recorded. In addition, for 2 children, mothers' complaints were recorded after each store visit. Mothers also rated satisfaction with their child's behavior. Last, verbal interactions were obtained via a cassette tape recorder for one mother–child pair (coded as positive, negative, or neutral verbalizations). (See Chapters 3 and 4 for measurement examples.)

Before the store visit, the experimenter described the appropriate be-haviors and modeled them in the home. The child then practiced the ap-propriate behaviors and received praise and verbal feedback about his performance. Each mother was instructed to award one point at periodic intervals (two or three times per store aisle) when the child was within her reach and to subtract two points when he was not. Each mother also was instructed to give descriptive verbal feedback to the child about his behav-ior (e.g., "That's a point; you're here with me." "That's too far ahead; I'll have to take two off."). Similar procedures were used for product distur-bance. The mothers carried pencils and point cards, and at the end of each visit, each mother announced the number of points earned and lost to the child. The balance of points was added to the child's home balance and was exchangeable for goods or privileges.

The results indicated the treatment package was effective for all 3 children. Follow-up measures demonstrated that the behaviors were main-tained at very high levels for 2 children; outcomes for the third child were variable. The evaluation of caregiver satisfaction found reduced com-plaints about shopping behaviors. Verbal interactions recorded for 1 child demonstrated that positive talk increased during the treatment and was maintained at a level higher than baseline. Negative comments dropped to a low level during treatment and to zero during follow-up. The results also suggest the importance of training for skills in the setting in which they occur. The researchers suggest that parents may be able to use these procedures "without prior home training" (Barnard, Christophersen, & Wolf, 1977, p. 59).

Clark and colleagues (1977) developed an extensive intervention package to help with family shopping problems, reported in three interrelated studies. The objectives were to "develop and maintain children's courteous behavior and enhance family interactions on shopping trips" (p. 607). The program components were described in the following way:

1. The management component consisted of a response–cost system. Children were allotted a 50-cent allowance at the outset of the shopping trip. Each time a child violated a guideline (made a distracting comment or engaged in a distracting behavior), a nickel was withheld from the child's shopping allowance.

2. The enhancement component consisted of parental instructions "to prompt and encourage interesting conversation about shopping and other topics to involve the children" in the family activity. (p. 607)

The first study evaluated the contribution of the components. The children, ages 7–10, were from group homes for neglected children. The "parents" in this initial study were surrogates involved in training as a "teaching parent." Observations were conducted in stores located in a shopping center.

The following procedures were implemented during the baseline condition and the two intervention phases. On the way to the shopping center, the parent described the guidelines to the child, which included staying close enough to the parent that they could touch and talk to one another, and not touching items for sale or things such as cash registers; explained to the child that running, yelling, and so on, would bother people and slow down the shopping trip, and that the parent had many errands to complete, and the child should not distract the parent by asking for things or tattling on others. The children were then required to repeat a briefer version of the guidelines, and they were told they would have 50 cents of their allowance to spend during "their" 10-minute shopping at the end of the trip. Any time a child did not follow the guidelines, the parent would hold back 5 cents of the child's allowance. If the child failed to follow the guidelines again, another 5 cents was withheld.

In a management plus enhancement condition, the procedures were the same, except that parents were instructed to talk to the children about their shopping as they were going through the store, including prices, quality, and so on. After the shopping trip, parents told children how much money could be spent, and the children were allowed to shop.

In the initial study, money withheld under the response–cost procedure could be spent during the next shopping trip if the child qualified as a "good shopper." However, this step was later eliminated from the treatment package because of the additional complexity (H. B. Clark, personal communication, March 29, 1991).

Comprehensive measures were taken of children's distracting behaviors and comments, children's social and educational comments, parents' teaching comments, and parents' coercive comments. In addition, parental consequences for behaviors were measured (such as parental description of why 5 cents was being withheld). The comments were tape recorded. The results were stated succinctly by Clark and colleagues (1977): "The management component significantly reduced distracting behavior and distracting comments but *also reduced social and educational comments*. However, adding the enhancement component increased social and educational comments to well above baseline levels" (p. 610, emphasis added).

A second study replicated the package with natural families and with younger children (ages ranged from 4 to 9). The parents in the second study were paid $4 for their participation plus a bonus for meeting scheduled appointments. In addition, a four-part "advice package" was developed to describe the components identified earlier to the parents. The first part described how to use the procedures. The second part included three quizzes on the components and scripts of shopping trips based on the "advice package." The third part included a form for the following: "space for a shopping list, a tally for keeping track of the nickels withheld . . . , and five self-feedback Yes/No questions for the mother to answer at specific intervals" (Clark et al., 1977, p. 613). The last part included a simplified version to help parents explain the new procedures for shopping trips to their children. There were 4 days of practice to teach the mothers to use the procedures.

The effectiveness of the advice package was demonstrated, and social validity evaluations were positive. Mothers reported that the advice package resulted in "more pleasurable and frequent shopping trips" (p. 617). They reported that the shopping trip was a better learning experience for the children. Three mothers reported spending *less* than usual for their children when using the procedures. Ratings on parental effort were mixed, although the mothers who thought that the procedure required more effort still thought that it was worthwhile. A third study replicated a slightly modified shopping advice package without professional intervention.

Together, the three studies convincingly demonstrated the potential use of behavioral techniques in the community to help make family outings more enjoyable and more of a learning experience. The authors discussed a *graduated practice procedure* as an important feature of the program. Initially, families shopped for only half of their usual time to help ensure that the children would be able to follow the guidelines and be reinforced. Otherwise, because of the response–cost procedure, children could lose all of their spending money despite improved behavior. Also, the briefer shopping trips at the beginning were likely to reduce the strain associated with the parents' newly learned behaviors. A booklet written for use by parents is available (Greene, Clark, & Risley, 1977).

Dinnertime Conversations

Parent advice packages have been developed for mealtime and dining out (Bauman, Reiss, Rogers, & Bailey, 1983; McManmon, Peterson, Metelenis, McWhirter, & Clark, 1982). From Bauman et al., (1983), steps for such interventions include (1) identifying appropriate restaurant behavior for children; (2) finding a table or booth away from the crowd; (3) sitting children next to a wall and separating them; (4) providing children with a premeal snack such as crackers; (5) ordering food children like; (6) providing toys while waiting for the food and removing the toys once it arrived; (7) moving utensils away from children; and (8) praising children for appropriate behavior. A study by Green, Hardison, and Greene (1984) used special place mats to stimulate family conversation during restaurant meals.

Correspondence training was used to enhance dinnertime conversation for preschool children, making it "more mutually interesting" (Jewett & Clark, 1979, p. 590). The locus of the intervention was in the preschool. The central features of the study were (1) the taped dinnertime conversations between family members, returned each morning to the school; (2) the simulated family meal held by the preschool teacher; (3) dinner conversation training sessions; and (4) the feedback sessions to check correspondence between what each child reported doing at dinner the previous evening and what he or she actually did. Conversational comments included initiating a topic, continuing a topic, or restating a comment. Conversational comments were taught using prompting, modeling, practice, and social reinforcement. The experimental conditions convincingly demonstrated the effectiveness of the intervention across all children. The authors wrote, "Conversational participation was apparently being maintained by natural consequences, such as parental attention, increased interaction with family members, and interesting new topics of discussion" (p. 601). A resource that evolved from this research is available for parents and practitioners (Clark, McManmon, Smith-Tuten, & Smith, 1985).

Sibling Interventions

Without a doubt, sibling interactions are a socializing force for many children. Also, many parents request specific help for problem behaviors between siblings. Powell and Ogle (1985) reviewed the topic of siblings and exceptionalities within a family context, and wrote, "If the sibling and the child with a handicap do not socially interact with each other, the loss of the benefits of such interaction will be more detrimental for the handicapped child than a nonhandicapped child" (p. 107). Conversely, improved interactions enable expanded interactions with normal children.

A study by James and Egel (1986) evaluated direct prompting as a way of increasing reciprocal interactions between siblings. The authors also were interested in generalizations to peer play and interactions across settings. The children targeted for the intervention were 2 girls and 1 boy (all age 4) in a noncategorical special education program. They were selected because of limited interactions with siblings or peers. Two of the children had cerebral palsy; 1 was nonambulatory and required a wheelchair. The other child was diagnosed with mental retardation and displayed a number of maladaptive behaviors such as body rocking. The siblings without disabilities ranged from ages 6 to 8. Based on parental report, the older siblings "occasionally" initiated play, but the young child with disabilities "rarely initiated or responded to interactions" (p. 174). In addition, two friends of the older siblings participated in the study, both age 7. The third child lived in a rural location, and no peers were available to participate in the study.

The intervention setting for 2 children (for play, training, and generalization) was in the usual play area in the home, containing household furnishings including a television set. The generalization setting for the third participant was an outside porch. The experimenters also conducted a "toy preference assessment" to choose reinforcing toys. The duration of toy play was recorded during brief structured observations.

The training of siblings was conducted in the home play area. Session lengths ranged from 12 to 15 minutes and were held an average of 5 days per week, with no more than two per day, 4–6 hours apart. The experimenter first modeled for the older sibling initiation of the interactions, prompts, and reinforcement of responses, as the child with a disability played with a preferred toy. For example, the experimenter would say, "Let's play cars," and would push the toy car toward the child with a disability. If the child responded, the experimenter provided social praise to the child. If the child did not respond, the experimenter used physical guidance in order to have the child push the car. A minimum of four interactions were modeled, and explanations were given to the sibling. Practice with feedback sessions was then conducted. The experimenter asked the sibling to use the strategies demonstrated in the modeling sessions to get the child with a disability to play. The experimenter gave verbal instructional cues and feedback to the sibling for 5 minutes while observing. If no positive social behaviors were observed for a 10-second interval, the experimenter prompted the older sibling to initiate an interaction. Prompts varying in obtrusiveness were used (i.e., "Make sure he is watching"; "Put his hands on the car") and social reinforcement was given. If the sibling did not respond within 10 seconds of the cue, or if it was incorrect, the verbal cue was repeated, the response was prompted, and reinforcement was provided.

Additional procedures were added to increase the targeted child's initiations if the rate of initiations was low. Using incidental teaching and time delay, the sibling held a desired toy and waited for the targeted child "to initiate" using verbal requests, signs, or gestures (p. 177). Mothers prompted interactions when observations showed that interactions were occurring in less than half of the intervals for two targeted children and their siblings.

The results indicated low levels of interactions during baseline. For each target child–sibling dyad, substantial increases in reciprocal interactions were found during the intervention. Follow-up data obtained 6 months after the study indicated that the reciprocal interactions had increased. Evidence for generalization to the groups with a friend of the child also was found, although the probes for assessing generalization were limited to 2 children within the same setting used for training.

Social validity of the intervention was assessed. Parents gave generally favorable ratings to items concerning increases in positive interactions and the responsiveness of the targeted child. There was some agreement that the targeted child was more likely to initiate interactions. The siblings did not express negative statements concerning interactions.

Schreibman, O'Neill, and Koegel (1983) trained sibling pairs to teach specific tasks to brothers or sisters with autism. In one of the three cases, an 8-year-old girl was trained to teach her 5-year-old brother. The tasks included (1) concepts of before–after and first–last; (2) coin identification; (3) classification of picture cards (e.g., animals, clothes); (4) pronoun concepts of "I have" and "you have"; (5) one-to-one correspondence; (6) capital letters; and (7) responses to short-term memory questions ("Who went to the store?").

The training and teaching sessions took place in the home. Two generalization probes were conducted at a research site resembling a living room. The sibling was taught reinforcement techniques, shaping, chaining, and discrete trial strategies through a videotaped presentation, after which the older sibling and the trainer discussed the various techniques.

The trainer also provided examples of how the techniques could be used in situations other than those described on the tape, and how the techniques could be applied to everyday problem behaviors and situations.

During the next phase, the sibling worked on one of the specified target behaviors with her younger brother for 30 minutes while the trainer observed. The trainer interrupted periodically to provide corrective and positive feedback to the sibling. When the sibling had difficulty performing specific techniques, the trainer modeled the procedure and asked the sibling to try it again. After each training session, a new task was selected and the sibling worked another 15 minutes without interruption from the trainer. Probes were taken during this period to determine the extent of skills generalization. A total of eight training sessions was conducted.

The results of the study indicated that the sibling used the strategies 73% of the time during baseline and increased her performance to 100% with training. The child's responses increased from 15% at baseline to 45% during training. Setting generalization probes indicated maintenance of performance for both children.

Other studies report the successful training of siblings in teaching one skill to a sibling with disabilities (Bennett, 1973; Cash & Evans, 1975; Colletti & Harris, 1977; Miller & Cantwell, 1976). Hancock and Kaiser (1996) report the effective use of milieu language interventions by children with younger siblings having expressive language delays.

James and Egel (1986) caution that long-term effects of sibling training programs have not been assessed sufficiently, especially outcomes for the siblings. Numerous factors may affect the success of such interventions. Issues in implementation include the organization and length of the sessions and training methods (i.e., incidental teaching, modeling, prompting). Training also requires the establishment of family rules. For example, if family members observe another member not carrying out the intervention, the behavior may be discussed with a professional. Miller and Cantwell (1976) presented a case in which a sibling observed and reported a father spanking the target child rather than following the intervention procedures, resulting in the father's anger toward the sibling. Following through is necessary in order for the parent to monitor the sibling's behavior to ensure that the intervention is being carried out as planned. Family dynamics (i.e., a shy child, domineering parent) may require intervention modifications. Activities need to be planned, and many promote sibling interactions at the preschool-age level, such as playing with balls, dolls, or acting out stories or themes (Powell & Ogle, 1985). From Powell and Ogle, other guidelines for a sibling teaching program include seeking voluntary participation and rewarding both children for participation. A 2-year age advantage for the sibling teacher usually is recommended. Sibling rivalry may undermine such efforts, and strategies to reduce jealousy and competition may be necessary.

PROBLEM BEHAVIORS

Bed-Wetting

The treatment of bed-wetting, or enuresis, has one of the most extensive literatures in behavioral psychology (Friman & Jones, 1998). A review reveals a wide range of treatments including drug therapy, surgery, various forms of psychotherapy, training in bladder control, the buzzer and pad techniques, and a multicomponent procedure termed *dry-bed training* (DBT).

A medical evaluation is advised as a standard practice. However, a review of the literature suggests two additional considerations. First, organic causes are estimated to be less than 1% (Forsythe & Redmond, 1974). Second, behavioral interventions may succeed even when other more radical or drastic treatments have failed. In many studies that demonstrated success with behavioral interventions, from 30% to 100% of the children had received prior medical treatment, including drugs or surgery.

Neither ignoring enuresis, nor radical medical treatment seem to be sound advice with a large proportion of enuretic children age 5 and older. Although "spontaneous cures" sometimes occur (Forsythe & Redmond, 1974), the result is not predictable for specific children; wetting is likely to persist through the childhood years for many, and into adulthood for some. Before age 5, intervention for enuresis is questionable (Doleys, 1979; Walker, Kenning, & Faust-Campanile, 1989). One factor leading to a possible decision to intervene is a sustained prior history of dry nights followed by wetting.

The multicomponent strategy of DBT for functional (vs. organic) enuresis builds on many basic interventions introduced earlier and has considerable research support. Many of the component strategies, such as self-monitoring, reinforcement for dry nights, and the supplemental use of a urine alarm, have been demonstrated to be successful as independent interventions (Walker et al., 1989).

As an overview, DBT (Azrin & Besalel, 1979) includes training in inhibiting urination and increasing functional bladder capacity, self-correcting of accidents, self-recording of successes and failures, using tangible and social reinforcers, and training specific habits in rapid awakening and urination (described as most important by Azrin & Besalel, 1979). Self-regulation, positive practice, and reinforcement are the basic procedures.

The treatment package has gone through many years of development. Major changes have occurred, especially recommendations about reduced professional involvement. However, while the program was written for parents, professional assistance is likely to increase chances for success.

The DBT program requires complete parent commitment for the duration of the training. A supportive emotional family climate is important. The three training phases are outlined as follows.

The Intensive Training Day

This includes a special shopping trip to buy salty food snacks, favorite drinks, and a 16-ounce graduated measuring cup. In the early afternoon, after all procedures have been carefully explained to the child, the child is encouraged to drink as much fluid as possible. This increases opportunities for intensive practice.

Every half hour, training in bladder control is carried out. If the child reports a need to urinate, he or she is encouraged to "hold back" as long as possible. If the need to urinate does not pass, the child is asked to pretend to sleep. An attempt is made to increase the duration of "holding back." Instead of the toilet, the child urinates in the measuring cup kept in the bathroom. The amount of urine is recorded and the child tries to beat earlier marks.

Also, as a part of the training day, parents teach children, even 3- and 4-year-olds, how to change bed sheets. Disposing of wet sheets and clothing, and getting fresh ones, are rehearsed.

The next major facet of the training day is referred to as "getting-up practice." This consists of 20 trials of (1) pretending sleep, (2) concentrating on bladder sensations, and (3) hurriedly arising from bed to urinate. The child pretends to sleep for about 1 minute. The room is darkened to make practice similar to bedtime. Just before the pretended bedtime, the parents review the procedures with the child and give encouragement. The positive practice is especially important after the first day. The 20 trials are instituted after a child wets (after changing sheets and nightclothes), and before bedtime of the succeeding evening if wet the night before.

The last major feature of the training day is the hourly awakenings after the child is asleep. If the child is asleep at 8:00 P.M. on the training day, the child will be awakened every hour until 1:00 A.M. First, the parents check the sheets. If dry, the child is gently awakened and is asked to concentrate on bladder sensations. The child makes the choice of either going to the toilet or waiting until the next hourly awakening. Praise is given and more drinks are offered (terminated before the last two awakenings). If wetting occurs during the training night, the child has already practiced the procedures during the day: changing the bed and self, and completing the 20 getting-up exercises.

The Posttraining Day Program

Three major features from the training day are maintained: attempts at increasing bladder capacity via urinating in the measuring cup, the "getting-up" practice, and the child's responsibility for correcting wetting accidents. Bedtime review of the program and progress, and encouragement for success or effort continue throughout.

The nightly awakenings are simplified. On the second night, the child is awakened once at the parent's bedtime instead of on the hourly schedule. If the child is dry, the nightly awakening is moved forward on the next night one-half hour, until it is eventually discontinued. If wet, the awakening is kept the same.

The child is shown how to self-record or chart progress. Also, a system of rewards is used. For example, a kitchen drawer near the chart may be filled with treats and small toys, giving the child a choice of rewards for dry nights. Social rewards also may be significant.

Phasing-Out Procedures

The procedure is maintained for 2 weeks. After that time, nighttime control has probably been acquired. Wetting is likely to reoccur for some children (about 25%). If so, the getting-up practice and responsibility for changing wet bedsheets and clothing are reimplemented.

Other Problems of Elimination

A successful multicomponent toilet-training approach has been developed by Azrin and Foxx (1974; Foxx & Azrin, 1973). Daytime wetting often may be treated successfully with frequent checks for dry pants, cleanliness training, frequent toileting, positive practice, differential reinforcement of communication (DRC), and reinforcement.

For functional encopresis (soiling), many of the basics that have been discussed apply. Medical conditions that may contribute to encopresis should be checked first (Boon & Singh, 1991; Friman & Jones, 1998). Crowley and Armstrong (1977) reported details of a successful home-based treatment of encopresis using positive practice, overcorrection, and behavior rehearsal procedures. Reimers (1996) reported successful results by using a stool softener, positive reinforcement, plus a restitution routine contingent on soiling (termed response–cost in the article; removing and washing clothing, cleaning him- or herself, and dressing).

Sleep Disturbances

Sleep disturbances, including difficulties getting to sleep and frequent awakenings, are prevalent with young children and may be highly disturbing to both children and other family members. Surprisingly, many young children are medicated for sleep disturbances, but such treatments may be contraindicated. Behavioral interventions that have been used include extinction (for crying or tantrums), positive reinforcement for desired behavior, shaping by gradually making the bedtime earlier, and cueing through bedtime routines (Durand, 1998).

As an example, Durand and Mindell (1990) modified an intervention suggested by Ferber (1985) for a 14-month-old girl who had difficulties going to sleep (tantrums), and who was waking up from one to three times during the night. The intervention, described as graduated extinction, was effective for the sleep problems and had positive outcomes for the parents in terms of marital satisfaction and maternal depression. The steps are outlined as follows:

1. One of the child's parents entered the room for a brief period (15–30 seconds) upon the child's waking. The parent was instructed to provide reassurance (such as saying, "It's okay, go to sleep now" in a neutral voice; p. 40), and to check for problems.

2. The parents were instructed to wait for progressively longer periods of time before entering the child's room on subsequent nights (increased by 5-minute increments). The longest period in the intervention was a delay of 20 minutes.

3. Two weeks later, the same basic intervention was applied to tantrum behaviors. The child required parental presence before going to bed. A parent put the child to bed and waited for progressively longer time periods before entering her room for a tantrum. Parents provided brief but neutral reassurance.

Seymour (1987) studied the effects of a comprehensive treatment for sleep difficulties across 4 families. The program included the following components: (1) explaining night waking to parents in terms of habit formation; (2) describing ways that parents accidentally maintain night waking (such as insufficient routines prior to bedtime, rewarding consequences for children's maladaptive behavior); (3) assessing the physical sleeping arrangements; (4) setting routines for before bedtime and for bedtime (meals, baths, story, cuddling); (5) ignoring crying after bedtime or giving minimal attention if needed; and (6) returning children to bed without cuddling or anger. Parents also were instructed to set daytime naps in a similar manner. Reinforcement was given to children when they slept through the night. A treatment program for children with severe disabilities and multiple sleep problems was described by Piazza and Fisher (1991).

Thumb-Sucking

Habits that persist and cause undue negative social or parental attention merit intervention consideration. Thumb-sucking may have these attributes and also may interfere with responding during free-play and structured learning situations. In addition, thumb-sucking may result in dental problems.

Many interventions have been recommended to parents to help with children's thumb-sucking; most have been insufficiently evaluated. Christensen and Sanders (1987) compared the effects of habit reversal and differential reinforcement of other behavior (DRO) for treating this behavior with 30 parents and their children (ages 4–9). Key issues were intervention effectiveness, generality and maintenance of change, undesirable outcomes or side effects, and acceptability of the intervention by parents.

The authors of the study had the parents select one training setting (such as watching television) and two generalization settings (such as bedtime). Observations included thumb-sucking, noncompliance, complaints (whining, screaming), aversive mands, aggression, oppositional behavior (rule breaking), and appropriate interactions and play.

The *habit-reversal* procedure was developed by Azrin and colleagues (Azrin, Nunn, & Frantz-Renshaw, 1980). The first phase included discussion about (1) working together to stop thumb-sucking, (2) identifying the stimulus conditions for the behavior and cues for the onset of the behavior, and (3) modeling and feedback for performing the alternative and competing response. The procedure "involved clenching both fists, ensuring that the thumb was enclosed by the fingers, and slowly counting to 20" (Christensen & Sanders, 1987, p. 286). The procedure was repeated three times if thumb-sucking occurred in the training setting. Parental counting was faded. The second phase required that the child remain in close proximity to the parent in the training setting for 30 minutes. Parents asked children to take the thumb or finger from the mouth and prompted the previously mentioned procedure contingent upon thumb-sucking, using manual guidance if necessary.

The training session was repeated in the third phase. The child was "reminded to become aware of the earliest sign of thumb sucking and to perform the exercise and counting" (Christensen & Sanders, 1987, p.

286). Children were reminded by parents to not thumb-suck outside the training sessions as well. Children were requested to perform the exercise (fist clenching and counting) contingent upon thumb-sucking or the agreed-upon early cue that signaled the behavior. Parents were requested to observe as closely as possible and cue the child once if thumb-sucking occurred.

The DRO training format was identical. The procedure was implemented in two phases. In phase one, a token system and rules were explained to the child. In the second phase, the parent implemented the training procedure. Children examined the tokens and selected possible rewards. The DRO involved an "escalating schedule." First, five rules were established, and each rule was applied for 2 or more days (if needed). Each rule specified a set number of tokens the child could earn, contingent on the absence of thumb-sucking for a specified period of time. If the child was not successful in 80% of the intervals for 2 days, the same rule was applied the following day. Each rule increased the interval between reinforcements (i.e., for Rule 1, sessions resulting in possible reinforcement were 3 minutes in length and increased to 30 minutes for Rule 5). The contingencies and intervals were explained to the child via a clock face. Parents were told to unobtrusively observe the child, and if thumb-sucking did not occur during the interval, the child was given a token and a mark was recorded on a record sheet. If the contingency was not met, the parent told the child that no token was earned and the record sheet was marked accordingly. After the 30-minute period, the parent and child counted the tokens, and if the criterion was met, the child earned the reward. Parents were encouraged to divide the day into 30-minute periods and observe as often as possible. Children also were able to earn other privileges at other times throughout the day.

Both interventions lasted for 10 days, and both were effective in reducing thumb-sucking in comparison to a control group. In addition, both interventions generalized to the other settings. Intervention effects were also noted during 3-month follow-up observations. An increase in oppositional behavior was observed during the intervention but was not evident during follow-up. Both procedures were judged as acceptable by most parents. Overall, the authors reported that the habit-reversal procedure may hold some clinical advantages in comparison to DRO: increased collaborative efforts and fewer negative side effects. Other possible treatments include increasing children's engagement in interesting activities to reduce opportunities for self-stimulation (differential reinforcement of incompatible behavior).

We have used self-control procedures in case studies with parent-reported success. The child is taught to discriminate the behavior, and prearranged "silent signals" are used to cue the child to self-record occurrences of thumb-sucking. Improvements in daily performances are cocharted with the child and earn rewards (see differential reinforcement of diminishing rates in Chapter 7).

Fears and Phobias

Early investigations of irrational fears are an important part of the history of psychology, but fears and phobias in young children account only for about 5% of all referrals for intervention (Ollendick & Francis, 1988). Behavioral interventions have been used with success in the treatment of many childrens' fears and phobias (Morris, Kratochwill, & Aldridge, 1988). There are two general tactics. First, Jersild and Holmes (1935) anticipated many current interventions by stressing that effective techniques "help the child to become more competent and skillful and . . . encourage him to undertake active dealings with the thing that he fears" (p. 102). Second, fears are maintained because attention by caregivers is given to children when they are fearful. Many successful interventions include combinations of strategies such as modeling coping behaviors and desensitization to the feared object or event, self-instruction, and contingency management.

SUMMARY AND CONCLUSIONS

Family systems issues are of primary importance for several reasons. First, they help define the quality of social and cognitive learning experiences provided to children. Second, family realities are related to intervention decisions. The role of the parent as change agent is dependent on many aspects of parental functioning apart from parent–child relationships.

In this chapter, we examined the role of parent as teacher and change agent within the context of family systems, the basics of home–school interventions, strategies to expand learning opportunities, and interventions for relatively common problem behaviors. The chapter builds on parent–professional collaboration and assessment strategies, targets for intervention, and basic interventions presented in earlier chapters. Chapter 9 continues the discussion of family interventions in the context of severe challenges and problem behaviors.

CHAPTER 9

♦♦♦

Parent Interventions for Severe and Risk-Related Problem Behaviors

♦

This chapter focuses on severe problems of children and situations associated with risk. Many parents are raising children under perilous economic, personal, and social circumstances. These factors directly and indirectly influence the care given to children and intervention decisions on their behalf. Children's developmental characteristics may place severe demands on family resources. In some problem situations such as abuse or neglect, the parents themselves are targets of intervention efforts.

PROBLEM BEHAVIOR IN THE HOME AND COMMUNITY

There are many potential obstacles to successful parent–child relationships. Major barriers include factors related to the adults' world that may create or exacerbate difficult child behaviors or demands.

Developmental Characteristics and Family Resource Demands

Significant effort and conflict may be involved in child care, depending on child characteristics and parental circumstances. Parents of young children with identified disabilities share the typical childrearing demands and scheduling challenges faced by all families. In addition, they report being unprepared and overwhelmed at the sudden need for specialized parenting skills, environmental modifications, and related intervention services (Bell, 1997; Miller, 1994). Excessive time spent in daily caregiving activities (e.g., feeding, bathing, dressing) can lead to physical and emotional exhaustion (Brotherson & Goldstein, 1992; Mahoney, O'Sullivan, & Robinson, 1990; McLinden, 1990).

Caregiving demands further increase with the severity of the child's disability and the fragility of the child's health (Mahoney et al., 1990; Rimmerman & Duvdevani, 1996). Problematic child behaviors, along with limited communication and social skills, may tax parent coping strategies and limit child care alternatives and social activities (Fox, Dunlap, & Philbrick, 1997; Hanson & Hanline, 1990; Seligman & Darling, 1997; Volkmar, 1993). These demands of daily living may make it difficult for parents to participate in intervention-related activities (Macmillan & Turnbull, 1983; Thurman & Widerstrom, 1990). Early-childhood professionals are challenged to collaborate with parents to develop effective intervention strategies that can ameliorate child behavioral difficulties and promote developmental skills leading to increased independence.

Insularity

The term "insularity" is used to describe mothers who are "'cut off' from social contact," and who view the limited contacts they do experience as unsolicited, or aversive (Wahler, 1980, p. 208). Wahler and his associates (Panaccione & Wahler, 1986; Wahler, 1980; Wahler & Afton, 1980; Wahler & Dumas, 1986) have examined the hypothesis that extrafamily contacts, especially when they are few or aversive, significantly affect childrearing practices. In these situations, the demands of parenting may lead to neglectful or coercive parent–child interactions.

Insular mothers also are at increased risk of treatment failure. The absence of problem-solving discussions between insular mothers and family members, friends, or professionals has been hypothesized as a keystone behavior that may help explain why these parents have problems with parenting skills (Wahler & Hann, 1984).

The findings by Wahler and his associates suggest that points of assessment must include more than child characteristics or those of the parent–child dyad. Interventions need to have positive outcomes for parents in their relationships with their children, and perhaps in their adult lives as well. If family needs are not addressed, parent–child interventions are more likely to fail.

Compliance Training

Noncompliance—ignoring parent (or teacher) requests—is considered to be a *keystone behavior* that merits intervention in many home and school situations. Generally, noncompliance occurs as a part of a constellation of behaviors: whining, tantrums, aggressive behaviors, "talking back," aversive demands ("I want it now!"), and other behaviors related to conduct disorders.

An important foundation is Patterson's *coercion model.* The central idea is that antisocial behaviors stem from deficits in parenting skills *and* maladaptive child behaviors: an unskilled parent interacting with a temperamentally difficult child. Patterson's coercion model is defined by three components: (1) learning antisocial behaviors through family interactions, (2) "stress amplifier effects" (such as economic stress or divorce), and (3) possible generalization to the school (Patterson & Bank, 1986).

Ineffective discipline is a key variable. Patterson's research group found that parents of antisocial boys tended to "scold, threaten, and nag as a reaction to both trivial and significant behaviors. Most significant . . . was their failure to back up their threats consistently" (Patterson & Bank, 1986, p. 57). Parents may comply with the child's refusals to obey commands. Extreme forms of punishment, or explosive discipline, also were characteristic of the parents.

A second major variable is that of *parental monitoring.* This construct has less adequate convergent validity than the other constructs proposed by Patterson and needs to be revised for younger children. Examples include increased "unsupervised street time" and failure to "believe" that children engage in major antisocial acts outside the home (Patterson & Bank, 1986, p. 58). Patterson and Bank hypothesized that monitoring has a relatively minor role in the early progression of antisocial behavior.

However, based on numerous research studies, and an alternative definition, we consider this construct highly promising. Sansbury and Wahler (1992) defined maternal monitoring in a different way by noting a mother's ability to detect instances of child aversive responses. Mothers characterized as using maladaptive parenting methods underreported these occurrences and tended to comply with their child's refusals to obey. Sansbury and Wahler found inconsistency to be a complicated function of biased maternal reporting and ecosystem quality. In summary, when conduct disorder behaviors are of concern at home, measurement constructs include parental responsiveness to reports of adaptive or maladaptive behaviors outside the home, monitoring child behaviors in the home, and responses to these behaviors. We also have used this construct to help guide assessment and intervention design for behaviors associated with other severe behaviors such as fire setting.

A third variable, termed "coercive child," refers to a reciprocal process where family members "train" each other to elicit coercive behaviors. For example, a three-part sequence might include an aversive behavior by a parent (such as an unpleasant request for bedtime), a coercive reaction by the child (whining), and the termination of the initial parental behavior. Very high levels of noncompliance can be produced quickly through such interactions. "The child learned that he could react aversively to demands made on him, and that if he persisted, probably 'won.' The child also learned that he could use a wide range of coercive means to produce rapid changes in the behavior of other people" (Patterson & Bank, 1986, p. 59).

Patterson and his associates have developed an extensive program based on social learning principles: It has both family and school components (Patterson, Reid, Jones, & Conger, 1975). The major features of the treatment program are outlined in Table 9.1. The program, intended for children ages 3 to 12, has been well researched. The strategies are to teach parents of antisocial children more effective ways for dealing with coercive behaviors and to reinforce socially appropriate behaviors. A key feature is training parents (as well as professionals) to observe behavior. Patterson (1975b) noted that without careful observations by parents or teachers, it is likely that they will experience difficulty in changing behavior.

Forehand and McMahon (1981) provided a detailed description of an intervention program for noncompliant children based on considerable research, primarily with children ages 3 to 8. The program was originally developed by Constance Hanf at the University of Oregon. The intervention has similarities to the program developed by Patterson and earlier work by Wahler and colleagues (Wahler, Winkel, Peterson, & Morrison, 1965). An outline of their treatment program is presented in Table 9.2.

The most salient features are two stages used to address parent–child issues. In the first stage, the parent is taught to effectively attend to appropriate child behaviors and to ignore inappropriate behavior. In other words, the parent is taught to be "a more effective reinforcing agent" (Forehand & McMahon, 1981, p. 51). The parent is trained to monitor effectively the child's appropriate behaviors and to stop the use of ineffective

---

TABLE 9.1.   Some Features of Patterson's Program for Aggressive Children

1. The parents are assigned a text written expressly for parents in order to provide the necessary background for skills training (*Living with Children* or *Families*). The target child is included in interviews and discussion.

2. Parents are trained to pinpoint two problem behaviors and two prosocial behaviors, and to track the behavior. Parents monitor two to three target behaviors for a 1-hour period for 3 days. Frequent phone calls are used by the professional to monitor the data.

3. Parents are trained in the use of a positive reinforcement system that include praise and tangibles (a simplified token economy). Contingency contracts are used.

4. A time-out procedure is introduced. Response cost also may be used.

5. Training in problem solving and negotiation are subsequently provided to parents through contracting.

6. Classroom intervention may be necessary, including (a) reduction of disruptive behavior, (b) home–school communication, and (c) help with academic skills.

TABLE 9.2.   Characteristics of a Compliance Training Program (10 sessions)

Phase I: Differential attention

1. The parent is taught to be a more effective reinforcing agent.

2. The parent is trained to increase the frequency and range of social rewards and eliminate verbal behaviors that are associated with deviant child behavior.

   a. The parent is taught to attend to and describe the child's appropriate behavior.

   b. The parent is required to eliminate all commands, questions, and criticisms directed to the child during the training sessions.

   c. The parent is trained to use rewards contingent upon compliance and other appropriate behaviors (e.g., use praise statements in which the child's behavior is labeled—"You are a good boy for picking up those blocks").

   d. The parent is taught to ignore minor inappropriate behaviors.

   e. In the home, the parent is required to structure brief (10–15 minute) "Child's Games" to practice skills learned in the clinic.

      (1) The child chooses the activity.

      (2) Watch with interest what the child is doing.

      (3) Describe enthusiastically what the child is doing.

      (4) Participate in the activity without restructuring (e.g., handing materials, taking turns).

      (5) Do not ask questions or give commands.

      (6) Do not teach or test.

   f. With the aid of a therapist, the parent identifies lists of child behaviors to increase, discusses the use of attends and rewards, and develops a program to increase two child behaviors outside of the clinic.

Phase II: Decrease noncompliant behavior

1. The parent is trained to use appropriate commands and time out.

2. The parent is trained to give direct, single commands and to allow the child 5 seconds to initiate compliance.

3. If compliance is initiated within 5 seconds of the command, the parent is taught to reward or attend to the child within 5 seconds of the compliance initiation.

4. If compliance is not initiated, the parent is trained to use time out, as follows.

5. A warning is given that labels the time-out consequence ("If you do not ___, you will have to sit in the chair in the corner").

6. If the warning is ineffective within a 5-second interval, the child is placed in the chair.

7. The child must remain in the chair for 3 minutes and be quiet and still for the last 15 seconds.

8. The child is then returned to the uncompleted task and given the initial command.

9. Compliance is followed by contingent attention from the parent.

Note: Adapted from Forehand and McMahon (1981). Copyright 1981 by The Guilford Press. Adapted by permission.

"commands, questions and criticisms" that are linked to noncompliant behavior (p. 51). Also, parents are trained to use rewards to increase compliance and positive parent–child exchanges, and to ignore minor problem behaviors. A "child's game" is used in the home to practice parent–child play skills learned in the clinic. The second stage consists of specific procedures to increase compliance with parental commands. The parent is trained to use appropriate commands and mild time out.

In other research, adjuncts to the program have been studied. Positive effects are reported for including training parents in social learning principles and self-control. Zangwill (1984) reported a replication of Hanf's procedure; he also found that the parents expressed approval of a "bug-in-the-ear" technique that enabled immediate therapist–parent feedback in training sessions.

Effective and Ineffective Commands

Promising points of analysis for many caregivers are the qualities of the commands given to the child. The rationale for evaluating parental commands is straightforward. The evaluation of child misbehavior must include attention to settings, events, parental behavior, and child behavior. The appendix provided by Forehand and McMahon (1981) is excellent reading for professionals working with caregivers of noncompliant children and provides an extensive discussion of coding parent–child interactions. While we dwell on the analysis by Forehand and McMahon because of their research with conduct-disordered children, note that very different analyses of child compliance exist (e.g., Parpal & Maccoby, 1985).

Forehand and McMahon (1981) define an *alpha* command as "an order, suggestion, question, rule, or contingency to which a motoric or verbal response is appropriate and feasible" (p. 191). Often, these are in the form of imperatives such as "Come here," "Please stop making that noise," or "Pick up your toy." They also include under this category *indirect commands* ("See if you can be quiet"), *question commands* ("Why don't we sit here?"), *permission statements and rules* ("There will be no more fighting"), *If–then statements* ("If you don't stop running, you'll hurt yourself"), and *chain commands* ("Stand up, come here, and sit down").

Beta commands include those whereby child compliance is difficult or impossible. These include commands that are interrupted or ended in some way by the parent, so that the child is unable to comply in a reasonable time period, or commands that are carried out by the parent before the child is able to comply. The second type of beta command is those that result in confusion, so that the child is unable to determine what behavior is expected. These include *if–when* statements ("Put it up here if you want to"), and *vague* commands ("Just be good for a while longer"). Other problem areas for commands include frequent and intense commands, a lack of reasonable proximity or closeness to the child, and a high rate of repetition of the original command, which in our work has been a frequent keystone variable.

Forehand and McMahon note that effective commands are "specific and direct," "given one at a time," and "followed by a wait of 5 seconds" (Forehand & McMahon, 1981, p. 76). They also suggest five types of commands that have the effect of *lowering* child compliance (pp. 74–75): (1) chain commands; (2) vague commands; (3) question commands ("Would you like to take your bath now?"); (4) "Let's . . ." commands (e.g., "Let's pick up your toys"), when the parent actually has no wish or intent to be involved in the activity; and (5) commands followed by a rationale or other verbalization (the rationale should come *before* the command). When parent–child interactions are working well, children respond to more subtle forms of directives and implicit rules, but these are not good starting places for noncompliant or defiant behaviors.

We think that adult commands or requests to children serve as a significant focal point of a functional analysis in many situations, and the descriptions by Forehand and McMahon serve as a major contribution. However, the alpha and beta definitions may benefit from refinement. In applying the definitions to teachers' interactions with children, Bramlett (1990) found less than satisfactory agreement (.77 for alpha commands and .50 for beta commands).

Roberts and Powers (1988) described the extensive development of the "Compliance Test," which measures responses to standardized chorelike instructions from the parent. The need for the test was based on extending and clarifying the Forehand and McMahon procedures. A low degree of compliance may be related to ineffective commands or noncompliance, or both.

Defiant Children

Barkley (1997) has made available a treatment package building on the earlier work by Hanf and McMahon and Forehand. The program has been designed for children between ages 2 and 11, but he states that it may be possible to use the program with children as young as 18 months depending on language development. One major change from an earlier edition is that spanking has been eliminated (from noncompliance with the time-out procedure). Barkley also has enhanced the usability of the program for clinicians by providing a step-by-step workbook.

In Barkley's program, the following definitions have been applied to noncompliance behaviors.

1. The child does not initiate behaviors within a "reasonable time" or about 15 seconds after a request or command from an adult (p. 17). (Note: Forehand and McMahon used a 5-second guideline. For training parents in the use of time out, Barkley recommends a 5-second rule as a first warning. Shriver and Allen [1997] take a normative approach and suggest 10 or 14 seconds representing one or two standard deviations in latencies between request and compliance for a small clinic sample. We think that the delay interval is an issue of social validity and behavior context and thus may be an important point of parent consultation. Circumstances may indicate the need for flexibility in using these guidelines.)

2. The child does not sustain compliance until the stipulations in the request have been met.

3. Other established rules are not followed in the situation (aggressive behaviors are emitted).

Since many of the overall features are similar to those outlined in the program by Forehand and McMahon, only two steps are summarized here. One step focuses on anticipating misbehavior in public places (stores, restaurants, church), visiting friends, and during transitions (such as from play to bedtime). Parents are taught a strategy referred to as *think aloud—think ahead*, in which the plans for misbehavior are developed. The four facets are (1) establish, teach, and prompt rules for appropriate behavior (i.e., before shopping, rules might be reviewed such as "Stay close," "Do not touch items," "Do not ask for toys or candy," etc.); (2) plan incentives for compliance with the rules; (3) plan disciplinary procedures for noncompliance; and (4) plan to engage the child in an activity or assign a responsibility to the child for the outing. Another step deals with planning for *future* problem behaviors. The parents are required to anticipate "new" problem behaviors and to learn how the basic procedures may be applied. The parents are expected to be able to "design" a behavior program based on the methods described in the overall program. We share similar procedures described as planned activity training later in the chapter. Last, Barkley's program also includes optional daily-school-behavior report cards.

Errorless Compliance Training

Ducharme (1996) presents a comprehensive program based on errorless learning and other principles discussed earlier. The program also has been applied to parent groups. Potential benefits include avoiding more aversive and stressful techniques such as time out. We outline some of the key components.

1. A range of typical parental requests is organized hierarchically based on probability of compliance. These are refined through a questionnaire and observation. Parent training includes observation assessment, delivering requests (Forehand & McMahon, 1981), and data collection.
2. In a structured fashion, parents give requests that are likely to have a high degree of compliance and provide reinforcement following compliance.
3. Requests with less likelihood of compliance are gradually introduced.

Other programs have been extensively developed for parents and young children with conduct problems. Webster-Stratton (1981a, 1981b, 1982) has developed a videotaped modeling program. Three conditions were compared: (1) self-administered, including 10–12 sessions of over 200 videotaped parent–child interactions; (2) group discussion plus videotape modeling; and (3) group discussion only. While all programs were effective, the most effective program included videotapes and group discussion (Webster-Stratton, Hollingsworth, & Kolpacoff, 1989). The details of this program are well described and serve as a general source (Webster-Stratton & Herbert, 1993) as does the work by Sanders and Dadds (1993) and Harding et al. (1994; See Chapter 4). Breiner and Beck (1984) reviewed intervention programs for noncompliant behaviors of children with developmental delays (as opposed to children described as conduct-disordered).

Parental Self-Regulation

This component is intended to increase the generalization and maintenance of behavioral change. The core issues are that parents may not continue with effective intervention programs once contact with the professional ends, or they may not automatically apply the intervention program to new or untreated problem behaviors, different settings, or other children with problem behaviors. Furthermore, it is likely that different settings (home, stores, community, neighborhood) place different demands on parents and provoke different antecedents or cues that result in effective or ineffective parental responses. Sanders and Glynn commented that "some settings may be 'high risk' occasions for [treatment] program inaccuracy" (1981, p. 224). "Parents' ability to alter, control, and rearrange their own parenting environment so that the environment prompts and reinforces the continued application and extension of skills once therapist support is withdrawn may require different strategies from those currently used in training parents" (p. 224).

Sanders and colleagues (Sanders & Christensen, 1985; Sanders &

Dadds, 1982; Sanders & Plant, 1989; see also Huynen, Lutzker, Bigelow, Touchette, & Campbell, 1996) have investigated an intervention referred to as *planned activity training* to help with problems of generalization to home and community settings. Seven skills were introduced sequentially to the parents using discussion, modeling, role play, and feedback:

1. How to prepare for situations in advance by organizing and managing time more effectively.
2. How to discuss rules regarding desired and undesired behavior in a relaxed and noncoercive manner.
3. How to select engaging activities for children in specific home and community settings.
4. How to encourage and extend children's engagement in activities by the use of incidental teaching procedures.
5. How to select and apply practical incentives for motivating children's desired behavior in different childrearing situations.
6. How to select practical consequences for undesired behavior in the same settings.
7. How to hold discussions with children following an activity to give feedback on desired and undesired behavior. (Sanders & Christensen, 1985, pp. 108–109).

Sanders and Glynn (1981) demonstrated the effectiveness of teaching 5 two-parent families self-management skills using a treatment package when intervening with disruptive behavior. This intervention was effective overall, but it was not possible to determine the effectiveness of the self-management program alone, since multiple components were used.

The steps and components are summarized as follows:

1. After a baseline phase, each family was instructed in the use of behavior modification techniques during a 2-hour meeting. The strategies included (a) discussing baseline data and effects of parental attention; (b) pinpointing problem behaviors in training and generalization settings; (c) checking parental perceptions; (d) explaining consequences for appropriate and inappropriate behaviors; and (e) explaining the intervention program. Examples of ineffective parenting strategies were taken from baseline data. Target behaviors included demands, tantrums, aggression, arguing, and interrupting.

2. The treatment included giving examples of descriptive praise in addition to "other contingent consequences . . . to increase appropriate behavior," and techniques for "behavior correction" (p. 228). The instructions were as follows: "(a) gain the child's attention, (b) describe calmly what the child has done wrong, (c) describe and prompt the correct behav-

ior, (d) give a further prompt if required, (e) speak up and praise the correct behavior if it occurs, (f) if the problem continues or worsens, deliver a firm verbal reprimand describing the incorrect behavior and back this reprimand up with a natural consequence (e.g., remove troublesome toy and give a brief explanation)" (p. 228). In addition, if the child was noncompliant following the reprimand, given demanding, tantruming, aggressive, arguing, and interrupting behaviors, a brief time out (3 minutes) was used. Detailed instructions for each step were printed on cards. Also, the accuracy of implementation was assessed for five intervention components: giving social attention, prompting, instructing, ignoring, and providing consequences.

3. Feedback sessions were held two times a week for 10-minute periods during home observations. Written feedback included (a) percentage of appropriate child behavior observed, (b) number of praise comments, and (c) percent accuracy of implementation. Three samples of interactions were analyzed with the parents. In addition, part of the session focused on parental verbal behavior and expanding play activities.

4. Parents were introduced to self-management in addition to continuing these above procedures. Parents were provided with a rationale for self-management and were trained in goal setting, self-monitoring, and planning related to parenting skills. The skills were taught sequentially in two phases.

Phase 1: Parents were introduced to goal setting and self-monitoring. Parents recorded on a "self-change card" whether or not they had implemented the home program each day, and if they had applied the procedure in the generalization setting. In addition, the therapist "illustrated" problem solving for one setting.

The steps summarizing specific components for child management were listed on a "self-monitoring card," illustrated in Figure 9.1. The cards were used to cue parents for planning skills. After three successful trials using these procedures, the parents were introduced to the second phase.

Phase 2: Parents selected another community setting, devised a management plan, implemented the plan, and evaluated whether the goal had been reached over three occasions. The step was repeated for a third community setting.

5. Self-maintenance training was initiated. Prompts and cues provided by the therapist, home feedback sessions, self-monitoring cards, and checklists were withdrawn. Parents were asked to continue using the behavioral techniques in different settings.

Aspects of parent self-regulation also are addressed in the treatment programs described by Barkley (1997) and Forehand and McMahon

HANDLING DISRUPTIONS WHILE VISITING

Instructions: Each time you take your child visiting, mark Date and Time, Yes, No, or N.A. (not applicable) for each of the steps below.

Steps to be followed:					
1. Prepare the child for the outing by describing the expected behavior. Describe where you are going and how long it will take.					
2. When you arrive involve the child in an activity and make sure the child has something to do, and you have a snack available.					
3. Speak to, ask questions, and praise the child for desired behavior every so often.					
4. If a disruptive behavior occurs (e.g., grizzling, demanding, tantrums) gain the child's attention immediately.					
5. Describe the problem (i.e., the undesired behavior) and state the correct behavior (e.g., waiting).					
6. If the child obeys, speak up and praise child for doing what he/she is told.					
7. If the problem continues give a direct terminating instruction.					
8. If child does not comply, immediately provide back up consequences (i.e., a logical consequence, or time out).					
Number of steps completed correctly:					

FIGURE 9.1. An example of a self-monitoring form used during self-management training. From Sanders and Glynn (1981). Copyright 1981 by the Society for the Experimental Analysis of Behavior. Reprinted by permission.

(1981). Extensive discussions of self-regulation for adults are included in Karoly and Kanfer (1982), and in the very readable book by Watson and Tharp (1996). Also, there is some evidence that parenting skills generalize to siblings (Humphreys, Forehand, McMahon, & Roberts, 1978).

Parent-Administered Time Out

Time out was discussed in the chapter on basic interventions; here, we focus briefly on parent applications. While there is much research support for the use of parent-administered time out with oppositional child behavior, as pointed out earlier, it can be easily abused, and its use may be avoided (Ducharme, 1996). A noteworthy feature of the treatment packages here is that they advocate increasing positive experiences and training in the use of positive approaches to discipline before implementing aversive forms of discipline. The brevity of time-out periods also is significant (3 minutes in the program described by Forehand & McMahon, 1981; 3–5 minutes in Patterson's program; 1–2 minutes per year of the child's age, with a limit determined informally by the severity of the misconduct in the program described by Barkley). Many suggest a contingency: The child remains in time out until he or she is calm and behaving appropriately; but this procedure also has been questioned.

There are numerous studies of time out, various modifications, and training (Flanagan, Adams, & Forehand, 1979). Wahler and Fox (1980) used time out for aggressive and oppositional behavior whereby if the child violated a household rule or did not follow a parent's direction, the child was told to go to a designated room (i.e., bedroom). The child would remain in the room alone and quiet for 5 minutes. "Quiet" was defined as not engaging in loud behavior that could attract attention. Clark (1996) describes the alternative of timing-out a toy when misbehavior is centered on the toy, whereby the child is not allowed to play with the object for a brief time.

Roberts (1988; see also Roberts & Powers, 1990) has an extensive review of procedures that have been advocated when children do not stay in time out, and compared two different procedures when "chair" time outs fail. A "room" time out (sending children to their room), lasted 1 minute and was followed by a return to the chair time out. In the second procedure, control-group children were spanked if they escaped from chair time out. Both were effective, but, most important, the procedures for room time outs do not use physical violence and are brief. Thus, the alternative procedure fits national calls from professional organizations to eliminate corporal punishment. The parent stays by the door while monitoring the child's behavior. Parent consultation for the use of time out should include strategies to handle possible resistance to the procedures.

Walle, Hobbs, and Caldwell (1984) examined different sequences of interventions involving differential positive attention and time out. They found that the use of differential attention may enhance the subsequent effectiveness of time out.

Parental Use of Tokens

Use of tokens is mentioned often in the preschool literature, and they may be used in many ways. Christopherson, Arnold, Hill, and Quilitch (1972) provided an extensive description of the use of tokens by families. One family included a 9-year-old boy described as being truant, noncompliant, and "sassy"; an 8-year-old girl with cerebral palsy, who was also described as hyperactive and exhibited tantrums; and a 5-year-old boy described as "whiny." All three children "bickered," and both boys had difficulty with bedtime.

Target behaviors, including household chores, were explicitly defined for each child and were posted on the bedroom door. For example, the bedtime posting was the absence of disruptive interactions ". . . following 5 minutes in which to settle down" (p. 486). Whining was defined as "a verbal complaint conducted in a sing-song (wavering) manner in a pitch above that of the normal speaking voice" (p. 486). Tokens were earned for chores completed and other nonregular duties, and were lost (response cost) if chores were not completed, if completion did not meet the posted definition, or if behaviors such as whining or bickering occurred. A "point card" was used to keep a record of the points earned and lost. The total intervention time for the family was 10 hours.

The study details an extensive multicomponent parental training program including a film, written materials, discussion, home visits, and phone contacts. Parents were requested not to make any changes in the token "economy" without the therapist. While very effective for the families, parental motivation, cooperation, and involvement were critical for success.

Parental Praise

Praising children for appropriate behaviors is frequently offered to parents as advice for handling misbehaviors. However, in three interrelated studies, Roberts (1985) raised questions about the usefulness of parental praise to induce compliant behaviors, although it has other important functions. For severe noncompliant and disruptive behaviors, treatment packages developed by Patterson, Forehand and McMahon, or Barkley, recommended earlier, should be considered. Another demonstration of the contributions and limitations of social attention, and need for broader treatment components, was provided by Budd, Green, and Baer (1976).

An Example of a Home–School Intervention

A treatment package illustrative of home–school interventions was developed by Budd, Liebowitz, Riner, Mindell, and Goldfarb (1981). The intervention had three facets: (1) teacher monitoring of school performance across the school day, (2) feedback to children on performance, and (3) a note to parents communicating school performance. The school day was divided into about 12 periods, lasting 4–8 minutes. Home privileges were established through consultation with parents. Each child met with the teacher individually in order for the teacher to explain the intervention and when a different behavior was added to the contingencies. Target behaviors were described to the children along with examples of how to earn stickers. In addition, children needed to describe verbally the behaviors required to earn stickers and were prompted as necessary. If no target behaviors occurred during a period, each child received a sticker that was placed on a token card. The classroom aide monitored behaviors using a kitchen timer and recording form. Following each period, the aide reported the child's performance to the teacher, who provided praise and feedback about performance to each child. When a preset criterion was met, each child could exchange stickers for home privileges through the token card. Based on the child's performance, the criterion was increased over time. If the criterion was exceeded, the child received bonus stickers and praise. Parents were contacted frequently but informally to monitor progress and to assist them with difficulties implementing the program. Parents recorded the activity earned on the back of the token card daily and returned the card to school the following day.

Overall, the results demonstrated convincing evidence of the effectiveness of the procedure. However, 2 children in one group were unresponsive (out of a total of 18 children), but behaviors improved when school-based reinforcement was added to the intervention. It should be noted that the study was conducted in a special summer program.

Attentional Problems and Activity Level

We have had many referrals expressing parent's or teacher's concerns about children changing activities at very high rates. Sometimes these behaviors are associated with aggressive or other patterns of behaviors such as inappropriately responding to rules or caregiver expectations of classroom or home settings. Often, high rates of activity change are associated with disruptive classroom behaviors and failure to complete assigned or self-selected tasks. These patterns of behavior are often described by syndromes involving child difficulties in sustaining attention and controlling impulses. This constellation of behaviors is now most often referred to as "attention-deficit hyperactive disorder" (ADHD) (DSM-IV; American Psychiatric Association, 1994) along with various subtypes. All of the behaviors associated with ADHD may affect specific daily tasks encountered in home or school as well as social behaviors required for peer and caregiver interactions. Experiencing difficulties with both peers and adults results in children being cut off from normal socialization experiences.

While there is no question of the significance of these behaviors for young children and caregivers, many diagnostic and treatment approaches to this syndrome are controversial. Major problems with ADHD diagnosis include (1) the classification soundness of the *syndrome*, (2) the possibility and problems associated with multiple etiologies, (3) the question of unintended negative outcomes associated with labeling, (4) questions concerning intervention decisions and utility, and (5) inappropriateness of this diagnosis for young children because of the lack of attention to developmental trends (Barkley, 1996, Gresham & Gensle, 1992; Power & DuPaul, 1996; Taylor, 1988; Whalen, 1989). A significant theme of the research is the difficulty of causal analyses and separating out other influences such as classroom and family environments, which may be subtle. In fact, classification of young children using conventional observations and rating scales is likely to be quite tenuous given the situational variability of the behaviors and the frailties associated with the recommended measurement devices. The behavior of children described as having ADHD varies by the type and amount of structure in settings, in response to different caregivers, and to the novelty or demands of settings. Disorganized settings can create corresponding behaviors.

More to the point of this book, for young children, effective interventions may be designed without the use of an ADHD label. There are strong rationales and tactics for behavioral interventions for young children. First, interventions may improve the coping behaviors of parents. Second, if sustained attention and performance can be improved, so may "impulse control" and its associated behaviors. Third, behavioral interventions that focus on alterations in the antecedents and consequences of behavior teach these relationships to children, and this may be effective in rule learning. For all of these reasons, we recommend functional assessments for targeting behavior and designing interventions for children referred for attentional and activity-related concerns.

Combining treatments in sustained programs and across settings may be necessary. Many intervention efforts for older children have used multiple components: parent training, self-control training, social skills interventions, medication, and educational interventions.

A significant issue for assessment and intervention design is that attention-related behaviors may vary widely by tasks or situations. The nature of the tasks is of critical importance for intervention design (salience, interest level, rate of presentation, instructions to tasks, length, prior activities, setting events, contingencies for performance). These factors are related to stimulus control and functional analyses (Chapter 6).

For preschool children, one important assessment strategy is the analysis of activity changes and play or task engagement. Examination of task characteristics in which the child sustains engagement may provide significant information for intervention design to reduce unproductive activity changes. Interventions may have to be sustained over long time periods and across settings to help with severe attentional difficulties. Programming for response generalization and maintenance is critical.

Relatively little research has focused specifically on parent-training applications. Barriers to effective parenting stemming from family ecology and parental characteristics influence intervention decisions and outcomes. The strategies that have been used are based on behavioral principles (Anastopoulos & Barkley, 1990) and systems theory (Cunningham, 1990). Intervention programs for families of children described as ADHD are closely related to the work of Forehand and McMahon (1981) outlined in the section on compliance training, and they are not reviewed further here. The reasons for considering the programs described earlier for noncompliant children are fairly straightforward. First, the goal of the intervention is to improve parent–child relationships. As examples, objectives focus on parental positive attending to play, improving parental commands (stimulus control and consequences), and teaching rule-governed behaviors. Second, a significant number of children described as ADHD also have conduct-disordered types of behaviors (oppositional or defiant). Third, the programs deal with practical issues of family life (e.g., bedtime and other routines).

There has been more research on the effects of stimulant medication than any other treatment for childhood psychiatric disorders. Despite successes achieved through the use of stimulant and antidepressant drugs for some older children, the responses may be temporary, difficult to predict, and associated with a range of side effects. Stimulant medication should not be considered as sufficient for intervention, but should be viewed as "respite rather than as a solution" (Whalen, 1989, p. 160). Regardless, drugs typically are not recommended for younger children.

SAFETY- AND HEALTH-RELATED INTERVENTIONS

We identified evaluating the danger of situations and behaviors as a priority in selecting target variables. Helping to ensure a safe home environment is a primary goal. Unintentional injuries are the "leading cause of death of children" (Peterson, 1988, p. 593). Mori and Peterson (1986) wrote, "Preschoolers appear to be the group most vulnerable to injury due to their developmental limitations in dealing with stressful or dangerous situations" (p. 106).

In this section, we discuss interventions that may have value for individual work with parents. Barone, Greene, and Lutzker (1986) and Lutzker, Frame, and Rice (1982) describe a program to reduce home accidents in high-risk families.

Fire Setting

Fires are one of the leading causes of death for preschool children (Peterson, 1988). With regard to intervention decisions, three issues stand out. First, family dysfunction may be an important context for intervention decisions. Other factors, such as parental depression and stress, can contribute to the danger. Peer and family interest in fire-related activities also may be a significant factor. Among the many variables that may have intervention implications, especially important are parental monitoring of behaviors, rule enforcement and effective use of discipline (vs. detachment or noninvolvement, and ineffective discipline), and basic safety.

Second, fire setting frequently has been discussed as a behavior evidenced by at least some conduct-disordered children. Thus, the research-based interventions for noncompliant children, discussed earlier, have important implications.

Third, intervention programs often have an educational component concerning fire. It is frequently appropriate to deal with children's curiosity and safety in addition to parental and child behaviors related to conduct disorders. Naturalistic supervised opportunities for conducting such training include campfires, candles, and barbecues.

There is limited research-based information on the elements of intervention design specifically for young fire setters. Studies have methodological and sample limitations, and little follow-up data. Based on our review of the literature and experience with parent referrals for this problem behavior, we offer suggestions for intervention planning. However, the most important recommendation is to refer to professionals experienced in the treatment and education of fire setters. Local fire departments have been very helpful.

1. *Discuss with the parents the seriousness of the behavior and overall safety proofing of the home.* Establishing the dangerousness of the behavior is a central concern. Beyond the potential for death or disfigurement, parents need to be informed of potential civil and legal responsibilities for damages. Kolko and Kazdin (1989a, 1989b) describe a firesetting interview for parents, and one developed for use with children. A major point of an interview is to determine factors related to behavioral dysfunction and parental risk factors, as well as those related to curiosity about or interest in fire. The Federal Emergency Management Agency (1994) also has developed semistructured parent and child interviews, a parent questionnaire, and recommended school interviews to aid in the determination of risk. The handbook is intended for use by fire service personnel but has many suggestions for educational and psychological service providers.

Fire prevention and basic safety instruction form an important component of treatment. Included are a room-by-room inspection for fire sources and combustibles, use of smoke detectors and fire extinguishers, and emergency fire procedures such as an evacuation plan and telephone numbers.

2. *Develop a contract with the parents.* Key elements of a contract may include (a) childproofing the house or apartment, (b) parental training and vigilance in monitoring child behavior, (c) enlisting the aid of others who smoke (babysitters, visitors) in securing lighters and matches, (d) installing alarms and safety equipment, and (e) participating in a *structured multicomponent parent program* for noncompliant or defiant children, such as the programs by Barkley, Patterson, or Forehand and McMahon. If parents do not agree to the terms of the contract, they may be referred to another agency that has the authority to evoke protective services for the child.

3. *Consult with the parents about parental monitoring.* Parents must monitor the child's access to and contact with fire material. This may serve as negative reinforcement to get the behavior under control. Problem-solve steps to help with parental monitoring. For example, in a case study by Barnett, a young child was turning on burners and "torching" stuffed animals. Along with other procedures, the mother placed bright "safety" tape in the area in front of the stove to teach limits and to give herself more time to react. If the child crossed into the "safety zone," the mother used a brief and mild time out. Also, knobs may be removed from stoves. One parent who lived in a situation where matches and lighters were easily available outside the home effectively "frisked" her young child upon returning from play.

4. *Examine with the parent any sources of stress or parental functioning that may be interfering with monitoring the behavior.* We have had situations of severe marital conflict where an uncooperative spouse deliberately left lighters and matches in places available to the child. The interviews described in Chapter 3 (waking-day and problem solving) may help identify dangerous settings and time periods.

5. *Discuss other possible sources of support for the parent.* Older siblings, grandparents, or friends may assist with monitoring of behavior and implementing intervention plans.

6. *Maintain close contact with the parent.* While the programs for noncompliance generally involve weekly meetings, daily contact through telephone calls or brief office visits should be considered, especially for the first 2–3 days. Based on the contract, there should be no attempts at fire setting, because the child is closely monitored. The program should be immediately effective, or a referral to another agency should be made.

7. *Evaluate the potential utility of a range of interventions for fire setting.* In general, it may be important to examine settings, supervision, and parental responses to fire-setting attempts, and to design a multielement

treatment based on family realities and child problem behaviors. In addition to educational strategies, negative practice, as a part of a multistep intervention sequence, has been recommended (Federal Emergency Management Agency, 1994). The negative practice involves repeatedly striking matches while under close supervision. Restitution also is recommended. However, positive approaches should be examined first. Negative practice may lead to negative side effects.

Treatment programs using negative practice and overcorrection have been described by Carstens (1982); Kolko (1983), McGrath, Marshall, and Prior (1979), and Wolff (1984). Insufficient research has been carried out to recommend the procedure in terms of general applicability, but they appeared to have been helpful.

Kolko, Watson, and Faust (1991) reported positive outcomes for a fire safety program used with children 4 years and older hospitalized for psychiatric problems. Objectives included increasing fire safety and prevention knowledge, reducing curiosity or interest in fire-related materials, and eliminating the children's fire involvement. In developing the group procedures, Kolko (personal communication, January 14, 1998) was concerned about the possible lack of attention to educational and curiosity factors, the potential aversiveness of some fire-related interventions, and the dependence on the skills of primary caregivers in situations related to risk and possibly troubled family relationships. The fire safety program outlined in Table 9.3 is carried out in a group format and requires that children be able to stay in their seats for 30 minutes and follow two-step commands.

Assuming normal curiosity and strict parental supervision, *educational programs may be an important intervention or adjunct.* Rather than the admonishment, "Don't play with matches," which inadequately teaches children about the function and use of matches and lighters, step-by-step programs teach safe fire-related skills in a way that satisfies curiosity. One good program is *A Match Is a Tool* from the Shriners Burns Institute (202 Goodman Street, Cincinnati, OH 45219). Helping children develop an appropriate fear of the consequences of fires is also a part of educational programs.

In summary, fire-setting behavior is complicated and threatening for all involved. Many of our fire-setting interventions have included teaming with community professionals, including fire fighters, and the following components: (1) home inspections and fire safety plans; (2) family rule clarification and reinforcement to increase children's self-regulated behavior; (3) compliance training and perhaps other psychosocial training for children (e.g., problem solving; Kolko, 1996); (4) environmental modifications (e.g., child proofing stoves, securing lighters, and monitoring of play behavior); and (4) fire-related education.

TABLE 9.3. Group Treatment for Fire Safety/Prevention Skills

Session 1

1. The characteristics and functions of fire (how it can help or hurt people) were presented.
2. The importance of adult supervision was discussed.
3. The severity and dangers of fire (damages, injuries, and costs of fires in the children's town) were discussed.

Session 2

1. Children were taught the difference between safe objects and those that must be used under adult supervision.
2. Specific fire-related objects (i.e., matches, lighters, sparklers) and safety rules (i.e., for adult use) were reviewed.
3. Children discussed their experiences with fire.
4. Using a worksheet, children placed red stickers over items that are not okay for play.

Session 3

1. A hand puppet was used to introduce the use of matches (simulated with pretend matches).
2. The children role-played what to do if they found matches (or related material).
3. Worksheets were completed to learn and practice identifying safe and unsafe materials.

Session 4

1. The children were instructed about what to do if a fire occurs (i.e., leave the house, call for help, don't go back).
2. A firefighter described the functions, responsibilities, and hardships of being a firefighter through discussion and role play.
3. Children discussed how it feels to get burned.
4. A demonstration was held about what to do if children's clothes caught on fire.

Note: Adapted from Kolko, Watson, and Faust (1991). Copyright 1991 by Elsevier Science. Adapted by permission.

Car Behavior

Car misbehaviors may be quite severe and in need of immediate attention. Disruptions due to noncompliance with seat belt safety, opening car doors when in motion, tantrums, or bickering with other children can contribute to car accidents. We have had parents report that they simply have stopped taking their children places unless absolutely necessary. In either case, car behaviors are an important point of parent consultation. Fortunately, the basics of intervention design may be applied.

In a case reported by Niemeyer and Fox (1990), a 5-year-old boy with Down Syndrome attacked his mother and sister while riding in the family car. Disruptive behaviors included grabbing and pulling the mother's and sister's hair, hitting them, throwing objects at them, and refusing to wear a seat belt. Often the mother had to stop the car at the roadside to bring his behavior under control.

The sister was trained to collect and record data for the duration of the study. During the first phase of the DRO intervention, seat-belt behavior was targeted. If the child did not remove his seat belt during a 3-minute interval, he received a sticker and praise. Upon arrival home, he received a small toy and verbal praise if he obtained the required number of stickers to meet a set criterion.

Once the boy had been wearing his seat belt consistently for 2 days, aggressive behavior was targeted. The procedures were the same: stickers, praise, and back-up reinforcers, contingent upon the absence of aggression. Aggressive behavior was significantly reduced during eight intervention sessions.

The intervention was then faded. Intervals for obtaining rewards were gradually lengthened. Initially, intervals were increased to 5 minutes over three sessions and then to 10 minutes over two sessions. The final interval consisted of the entire ride (30–40 minutes). Upon arrival home, he received a small toy. Other school-based interventions for bus and car and behavior are reported in Chapter 11.

CHALLENGES AND DIFFICULTIES
IN WORKING WITH FAMILIES

The family is the foundation of early intervention efforts, especially the presence of a responsive and guiding caregiver. There are many challenges to ensuring this foundation. First, professionals working with families need to make certain that barriers to family intervention are not the result of clashes of style, cultures, or values. Very different situations are created when parents are not able to fulfill the normal roles for reasons such as illness, marital conflict or family dysfunction, parental adjustment problems, or psychopathology. In this section, we review interventions that may be necessary when parents are not acting in the best interests of their children.

Parental Adjustment Difficulties

Perhaps counterintuitively, except in extreme cases, *direct* links between family and parental difficulties and childrens' risk status or vulnerability are not always evident. Some children do seem to be less vulnerable than others (Garmezy, 1985; Weintraub, Winters, & Neale, 1986). Even so, the evidence for *indirect* links is substantial and includes both affective disorders (Panaccione & Wahler, 1986; Webster-Stratton & Hammond, 1988) and conduct disorders (Patterson & Bank, 1986; Wahler & Dumas, 1986). For example, maternal depression may be a significant variable in parental perceptions of their children's behavior (Friedlander, Weiss, & Traylor, 1986), the experiences that are provided to children, and opportunities for modeling various behaviors. In such cases, the school-based professional is likely to seek outside help for parents through referral to community or private resources for personal, family, or marital therapy.

Child Abuse and Neglect

The topic of child abuse and neglect is of growing concern to early childhood professionals. While every state has child protection and mandatory reporting laws, legal definitions of abuse differ, are frequently vague and imprecise, and are subject to varying interpretations (Portwood, Reppucci, & Mitchell, 1998). Seven *acts* have been identified to help define situations involving psychological maltreatment: rejection, degradation, terrorization, isolation, corruption, exploitation, and denial of emotional responses (Brassard & Gelardo, 1987; Wolfe & McEachran, 1997). This concept encompasses parental acts of omission which lead to emotional, cognitive, or educational neglect (Hart & Brassard, 1987).

Certainly, much needs to be learned about potentially very different types of abuse (psychological, physical, and sexual) and about responsiveness to interventions. Empirical evidence regarding intervention effectiveness is limited due to the heterogeneous nature of the population, the complexity of the problem, and the inability to randomly assign individuals to control or treatment groups (Hansen, Warner-Rogers, & Hecht, 1998; Kolko, 1998). Wolfe (1987) presented a three-stage model of abuse and neglectful behavior (Figure 9.2).

There are important limitations to behavioral interventions with abusive or neglective parents. However, these are best viewed as limitations of the scientific and professional understanding of the syndrome, and contexts of abuse and neglect, and not an indictment of behavioral interventions in such situations.

First, there may be limitations in child behavioral approaches with parents having severe forms of psychopathology or substance abuse (Kolko, 1998; McMillen, 1997). Second, involvement with the legal system may lead to questions, conflicts, and dilemmas for parents and professionals. For example, parents must have opportunities to practice new skills, but they may not have custody of the child because of abuse, or they may be allowed only brief visitations.

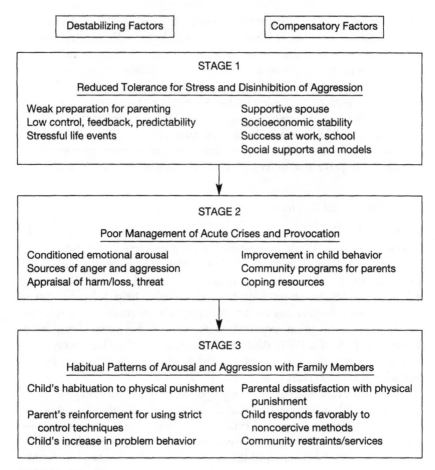

FIGURE 9.2. Transitional model of abuse and neglect. From Wolfe (1987). Copyright 1987 by Sage Publications. Reprinted by permission.

Also, it is important to use assessment data to develop and evaluate effective intervention strategies that can improve the quality of parenting (Greene & Kilili, 1998), but parents may be reluctant to give accurate reports because of their concern that the data may be used to help build a case against them. Since abuse is usually a private matter, data collection other than through indirect means is problematic. However, without strong data, treatment efficacy and recidivism are serious questions.

Third, interventions need to be sufficient in scope given a family's limited personal, social, and economic resources, and sometimes chaotic lives. Fourth, because of crisis situations, systematic solutions may not be sought. Fifth, often abusive parents do not refer themselves for treatment and may not view themselves as having a problem. High-risk families may find center-based treatment expensive, geographically distant, inflexible in scheduling of appointments, blaming and critical, and may fail to seek or drop out of treatment (Webster-Stratton, 1998). Sixth, prevention and early intervention are necessary. By the time that abuse is reported to child abuse workers, the situations may be so severe that children have been significantly harmed.

In earlier chapters, we included aspects of assessment and intervention design that are critical in these cases: determining danger and risk, general factors related to family ecology and problem identification, and assessing children's needs and behaviors. Of special importance are harsh verbal and physical discipline strategies, and emotional responses such as anger that may interfere with more adaptive plans for discipline. Anger-control interventions may be necessary (Hansen et al., 1998; Wolfe, 1994). Also of great importance are annoying, difficult, or disruptive child behaviors. Belsky (1993) describes a coercive parent–child interchange which escalates to physical aggression regardless of the type or severity of child behavior. Younger children are more likely to be targeted for physical abuse, as they spend more time with caregivers, are more physically dependent and vulnerable, and have more difficulty regulating their emotions, evoking harsh and punitive responses (Belsky, 1993). Systematic daily reports by parents of significant behaviors and emotional reactions may be critical.

Given these considerations, one of the most important aspects of decision making is parental motivation for intervention. Many suggestions have appeared in the literature to deal with this problem, but it may be necessary to develop individual strategies based, at least initially, on forming a treatment alliance (Weitzman, 1985). A basic approach is the use of behavioral contracts (Conger & Lahey, 1982; Reid, 1985). A sample contract is depicted in Figure 9.3.

Reid (1985) suggested initially framing the problem by "the daily problems the parent is experiencing with the child" and not by the abuse incident (p. 779). The consultant then may act as an advocate for the parent in dealings with protective service agencies and the courts as long as objectives in treatment are being met.

With regard to specific intervention approaches, a wide variety of techniques can be found. A thorough assessment is necessary to understand the idiosyncratic differences of each child and family, and individualized intervention approaches are essential (Kolko, 1998; Hansen et al., 1998). In addition, it is important to attend to ethnic and cultural issues when planning and carrying out interventions (Greene & Kilili, 1998; Webster-Stratton, 1998; Wolfe, 1994) as parenting and child-rearing beliefs and practices vary.

SERVICE CONTRACT

Between: _____ and _____

Date: _____

In undertaking to assist our family, [the therapist] agrees to help us explore the effectiveness of our parenting approaches with our son, and to improve in areas that are identified by ourselves and [the therapist]. In this manner, we hope to assist our son in developing more acceptable and desirable behavior at home.

We agree to attend scheduled appointments regularly (approximately once per week for 2 hours), and to follow through on suggestions provided by [the therapist]. We will provide [the therapist] with comments as to the problems and successes we may encounter along the way, to allow for a better "fit" between our style and [the therapist's] suggestions.

The goals of our involvement, as discussed between ourselves and [the therapist], focus on increasing the amount of time we spend with Ben, particularly in terms of active play, developmental stimulation, and positive attention. As well, we hope to improve our methods of discipline with Ben, in order to reduce our use of criticism, harsh punishment, and anger.

(If applicable or agreed to):

We agree to permit [the therapist] to discuss our progress with our case-worker, Ms. ___, for the purpose of assisting in case planning and fulfilling our agreement with the agency. A written report at the completion of the program will be provided to our caseworker by [the therapist]. *We will have the opportunity to discuss in full the contents of this report with [the therapist] prior to its being sent.*

We understand that any person with whom we may be involved in this program is obligated to report to the child welfare agency any *suspicions of harm or risk* concerning our child that they may have. Such concerns, whether minor or major, will be brought to our attention by [the therapist] in all cases, in an effort to improve on the situation.

All information from our contacts with this treatment program are treated as confidential, with the exception of information required by law or agreed to by our signature.

Signed, for family: Dated:

Signed, for agency:

FIGURE 9.3. Sample contract for child abuse interventions. From Wolfe (1991). Copyright 1991 by The Guilford Press. Reprinted by permission.

The approach developed by Patterson and his associates, described earlier, has been applied to abusive families (Reid, 1985). Interventions that are skill oriented include parent training in behavioral principles, anger control, stress management, and appropriate knowledge and expectations regarding child development (Hansen et al., 1998; Webster-Stratton, 1998). Techniques have included many of those described in earlier chapters, including modeling appropriate parent–child interactions and ways to handle disruptive behaviors, rehearsal, and feedback. Other points of analysis are the cognitive competencies in constructing alternative modes of behavior and belief systems of the parents (Mischel, 1981). Wolfe (1994) suggested that cognitive-behavioral, parent-focused interventions are particularly effective and less threatening to parents because of their concrete problem-solving focus (i.e., obvious focus on changes in parent–child interactions during everyday parenting situations). Safety-oriented approaches to abuse and neglect were described by Tertinger, Greene, and Lutzker (1984) and Hansen et al. (1998).

While a number of factors have been associated with increased risk for abuse (e.g., child born prematurely or with a disability, parental history of maltreatment, and unemployment), ecological models stress the situational nature of abuse (Altepeter & Walker, 1992; Belsky, 1993). Because abusive and neglectful situations are complex, multicomponent treatments that include parent and child interactions are perhaps the safest alternative (Isaacs, 1982). Effective program indicators include (1) early, intense, and individualized interventions, offered within the parent's home or community, focusing on parent–child interactions and increasing the child's functional language (Daro & McCurdy, 1994; Wasik, 1998); (2) developmentally appropriate day care to provide the parent respite and to teach the child adaptive, social, and regulatory skills to buffer abuse (Campbell & Taylor, 1996; Wasik, 1998); (3) intentional program efforts to increase the parent network of social support (Belsky, 1993; Daro & McCurdy, 1994; Kolko, 1998; Webster-Stratton, 1998); (4) intervention strategies to improve the parent's ability to cope with environmental stressors (McMillen, 1997); and (5) training efforts that incorporate videotaped vignettes of parenting situations and encourage active participation in applying concepts and strategies during role play, group discussion, or individual homework assignments (Lutzker, Bigelow, Doctor, Gershater, & Greene, 1998; Webster-Stratton, 1998).

Prevention efforts have focused on reaching high-risk families early in their parenting experience and connecting them with parent mentors and professionals for training and support. Two programs have utilized Head Start settings for prevention efforts. The Partners program (Webster-Stratton, 1998a, 1998b) randomly assigned Head Start centers to an intensive parent training and support program associated with Head Start enrollment or Head Start alone. Parents were offered monetary incentives, meals, and child care for participation in the training, and the program included a response-cost for missed sessions. The Partners program (Webster-Stratton, 1998a) taught behavior management, play facilitation, and problem solving using videotaped vignettes, group discussions, and homework assignments, and offered social support through weekly group participation and group member (rotating "peer buddies") and/or trainer telephone calls. Individualized interventions were suggested to fit parenting situations described within the group sessions or individual contacts. Outcome data were pretest–posttest for the intervention and control conditions, and included teacher reports of child behaviors, independent observations of children at home and in school, and consumer satisfaction data. Parents reported positive to very positive satisfaction with the intervention (Webster-Stratton, 1998b). Independent observers found fewer negative behaviors, increased compliance, and more prosocial behaviors for the children whose parents had undergone intervention. Observers also reported less critical remarks and physically negative discipline, and more positive, appropriate, and consistent discipline. Teachers reported higher levels of involvement for the Partners group.

Fantuzzo and associates (Fantuzzo, Stevenson, Weiss, Hampton, & Noone, 1997; Fantuzzo, Weiss, & Coolahan, 1998) describe a trilevel intervention program associated with Head Start enrollment. In the first component, Reach Out, Head Start recruiters collaborated with child protective services agencies to facilitate enrollment of high-risk families (e.g., home visitations for enrollment, free medical screenings). The second component, Community Outreach through Parent Empowerment (COPE) involved these high-risk parents in structured training sessions and attempted to bring them into a supportive peer social network. The final component (Play Buddy) involved parent volunteers and confederate peers to engage the child of at-risk parents in play situations. Outcome data revealed that formal parent training resulted in reduced stress, improved parenting skills, and increased involvement in the child's classroom. Teacher ratings and observational data revealed increased social play and decreased behavior problems in children involved in the Play Buddy intervention.

Most of the research pertains to physical abuse; Wolfe and Birt (1997) provide an analysis of sexual abuse. It is difficult to be a scientist-practitioner in cases of sexual abuse because of the limited research base for very young children. The results of assessments such as children's self-reports may be tenuous, and parental ratings may not be valid. The different intervention implications and long-term outcomes of intrafamilial (incest) and extrafamilial (i.e., babysitter) abuse are enormous. To complicate matters, the symptoms associated with abuse vary across so-called internalizing behaviors (anxiety, fear), externalizing (aggression, restlessness), and sexually acting-out behaviors. Furthermore, the symptoms may be combined and delayed in their expression.

As with many problem situations, prevention efforts for sexual abuse may be important. However, Wolfe (1994) reviewed outcomes of sexual abuse prevention programs and concluded that, while they increased child knowledge, there was no decreased risk for abuse. This highlights the critical nature of adult protection of young children. Characteristics of potentially effective sexual abuse prevention programs with young children include training modules incorporating (1) visually interesting and developmentally graduated videotaped presentations of sexual abuse prevention concepts; (2) behavioral rehearsals of prevention strategies with feedback; (3) general assertiveness, decision-making, and communication skills; (4) an emphasis on the need to tell others every time abuse occurs; and (5) information that can be incorporated into natural school curricula (Daro & McCurdy, 1994; Hulsey, Kerkman, & Pinon, 1997). At present, many questions also are being raised about prevention efforts.

Respite

Respite care is defined as short-term relief (day or night) for families of persons with developmental disabilities. Respite care may be a highly significant intervention for families. Potential benefits are (1) relief from emotional and economic stress; (2) accessibility of families to child care facilities, other appointments, and errands for periodic and emergency needs; (3) enjoyment; (4) prevention of abuse and neglect; and (5) elimination of need for out-of-home placement for difficult children. It may have direct personal, social, and economic benefits for parents and indirect benefits for children (Turnbull & Turnbull, 1986). Many interventions place increased demands on parents, but for some parents, "respite may be more important and beneficial than increased involvement" (White, 1985–1986, p. 413). Respite care providers also may be included in intervention plans.

However, there are many challenges to providing respite care. Although there are many alternative plans, including in-home, extended-family, and community-based programs, services available to families may vary widely, as may the training of community respite care providers. Many parents may not be comfortable having the individuals who are available to provide respite services in their home or responsible for their child.

There is little research on the topic. Rimmerman (1989) found that respite services of at least 6 hours per week provided to mothers of children with developmental disabilities resulted in ratings of enhancement of coping and less stress.

SUMMARY AND CONCLUSIONS

We discussed atypical problem behaviors in the home and community within the contexts of family systems and parenting behaviors. Noncompliance is a keystone behavior related to many interventions discussed in the chapter. Treatment programs for noncompliance focus on improving the quality of parent–child relationships and behavior management in the home and community. Parental planning is a significant component.

Another critical aspect of preschool services involves attention to dangerous behaviors. Special consideration was given to fire setting and abuse. For both of these situations, a contract serves as the basis of services, clearly delineating the parent and consultant roles. Interventions for both typically comprise multiple components that build on many topics considered throughout the book. Improving the relationship between parent and child, parental monitoring of behavior, and effective strategies for misbehavior are primary, but interventions also may need to deal more broadly with parental needs apart from child-related responsibilities.

CHAPTER 10

♦♦♦

The Classroom as Ecosystem[1]

♦

The range of preschool philosophies, theories, and curricula—and the potential controversies—is enormous. Preschool classrooms may be organized along many dimensions, depending in large part on the beliefs, values, and training of educators and the goals of the programs. At one extreme, preschool teachers may be highly child-directed and may focus on encouraging the child's interests or selecting experiences assumed to facilitate normal development. Others may be highly directive and prescriptive.

Some preschool classrooms are specifically tied to individual theoretical orientations (Montessori, Piaget). Bereiter and Englemann's (1966) curriculum is an example of the application of behavior principles to preschool education. However, even when a particular curriculum is adopted by an agency, implementation differences may be very great across classrooms. Moreover, it is likely that many preschool educators are guided by eclectic or unspecified personal theories or philosophies. Preschool programs related to children with disabilities are in a rapid state of development and are difficult to characterize.

Given these broad potential differences in philosophy and practice, we have elected to focus on possible roles of teachers and children in intervention design and to emphasize preschool classrooms as ecosystems. Hobbs wrote, "The group is important to the child. When a group is functioning well, it is extremely difficult for an individual child to behave in a disturbed way" (1966, p. 1112). Well-functioning classrooms teach adaptive skills and, along with appropriate curricular decisions, help prevent behavior problems (Dunlap & Kern, 1996; Nordquist & Twardosz, 1990).

---

[1]John Hall contributed to the writing of this chapter.

ORGANIZATIONAL AND SYSTEMS INTERVENTIONS

The philosophy, quality, organization, curriculum, and available services directly affect assessment and intervention decisions. There are numerous sources on model curriculum. One framework for early childhood programs is provided by the National Association for the Education of Young Children (NAEYC). Their guidelines for a curriculum are reproduced in Table 10.1.

The NAEYC provides guidelines for adult–child interactions, home–school relationships, and developmental evaluations. The interaction guidelines focus on responding to children's needs, encouraging learning

TABLE 10.1.   Guidelines for Developmentally Appropriate Practice

1. Developmentally appropriate curriculum provides for all areas of a child's development: physical, emotional, social, linguistic, aesthetic, and cognitive.

2. Curriculum includes a broad range of content across disciplines that is socially relevant, intellectually engaging, and personally meaningful for children.

3. Curriculum builds upon what children already know and are able to do (activating prior knowledge) to consolidate their learning and to foster their acquisition of new concepts and skills.

4. Effective curriculum plans frequently integrate across traditional subject matter divisions to help children make meaningful connections and provide opportunities for rich conceptual development; focusing on one subject is also a valid strategy at times.

5. Curriculum promotes the development of knowledge and understanding, processes, and skills, as well as the dispositions to use and apply skills and to go on learning.

6. Curriculum content has intellectual integrity, reflecting the key concepts and tools of inquiry of recognized disciplines in ways that are accessible and achievable for young children, ages 3 through 8 (e.g., Bredekamp & Rosegrant, 1992, 1995). Children directly participate in study of the disciplines, for instance, by conducting scientific experiments, writing, performing, solving mathematical problems, collecting and analyzing data, collecting oral history, and performing other roles of experts in the disciplines.

7. Curriculum provides opportunities to support children's home culture and language while also developing all children's abilities to participate in the shared culture of the program and the community.

8. Curriculum goals are realistic and attainable for most children in the designated age range for which they are designed.

9. When used, technology is physically and philosophically integrated in the classroom curriculum and teaching (See "NAEYC Position Statement: Technology and Young Children—Ages Three through Eight" [NAEYC 1996b]).

Note. From Bredekamp and Copple (1997). Copyright 1997 by the National Association for the Education of Young Children. Reprinted by permission.

and development, expanding opportunities to collaborate with peers, facilitating choice making and task completion, and detecting stress in children's behavior. Adult roles in the development of self-esteem and self-control are included, along with adult roles in developing children's independence. Parental rights in decision making, with the teacher in collaborative partnership with parents, and interagency communication are emphasized in the section on home-program relationships.

Early childhood special education professionals responded critically to NAEYC's original set of guidelines (1986) for developmentally appropriate practice with regard to children with special learning or behavioral needs. This excerpt from Carta, Schwartz, Atwater, and McConnell (1991) illustrates their concern as more children with identified special needs were included in developmentally appropriate early childhood programs:

> The philosophy of early education . . . proposes that preschool programs should be child centered, allowing children to make choices about what is to be learned. While this approach may be logical for typical young children, it falls short as a standard of effective programming for young children with disabilities. (p. 2)

These professionals emphasized the need for "specialized" teaching and instructional practices for children with special needs, including structured classroom experiences and research-based interventions for instructing and managing behavior. (See Bredekamp, 1993; Carta, 1995; Carta, Atwater, Schwartz, & McConnell, 1993; Fox, Hanline, Vail, & Galant, 1994; Wolery & Bredekamp, 1994; Wolery, Strain, & Bailey, 1992, for reviews of these debates and attempts at resolution.) This prompted the authors of the 1997 revision of the NAEYC guidelines for developmentally appropriate practice to include statements regarding strategies for effective instruction of children with identified disabilities or those who exhibit unusual habits or interests. Early childhood teachers are encouraged to choose from a range of instructional strategies (including modeling, prompting, reinforcement, and other behavioral interventions) to sustain a child's engagement in classroom activities and to promote the acquisition of necessary developmental skills. Our emphasis is on the soundness of individual intervention decisions reviewed in earlier chapters as was well captured by Safford (1989; see also Bredekamp, 1993) in describing the need for *individually appropriate practice*.

The first step in establishing educational and psychological services for children with learning and behavior problems is organizational assessment and development. A wide range of intervention alternatives may need to be examined to meet the desired goals for individual children. A likely initial focus of educational consultation is effective teaching and learning strategies that encompass a wide range of functional developmental skills. Functional skills emphasize the "usefulness of learned responses" (Bricker, 1986, p. 302). The goals of a functional curriculum are to expand opportunities and to facilitate independence and adaptability (Bricker, 1986; LeBlanc et al., 1978).

Furthermore, the social development of young children is enhanced by successful participation in well-functioning groups established and maintained in preschool classrooms. Social problem-solving skills are taught, modeled, prompted, and reinforced in ongoing interactions through the efforts of peers and teachers.

Classroom Ecologies

From the viewpoint of professional-practice decisions, it is helpful to view each preschool classroom as a natural ecosystem. Any change for individual children may affect other children's and teachers' behaviors in planned and unplanned ways. Thus, preschool classrooms are interdependent systems (Carta, Sainato, & Greenwood, 1988). The list of potential variables is vast, and relatively few empirical studies are available to guide practice (Burstein, 1986; Carta et al., 1988; Rogers-Warren, 1982). A special issue of *Education and Treatment of Children* was dedicated to this topic (McEvoy, 1990).

While it is not possible to separate the physical from the social aspects of the environment, these two major classes of variables serve as the basis for ecobehavioral analysis. First, physical, relatively fixed, or programmatic classroom attributes may be assessed. Examples of potentially modifiable variables include availability and arrangement of play and work (or curricular) materials, and spatial arrangements of classrooms. Many alternative physical and social arrangements are likely to promote personal and social competence among group members if core design principles are applied. We return to discussions of relatively fixed qualities of classrooms throughout this and the next chapter. Several examples of classroom organization have been developed to help facilitate social interaction and skills acquisition (Bailey, 1989; Bailey & Wolery, 1992; Nordquist, Twardosz, & McEvoy, 1991).

Another broad class of variables that falls under the relatively "fixed" category is *routines*. Several facets of routines are significant for intervention design. Routines provide children with predictable learning situations where cues and models of appropriate verbalizations and behaviors are consistently available. A wide variety of social and preacademic skills may be taught through the use of routines and rules for conduct. With increases in skills development, children are able to perform and learn how to anticipate the necessary behaviors (Rogers-Warren, 1982), and thus are able to perform more independently. Furthermore, routines are important for caregivers—efficient routines are time and energy savers. Thus, the behavior of children who are unsuccessfully adapting during classroom routines may be considered as targets for assessment and intervention.

The sequence of routines also may be an important variable. Krantz and Risley (1977) found that scheduling a quiet period, such as story time, after an active period resulted in more disruptions than the reverse order. One reason for the importance of the waking day interview described in Chapter 2 is that the preschool consultant can identify significant planned activities and routines (or absence of helpful routines) throughout the day, from awakening to bedtime.

A second class of variables, such as teachers' and children's behavior, is interactive or *dynamic*. Teacher behaviors include arranging daily learning activities, assigning play groups, managing activities, pacing instruction, and interacting on countless occasions in both obvious (attention, praise, reprimand) and subtle ways (eye contact, affective tone). The power of contingent positive attention for teaching and improving behaviors and for classroom management is unquestioned. The form of teacher requests is an important research topic (Atwater & Morris, 1988; Strain et al., 1983). Thus, environments have significant educational, social, and interactive qualities that merit analysis.

Considering the great number of variables that may need to be examined, an ecobehavioral framework has potential value for guiding both classroom design and consultative services to preschool teachers. Two major features of ecobehavioral classroom analysis follow.

1. *Necessity for child–environment fit.* The most obvious point of consultation is whether a child can receive instruction within a particular classroom, or whether some factors need to be modified to enable the fit. Examples of potential points of analysis include methods of instruction and effectiveness of classroom management, group size and composition, teacher tolerance, and support services for teachers.

2. *Necessity for kindergarten survival skills.* One of the important lessons from special programming for older children is that education in specialized settings may actually reduce chances for success in integrated or inclusive settings. The discrepancies between special and general education learning environments may increase problem behavior and decrease skill generalization in transition settings (Vincent et al., 1980). Special settings, in contrast to general education classrooms, are characterized by relatively greater teacher effort in supervising and monitoring behavior of individual children with special needs and reducing the complexity of tasks for children. Thus, it may be important to teach directly the skills needed in

anticipated environments. Examples of relevant skills include independent work habits and appropriate responses in group instruction.

Many measures of various aspects of preschool ecologies have been developed. One of the best researched is the Ecobehavioral System for Complex Assessment of Preschool Environments (ESCAPE) (Carta et al., 1985, 1988). Harms, Clifford, and Cryer (1998) present a rating scale for early educational environments. Another environmental assessment scale is described by Dunst, McWilliam, and Holbert (1986; Project Sunrise, 1989). Earlier, template matching was presented as a strategy to assess both skills and environmental demands.

Curriculum-Based Intervention

One of the most important aspects of early intervention is inherent in the design and execution of a preschool curriculum. An ecologically based curriculum for young children includes the continuous assessment of skills in ways that are linked to teaching. Curriculum-based assessment also includes the assessment of the classroom ecology (Fuchs & Fuchs, 1986) to enable observations of children's performance in preacademic, social, and other developmental areas. The assessment should yield information to help delineate the conditions necessary for competent performance. There are currently many alternative preschool (or day care) curricula, and we highlight several to illustrate differences.

The Carolina Curriculum for Preschoolers with Special Needs (CCPSN; Johnson-Martin, Attermeier, & Hacker, 1990) is an extension of a curriculum for infants. The CCPSN divides developmental domains into teaching sequences that may be used within home, preschool, or day care settings. The domains include cognition, communication, social adaptation, and fine and gross motor skills. Curriculum sequences referred to as "areas" are embedded within the domains. For example, *Cognition* contains attention and memory, concepts, symbolic play, reasoning, and visual perception.

The CCPSN has many important features. Characteristics of the setting are considered: the physical setting (areas for pretend, "messy," quiet, constructive, manipulative, visual–motor, active play), the structure of the day, strategies to optimize appropriate behavior, and the importance of story time. The authors review a wide range of disabling conditions, with strategies to facilitate instruction. Also, they emphasize skill *sequences*, not individual items. Testing and teaching (both individual and group) activities are described for each skill.

Entry into the curriculum is based on an *assessment log* that serves as a criterion-referenced instrument. Item selection is based on clinical experience, research, and traditional developmental scales. The assessment log is completed through naturalistic classroom observations that occur over time (1 day to several weeks). Both emerging and mastered skills are recorded on a developmental progress chart.

Activity-based intervention (Bricker & Woods Cripe, 1992; Bricker, Pretti-Frontczak, & McComas, 1998) concentrates on ways to achieve child-related objectives in routines, planned activities, and child-initiated activities. Important characteristics of the model include the use of logically occurring antecedents and consequences, progress monitoring, and emphasis on functional and generative skills. (A generative skill requires that the child adapt responses to novel or changing situations.) Learning activities are specifically designed to interest children and promote multiple developmental goals within specific activities. Examples include planting seeds, acting out a song, or playing circus.

Curriculum development also may be related to specific content areas (language development, social skills, etc.). Bracken and Myers (1986) provide a program for teaching 250 basic concepts, including the following subdomains: color, comparisons, shapes, direction/position, social/emotional, size, texture and materials, quantity, time and sequence, letter, numbers and counting. McGinnis and Goldstein (1990) have downwardly extended a comprehensive intervention for teaching social skills to young children. Abraham, Morris, and Wald (1993) describe a model for inclusive early childhood education.

In summary, curriculum-based assessment provides information concerning a child's educational and developmental levels, characteristics of current learning environments, and the effects of instructional interventions. A well-developed curriculum (1) includes a wide range of functional, developmentally sequenced tasks; (2) enables ongoing measurement; and (3) facilitates the use of a variety of teaching and learning strategies. Curriculum-based assessment is fundamental to preschool service delivery and facilitates screening and assessment for intervention purposes. The overall curriculum should focus on preacademic, personal, and social outcomes. Specialized or focused curricula that may be useful for intensive interventions in such areas as language or social skills have been developed.

Improving Preacademic Skills

The elements of good instruction apply. These include the appropriateness of objectives and instructional techniques, frequent opportunities to practice skills, feedback related to performance, progress monitoring, and contingencies for improved performance (Lentz, Allen, & Ehrhardt, 1996).

Preattending

For many children, preattending skills are an important point of assessment and intervention. Preattending skills include looking at the materials and listening to instructions (Chapter 6).

Opportunities to Respond

Giving children frequent chances to practice is fundamentally related to skills acquisition. In many preschool classrooms, such opportunities may occur less often than expected. As reported in Carta et al. (1988), transitions and unoccupied time actually may be more prevalent than "engaged" learning time in preschool environments. Bricker and Woods Cripe (1992) discuss many ways to increase opportunities to respond in natural settings. An application of the concept of "opportunities to respond" is provided by Sainato, Strain, and Lyon (1987) in a study of choral responding in a preschool classroom for children with disabilities.

Language and Early Literacy Skills

Schwartz, Carta, and Grant (1996) discussed the relationship between ecologically based language interventions and children's gains in performance. Not surprisingly, children with greater gains in communication skills were in classrooms with greater evidence of language instruction and intervention. Powerful classroom strategies include using natural settings for language instruction, sharing the control of topics with children, being responsive to children's language use, using a variety of teaching materials and tasks, giving feedback, using a variety of natural positive consequences or reinforcers (other than praise), and making some materials accessible contingent on communication attempts.

Early literacy refers to prerequisite skills for reading and writing (Snow, Burns, & Griffin, 1998). Language is one of the significant early literacy skills. A subset of language skills is phonological awareness, which refers to recognition of the sounds in words (or phonological components), and skills in manipulating phonological units (Kaminski & Good, 1996). Examples include rhyming, segmenting words into phonemes (e.g., mat into /m/ /a/ /t/), and pronouncing words if the initial phoneme is removed (e.g., hill/ill). Accuracy and fluency in naming letters is another key skill related to future reading success that may need to build on phonological awareness. Preschool classroom design also has focused on facilitating early literacy through play (Katims & Pierce, 1995; Morrow & Rand, 1991).

Delayed prompting is a form of errorless learning based on stimulus control. The basic procedure involves transferring control from a prompt (or assistance) to the natural stimulus by using a systematic time delay. The intervention has been used with young children who have difficulty acquiring preacademic skills such as letters, numbers, colors, shapes (Bradley-Johnson, Sunderman, & Johnson, 1983), and sight words (Alig-Cybriwsky, Wolery, & Gast, 1990). In the study by Bradley-Johnson et al. (1983), clear benefits were shown over a fading procedure. Alig-Cybriwsky, Wolery, and Gast (1990) presented a procedure to use time delay in an instructional group. The description of the procedures is complicated, but salient features are included in Table 10.2. Schuster and Griffin (1990) describe the use of errorless learning with task analysis and chained (multi-step) tasks.

TABLE 10.2.   A Group Time-Delay Procedure

1. A small group of children (i.e., 4) were selected to participate. Children selected were able to "(a) sit and attend to the trainer and materials with three other children present for 15 minutes; (b) verbally imitate letter and word names; (c) match all words used in the study; (d) wait 3 seconds for a prompt [this was trained . . . if children did not wait]; (e) comply with verbal directions, 'Let's say the letters,'. . . ; and (f) select a reinforcer from a provided array" (p. 101).

2. Six unknown target sight words were identified for each child.

3. During the first session, two of six words were selected for each child, and six trials were provided for each word (i.e., 12 trials per child).

4. General attentional cues (i.e., "Look"), and specific attentional cues (i.e., "Let's say the letters") were given. Children's performance was assessed in probe sessions. As each word was presented in a flashcard format, the teacher cued the child saying, "[Child's name], what word?"

5. A "no delay" procedure was used for the first session of each instructional condition. Subsequent sessions used the 3-second delay as follows.

6. If the child did not respond within 3 seconds, the teacher modeled the correct response (e.g., "This word is red") and waited another 3 seconds for a response.

7. When the child correctly anticipated and waited for the model, the child was praised and received reinforcement first given on a continuous schedule but thinned to every third response.

8. If the child responded incorrectly within the first 3 seconds (prior to the model) the teacher said, "No. The word is ___; remember to wait if you don't know."

9. If the child responded incorrectly after the delay and model, the teacher said, "No, the word is ___."

10. If another child responded before the target child, the teacher said, "Only say the answer when it's your turn."

11. Review trials at the beginning of instructional sessions were included for previously learned words.

Note. Adapted from Alig-Cybriwsky, Wolery, and Gast (1990). Copyright 1990 by The Division for Early Childhood of the Council for Exceptional Children. Reprinted by permission.

Sociodramatic Play

Sociodramatic play is ubiquitous in preschool settings and in preschool curriculum discussions (Petrakos & Howe, 1996). Still, its power as an intervention may be overlooked. Rosen (1974) characterized sociodramatic play in the following way:

> Sociodramatic play . . . occurs when several children take on different roles and interact with each other in terms of a situation that they have spontaneously created (e.g., a doctor's office). . . . Sociodramatic play, being complex, activates the emotional, social, and intellectual resources of the child. (p. 920)

Evidence suggests that sociodramatic play can be taught, and that potential gains may include cognitive and social problem-solving skills (Rosen, 1974; Saltz, Dixon, & Johnson, 1977; Saltz & Johnson, 1974; Smilansky, 1968). There are important individual, social, cultural, and environmental aspects of play that, unfortunately, are beyond the scope of our review. Many interventions employ aspects of sociodramatic play, and they are discussed at various points in the chapter.

In the study reported by Saltz and Johnson (1974), children enacted folk tales such as the Billy Goats Gruff. Children listened to stories, were assigned roles, and with teacher prompts, narration, and at times, role taking, they dramatized the story. Successive sessions enabled children to play various roles. Children also discussed the story plots. The results showed an increase in spontaneous sociodramatic play and some preliminary evidence for cognitive growth.

CLASSROOM MANAGEMENT

Strategies for classroom management are necessary for providing learning activities and developing well-functioning groups. Here, we discuss several aspects of classroom management that have been of special significance in our consultations with preschool teachers.

Building Activity Centers

Activity centers are interesting for children and are linked to learning objectives in curriculum. Numerous sources describe in detail the development of activities to promote learning objectives (Bricker & Woods Cripe, 1992; Odom et al., 1988). Our purpose for mentioning the topic here is to emphasize the relationship between enriched classrooms that hold children's interest and classroom management. Peters (1995) found that appropriate social engagement improved in *all* activity centers as a result of introducing novel centers (e.g., *Head Start Pet Shop*, and *A Day at the Ocean*), developing rules and contingencies for play, and monitoring and prompting appropriate behaviors. In addition, teaching children theme- and play-related scripts may help children with play skills (Goldstein & Cisar, 1992). Stollar, Dye Collins, and Barnett (1994) built on activity centers to reduce disruptive activity changes.

Classroom Rules and Limits

Rules and situationally-based limits (Bredekamp & Copple, 1997) are used to communicate expectations for behavior in the classroom. "Only by actively teaching . . . rules . . . and how to follow them can teachers be fair in their classroom management efforts" (Paine et al., 1983, p. 55). Rules also are used as a basis for determining successes and criteria for positive attention when teachers "catch" children being "good." The use of effective rules is common to most studies evaluating classroom management procedures. Rule learning is one foundation for self-regulated behaviors.

Paine and colleagues (1983) suggested many strategies for classroom management with rule development serving as a keystone. Except as noted, the following principles for developing effective rules are abstracted from this source (pp. 55–58, 63).

1. *Developing rules.* Use as few rules as possible for classroom situations; use developmentally appropriate wording; use positive statements or guides (do's rather than don'ts); post the rules or limits prominently and in a way comprehensible to children, such as with pictures. Rules can include developmentally appropriate outcomes such as task completion (Fowler, 1986).

2. *Establishing rules and limits.* Plan rules prior to the first day of school; decide rules (and behavior) appropriate for each activity; teach rules and limits and their rationales immediately (for expectations, fairness, safety, and discipline); have children participate, if possible, in developing and discussing classroom limits.

3. *Implementing rules.* Use brief mini-teaching sessions to train rules before activities; give "rule-following practice"; use positive attention for rule-following behavior; encourage children to help each other in following rules.

4. *Maintaining rules.* Gradually reduce teacher prompts and feedback based on desired behavior for activities (Fowler, 1986). This may be accomplished in many systematic ways. For example, on Mondays, during the first several weeks of school, after vacations or holidays, or when nec-

essary, review rules and limits; periodically (several times a day), catch children following rules and use positive attention; continue to develop peer support for rule following. Essentially, rule behavior may be governed by the task and activity, and, ultimately, by peers with teacher supervision (e.g., Fowler, 1986). External cues are faded as children respond to more subtle cues, and behavior becomes increasingly self-regulated.

Excessive Activity Changes

Early studies by Jacobson, Bushell, and Risley (1969) illustrated several valuable components of preschool interventions. The studies also are noteworthy because they were conducted by parents who functioned as staff members in the Head Start classrooms. The research focused on "excessive switching" from task to task by the children—a frequent concern of preschool teachers.

The major feature of the intervention involved a *switching system*. The system included (1) the definition of activity areas (blocks, manipulative toys, creative area) and (2) a "switching task." At the beginning of the intervention, the children were free to enter any activity area of their choice. Each area was defined by boundaries (i.e., block area). To change activities, the child had to engage in a "switching task" whereby he or she would stop at a special table and complete a task (matching, preacademics). Upon completion of the task, the child received a "ticket" to enter another area and could stay as long as he or she wanted. The child's name was written on the ticket, and the time was noted to keep track of the activity changes. In order to move to another activity, the child again had to go to the special table, complete a switching task, and obtain a ticket. The results indicated a reduced rate of switching as expected (see micronorms, Chapters 3 and 5, for individual goal settings).

The use of switching tasks offers potential advantages. First, a switching task may help reduce unproductive movement during activity periods. Second, it may help introduce activities that may not be well attended by some children because of other interests (writing centers vs. playing with blocks). As Jacobson et al. (1969) suggested, a switching task may reduce teachers' attempts to get children to try learning activities. For some children, the rate of activity change may be an important target behavior, which may be modified through a switching task. One potential negative outcome is that by making the switching requirement too difficult, children may elect to remain in an activity area and use the time unproductively.

Given the high number of referrals for activity level, surprisingly few studies can be found that directly address activity changes. Stollar, Dye Collins, and Barnett (1994) described a multicomponent intervention that achieved reductions in disruptive activity changes through environmental changes, building on the idea of switching events. Key features of the intervention included (1) opening new high-interest activity centers; (2) clarifying and teaching classroom rules; (3) restricting access to the high-interest centers by setting reasonable time limits (Sulzer-Azaroff & Mayer, 1991); and (4) using a response–cost lottery (Witt & Elliott, 1982) whereby appropriate behavior in an activity center allowed for choices in the new centers during the next play period.

Studies by Rowbury, Baer, and Baer (1976) also examined access to more desirable activities through the completion of required preacademic activities. The emphasis of their study has several important facets. First, a "natural classroom reinforcement system" (p. 87) was established. Natural reinforcers included such activities as play and free time, supported by interesting materials. Second, the focus was on both learning and maintaining preacademic skills for children described as having severe and diverse problems. The children had been referred to a special preschool classroom because of comprehensive behavior problems including short attention span, hyperactivity, disruptive and aggressive behaviors, bizarre or eccentric mannerisms, and language and cognitive deficits. The researchers reported the use of token reinforcement to mediate access to the play area contingent upon completion of preacademic tasks. A second study analyzed the functions of teacher attention and guidance within the token system of management.

In the first study, the classroom was divided into two areas: a work area equipped with preacademic learning materials, and a play area with enjoyable activities. The work area contained 14 preacademic tasks taken from preschool curricular materials (seven tasks were used at any one time). Dividers were used to separate the areas, but passages enabled movement between areas. Tokens were available in the work area, and timers for each child were present in the play area to control for the length of play time. In the preacademic work area, tasks were arranged on tables or on the floor. The "work area" teachers announced to the children that it was time to work, and the children were led to the area if necessary. Children were then invited by the teacher to complete an activity, and they were free to select one out of seven tasks. Throughout the work time the teacher remained available to help children by demonstrating, assisting, instructing, or praising appropriate work. If a child met the criterion for a task, he or she received praise and a token, and the timer was set for 5 minutes. A snack was given to the child if requested. The child was allowed to select the play activity, which included at least one activity highly preferred by the child. The "play area" teacher provided materials and interacted with the children as they played. When the time was up, the teacher announced it was "token time" and the child returned to the work area, where the sequence was repeated. The entire sequence was in effect for 1 ½ hours per day. The experimenters also manipulated the number of completions required for reinforcement (one, two, or three).

The results of the first study indicated that the system was effective in creating and maintaining high levels of work completion, and that increasing the requirement for completions necessary for reinforcement brought corresponding increases in completion levels. When access to play was not contingent upon work completion, levels of work completion dropped.

The second study, reported in Rowbury et al. (1976), focused on the teacher's role within the token system, including teacher guidance for preacademic tasks. Teacher behaviors included prompts, guidance, explanation, and praise. The results indicated that teacher guidance appeared to be a vital component in the development of preacademic skills.

"Do I Have to Be Good All Day?"

Another problem frequently encountered in managing classroom behavior is the timing of reinforcement. This issue was examined by Fowler and Baer (1981), who wrote,

> Social and economic factors often limit the frequency and immediacy with which behaviors, once established, can be reinforced. Thus, the ability to tolerate inconsistent schedules of reinforcement and delays in reinforcement often becomes critical for maintenance of specific behavior changes, as well as for generally successful functioning in society. (p. 13)

While delayed reinforcement is not typically effective as a means of changing behavior, it may be helpful in *maintaining* behavior. As Fowler and Baer point out, the delay of reinforcement may also assist with efforts to promote generalization.

Seven children participated in the study reported by Fowler and Baer (1981). Two had behavior problems (noncompliance and tantrums); the others were considered to be typically developing children. Target behaviors were individually selected: sharing, cooperative play, positive comments about classroom activities, in-seat behavior, and conversation with peers. The teachers' use of prompts and praise also was recorded. The study was carried out in the preschool classroom, and training sessions were conducted in an adjacent room. Two procedures were compared: (1) an early feedback and reinforcement condition, which occurred directly after the period during which the behavior occurred; and (2) a late-feedback and reinforcement condition (with intervening class periods).

First, a brief training session (2–5 minutes) was held to rehearse the target behavior and to remind "the child to perform the behaviors the criterion number of times in the classroom" (p. 17). A second session (held either early or late) was used to provide feedback about behaviors and to give reinforcement. Stickers or points were used to obtain an immediately available small toy, or they were saved and later exchanged for a larger prize.

The late-reinforcement condition helped promote generalization "for children whose behavior did not generalize spontaneously" (p. 20). The authors of the study suggest that monitoring one activity period and providing reinforcement at the end of the day may help maintain behaviors and increase generalized results. They explain the results through the use of *indiscriminable contingencies*, whereby children are unaware of "the time or setting" during which the appropriate behavior is reinforced (p. 20; see generalization principles in Chapter 5). For example, two children asked, "Do I need to share all day?" Once generalization is established, the timing may be less critical.

Fowler and Baer (1981) concluded that "reinforcement delays should be considered routinely for teaching programs, both for maintaining appropriate social behavior . . . and for maintaining academic performance" (p. 23). The procedure may have practical benefits for teachers.

Recruiting "Natural Communities of Reinforcement"

Children in some settings may not receive sufficient positive attention for their learning successes. Also, the generalization of skills is a major concern for behavior-change programs. Furthermore, one of the primary objectives for typically developing young children, children with disabilities, or those at risk, is teaching independent work behaviors. Skill in recruiting positive attention from teachers may be critical for success in later inclusionary settings for children with disabilities. In two interrelated studies reported by Stokes et al. (1978), children were taught to evaluate their work and appropriately gain the teacher's attention for praise. Thus, the studies illustrate possibilities of training children to adapt to classrooms.

Participants in the first study were 4 typically developing children. The 4 children in the second study were described as having comprehensive academic and behavior problems. The studies were conducted in the regular preschool classroom and during a remedial summer class.

The studies focused on the effects of teaching the children independent work skills and methods for prompting teacher comments regarding their work. In a training condition, children were taught the dimensions of good work, such as working consistently and quietly. The children also were taught to prompt or cue for evaluative comments from teachers following self-evaluation. The children's skill in *cueing* was the major dependent variable. Cues were defined as the child's statements "inviting favorable comments or positive evaluations of . . . work or general behavior, e.g., 'Look how much I've done'" (p. 287). The children's work involved tracing lines and letters. The cues were taught through "instructions, role-playing, feedback, and praise" (p. 288). The following behaviors were taught: "Do good work, then evaluate the quality of that work, and, when the quality of the work was good, cue the trainer to evaluate that work" (p. 288). Children were reinforced by the trainer for following the instructions in their regular classrooms.

In summary, the results of the study successfully demonstrated the influence of the children's behaviors on adult behaviors for both typically developing children and those with problem behaviors. Stokes et al. (1978) discussed the importance of the results in terms of children becoming active change agents in their own environments. They suggest that such intervention may be "important to young children who find themselves bereft of attention in classrooms, perhaps because they are labelled deviant, or perhaps because they do not represent a problem to their teachers" (p. 287). The social realities were addressed: Children were taught to "ask . . . a few times about the quality of their work, but do not ask too often" (p. 289). Appropriately low rates of behaviors for cueing teachers are desirable. A rate of two to four cues per 10-minute session was the authors' goal based on the opinions of preschool teachers. To effectively deal with the potential problem of children using the same repetitive cues, the use of diverse cues and prompts was stressed ("Try to say something different each time" [p. 292]). Skills related to judging the proximity of teachers also were necessary.

Transitions between Activities

Transitions may be difficult for both children and teachers. We review general principles adapted from the Juniper Gardens Children's Project (Carta, n.d., pp. 6–19) based on research by Sainato, Strain, Lefebvre, and Rapp (1987), and offer several interventions for improving planned activity changes.

1. *Develop, teach, and practice transition rules.* Building on our earlier discussion of rules, some rules may apply to the entire day, whereas others may be developed for transitions (i.e., "Walk in the classroom," "Help your neighbor"). Consider picture prompts for teaching and displaying rules.
2. *Plan contingencies for rules.* Contingencies may include positive attention for rule following, corrective feedback, and an opportunity to

correct behavior. Consider prompts to help reduce the need for corrective feedback.

3. *Set teaching goals to increase children's independence.* Effective transitions will decrease (a) unproductive transition times, (b) close monitoring of children's behavior, and (c) prompting of behavior.

4. *Assess children's behavior during transitions.* Likely individual behaviors of concern to teachers include wandering, disrupting, or needing repetitions of requests for compliant behaviors.

5. *Define appropriate behaviors for transitions.* Examples of expectancies for behaviors that need to be defined and taught to children may include moving to activities, getting materials, cleaning activity centers, or asking for help.

6. *Consider different interventions to improve transitions.* Interventions include clear instructions (short, concise, positively stated, with sufficient wait time), "beat the buzzer" to reduce time in transitions, peer helpers, or ending transitions with brief activity reinforcers.

7. *Consider rearranging the environment.* Ideas include eliminating physical obstacles and providing materials to increase independence.

8. *Teach, monitor and maintain transition behaviors.* Prioritize transitions targeted for intervention by the amount of teacher time and energy spent during that particular time period. Have children practice. As children become more skilled, fade prompts and instructions to make transitions more challenging and natural.

9. *Add fun and creative instructional tasks.* Examples include varying silent versus whispering transitions, or giving transition instructions in different ways.

Carden Smith and Fowler (1984) compared teacher-monitored and peer-monitored token systems for reducing disruptive behavior during transitions. The setting was a special class designed for children with behavior problems. Three kindergartners who were the most disruptive during transition periods served as targets, and children were assigned to different teams each day.

In the teacher-monitoring phase, the teacher first explained the token system, role-played appropriate transition behavior, and questioned children about their understanding of the procedures (three sessions). Points were given for each appropriate transition behavior, and each team was directed to perform one of three transition activities: (1) cleanup (children received 1 point for helping to clean up the assigned space without disruption); (2) bathroom (children received 1 point for walking to the restroom, using it within a few minutes, and returning to class); and (3) waiting (children received 1 point for selecting a book, sitting on a mat without disturbing others, and returning the book on teacher request). Children who received the maximum number of points voted for a backup reinforcer (i.e., kite flying). Children obtaining 2 out of 3 points were allowed to participate in the backup reinforcer, and those children who obtained one or no points received a mild negative consequence. Note that some earlier interventions included positive as well as negative consequences as components. We report many of these studies because of their overall effectiveness, but also point out that the impact of aversive elements may be mitigated by many positive procedures discussed earlier.

For the peer-monitoring phase, the point system and backup reinforcers were maintained. Children were divided into teams, and team captains were selected, who awarded points and monitored performance, reminded peers of appropriate behavior, and participated in activities. Captains were regularly selected from those children who had obtained the maximum number of points the day before and a lottery was used if there were many children in this category. Team captains were reminded of their roles and awarded points to themselves and others following the performance of an activity. The peer monitor was assisted in awarding points by the teacher asking if team members had met transition responsibilities.

Results indicated that both teacher monitoring and peer monitoring were effective in reducing disruptions during transition periods. However, peer-monitoring procedures were superior. In addition, the level of participation by the target children during transition activities increased during both monitoring phases.

In a follow-up study involving 9 children attending a remedial kindergarten classroom, the initial teacher-monitoring procedure was eliminated. The children identified as monitors were trained in the token system, role-played the procedures, and practiced awarding points and providing corrective feedback. The results demonstrated that peer monitoring was effective in reducing disruptive behavior during transitions as well as increasing target childrens' participation in the activities.

The progressive use of teacher-monitoring strategies followed by peer monitoring and self monitoring for the management of transitions was investigated by Fowler (1986). This study replicated the peer-monitoring intervention by Carden Smith and Fowler (1984), and extended the analysis to the use of self-monitoring. Major features of the study are described here.

The transition periods included cleaning up learning centers, using the restroom, and waiting for a large-group activity on mats. While on the mats, children were allowed to look at books and eat snacks. Children targeted for the study, described as having behavior and learning problems, were assigned to teams. The behaviors of interest for 3 target children included participation or engagement in the transition activities, inappropriate behavior, and teacher and team-captain prompts for rule following. The behavior of the other class members also was monitored. Points were awarded for cleanup, restroom, book-time, and snack responsibilities.

Peer monitoring was introduced after three training sessions (each about 10 minutes), which were described as follows: "The teacher met with small groups of three or four children, reviewed the class rules with the children, role-played the duties of the team captain and teammates, and practiced point awards" (Fowler, 1986, p. 576). Photographs of children depicting completion of the routines for the activities were used for review and as reminders about expected behavior. In addition, the children received an oral quiz on appropriate transition behaviors. Classroom rules were reviewed daily throughout the condition in brief meetings just before the transition.

Children were assigned to groups, and team captains were appointed. Team captains had the tasks of helping teammates participate in transition activities, and prompting and praising participation. The pictures were posted as reminders for children. "Report cards" with pictures of activities and of each teammate were used for feedback purposes. Team captains also monitored their own behavior, thus building in self-monitoring practice.

> The teammates reported the activities in which they had participated appropriately to the team captain. If the team captain agreed with the report, he or she handed the report card to the teammate who made checkmarks next to the appropriate activities in the column under the teammate's picture. If the captain disagreed with a teammate's report, the captain was instructed to not hand over the report card and to say why he or she disagreed. In these cases, the team captain completed the report card. (Carden Smith & Fowler, 1984, p. 577)

The teacher supervised the discussions and point awards, and intervened if she disagreed with the point awards. The points were used in the following way. Children with 4 points could vote for and participate in an outdoor activity. They also were eligible to be the next day's team captain. Children with 3 points could participate but could not vote on the activity. Children with 2 points missed 5 minutes of the activity. Children with 1 or zero points remained indoors with other mild consequences (the reward system was structured so that this contingency was rarely needed).

In the *self-monitoring* condition, team captains passed out report cards and teammates checked activities with regard to appropriate participation. Team captains and the teacher did not change the points.

The results of the study demonstrated increased rates of participation for the 3 target children as well as reductions in inappropriate behavior across both the peer- and self-monitored conditions. However, the peer-monitoring condition may have been slightly more powerful. While the appropriateness of behavior tended to be overestimated through self-monitoring, the team captain or teacher corrected these inaccuracies in the peer-monitoring condition. In the self-monitoring condition, where corrections were not provided, errors ranged from 10% to 25%.

A peer-mediated strategy and an antecedent–prompt procedure for facilitating transition periods were compared by Sainato, Strain, Lefebvre, et al. (1987). The peer-mediated strategy involved assigning typically developing children to peers with disabilities as "buddies" during the transition period. The antecedent–prompt procedure consisted of instructing children with disabilities to ring a bell when the transition period was completed.

Six typically developing children and 3 children diagnosed with autism participated in the study. The setting was an integrated preschool classroom housed in an elementary school. Transition periods included (1) group circle to lesson, (2) snack to bathroom, and (3) group circle to a language activity. The rate at which children transitioned from one activity to the next was recorded, along with other child and teacher behaviors.

During an initial baseline phase, the teachers conducted transitions in the usual way. Stimulus cards representing three different conditions were present but were not explained to the children. Card 1, with a large stoplight showing a green light, represented a nontreatment setting; Card 2 represented the bell condition and had a large bell drawn on it; Card 3 represented the buddy condition, with a large "smile face" drawn on it. During a second baseline, teachers refrained from helping children through transitions (except for those children who were still "wandering" after 4 minutes).

During the peer-mediated strategy (a "buddy" system), the teacher showed Card 3 and told the children they would help their friends get to the next activity. The teacher then modeled taking a peer's hand and leading the child through the transition with prompts. For the second transition condition, children were shown Card 2. Each target child (with a disability) was given a specific direction to go to another area and ring the bell. The peers were instructed to "let their friends go by themselves" (p. 288). During the no-treatment transitions, the teacher showed Card 1 and then instructed each child to go to a designated area. The final phase involved the use of the bell across all transition periods.

Although the results indicated that the peer-mediated strategy was effective in reducing off-task behavior during transition periods, the bell procedure (Card 2) was superior in increasing the transition rate. In addition, verbal and physical prompts by the teacher were significantly reduced. The results suggest that the bell may have been reinforcing to the children, while the peer-mediated strategy provided no direct reinforcement, but relied on prompts. However, extensive use of a bell may be irritating to teachers (D. M. Sainato, personal communication, June 27, 1991).

A simple and effective intervention designed to improve cleanup routines was described by Wurtele and Drabman (1984). During baseline, kindergarten children took an average of 11.6 minutes for morning cleanup tasks. The children tended to ignore teacher prompts and encouragement during this time period. The intervention consisted of the following announcement:

> Boys and girls, today we are going to play a game. I am going to set this timer to ring in __ minutes, and I want to see if you can get the room cleaned up before the buzzer rings. All the areas must be cleaned and you must be sitting in the circle when the buzzer goes off. Get ready to beat the buzzer (set timer) . . . Go! (p. 405)

For the first 4 days of the study, the timer was set for 8, 6, 5, and 4 minutes; after that, the timer was always set for 4 minutes. No specific consequences were given for beating or not beating the timer. The average time for cleanup during the intervention was 4.3 minutes. Teacher acceptance was reported to be quite favorable.

Staff arrangements also may have important differential outcomes for transitions. In an often-cited study, LeLaurin and Risley (1972) found that assigning teachers to "zones" or activity areas was more efficient than assigning teachers to small groups of children. The study focused on transitions from lunch to naptime that included stops at the bathroom and a "shoe area."

INCLUDING CHILDREN WITH DISABILITIES

Mainstreaming, Integration, and Inclusion

Bricker (1995) describes the progressive use of the terms "mainstreaming," "integration," and "inclusion" as young children with disabilities spend increasing amounts of time in educational and community settings with typically developing peers. *Mainstreaming* refers to the reentry of children with mild disabilities into regular education settings and is viewed as less applicable to children with early identified disabilities (Bricker, 1995). *Integration* refers to the combining of children with disabilities and typically developing peers into classroom and community settings but does not necessarily imply that children attend neighborhood schools (McLean & Hanline, 1990; Snell, Lowman, & Canady, 1996).

Major professional associations have endorsed position statements advocating *inclusion* of children with special needs (Division for Early Childhood of the Council for Exceptional Children/National Association For the Education of Young Children, 1994; National Association of School Psychologists [NASP], 1993). Central to the concept of inclusion is the right of all children, regardless of type or severity of disabilities, to participate actively in natural settings within their neighborhoods and communities, and to engage in the same or similar activities and experiences as typically developing peers (Division for Early Childhood of the Council for Exceptional Children, 1994; McCormick, Noonan, & Heck, 1998; Snell et al., 1996; Wolery, Werts, Caldwell, Snyder, & Lisowski, 1995). The NASP (1993) position statement on inclusion identified inclusive programming for students with disabilities as incorporating individually appropriate instruction and related services within the context of the age-appropriate classroom of the neighborhood school.

Rationale for Integration and Inclusion

The practices of integration and inclusion are based on the belief that children with disabilities benefit from the proximity and interaction with typically developing peers (Fleming, Wolery, Weinzierl, Venn & Schroeder, 1991; Jenkins, Odom, & Speltz, 1989; McLean & Hanline, 1990). Legal foundations for these practices are found in the Individuals with Disabilities Education Act, PL 99-457, and the Americans with Disabilities Act (Bricker, 1995; Bruder, 1993; Eiserman, Shisler, & Healey, 1995; Gemmel-Crosby & Hanzlik, 1994). Havey (1998) reviews Federal law and court decisions that link inclusion to the legal mandates for "appropriate education" in the "least restrictive environment."

Parent Responses to Integration and Inclusion

The most important advantage of participation in inclusive settings was identified as opportunities to interact with typical children (Miller, Strain, Boyd, Hunsicker, McKinley, & Wu, 1992). However, parents of children with special needs may have concerns over inclusive educational settings (McLean & Hanline, 1990). One concern is the ability of inclusive programs to deliver specialized instruction or appropriate intensity of services (Rose & Smith, 1993). Parents also may fear for their child's safety in settings where teachers are inadequately trained and poorly paid (Bricker, 1995). Bennett, Lee, and Lueke (1998) interviewed parents of children with special needs regarding their decision to place their child in an inclusive setting. Parents sometimes opted for dual enrollment in inclusive and specialized settings in order to access social interaction with typical peers while continuing to receive intense and specialized services to maintain developmental progress. They found that several decision-making factors impacted parents' decisions to place their child within inclusive programs: (1) nature of their child's disability; (2) age of the child; (3) parental experience in the school system; (4) professional expectations; (5) desired level of parent's involvement in their child's education; and (6) the physical layout of the educational setting.

The Effects of Integration and Inclusion on Young Children with Disabilities

The most consistent positive outcomes for children with disabilities included in regular education settings are improvements in social and play skills, and increased time spent in positive interactions with typical peers (Brinker, 1985; Buysse & Bailey, 1993; Haymes, Fowler, & Cooper, 1994; McLean & Hanline, 1990). Jenkins et al. (1989) observed preschool children with disabilities in integrated and nonintegrated classrooms and found that children with disabilities receiving education with typical peers demonstrated improved levels of interactive play.

There is also evidence that inclusion can improve behavior and impact developmental gains. Bruder (1993) found that significant developmental and language gains for 30 children with disabilities were associated with children's participation in integrated settings. Jones and Carlier (1995) used team teaching and cooperative learning in an inclusive setting to impact social competence and to decrease behavioral concerns such as aggression and noncompliance.

These positive results extend to children with more serious disabilities as well. McGee, Paradis, and Feldman (1993) observed 29 children with autism integrated into a university-affiliated preschool setting, and found that levels of autistic behaviors decreased with close proximity of typical peers. McGee et al. (1992) found that levels of inappropriate behavior of 3 boys with autism declined in the presence of typical children. Hanline (1993) observed decreased social isolation and increased participation of 3 children with profound disabilities fully included in a preschool summer program. The authors attributed the program's success to (1) the curriculum emphasis on learning through play, (2) the presence of very responsive peers, and (3) the preparation of typical children in ways to understand and respond to the idiosyncratic behaviors of peers with profound disabilities. Lee and Odom (1996) observed 2 children with severe disabilities enrolled in an inclusive setting and found a relationship between increased interactions with typical peers, increased social engagement, increased motoric involvement in play, and decreased rates of stereotypical behaviors.

Reviews of integration- and inclusion-related research agree that regular education placement alone is generally insufficient to improve skills of children with disabilities (Buysse & Bailey, 1993; File & Kontos, 1993; Fleming et al., 1991; Hundert & Hopkins, 1992; Jenkins et al., 1989; McLean & Hanline, 1990). Novak, Olley, and Kearney (1980) observed children with disabilities in integrated and segregated settings, and found that, in both settings, children with disabilities played less with peers, spent less time in close proximity to other children, and initiated and received fewer social interactions than typical peers matched for gender, age, and socioeconomic level. Fewell and Oelwein (1990) compared children in three levels of integrated settings (zero minutes, 1 to 300 minutes, and over 301 minutes per week in an integrated setting) and found that the classroom curriculum and the quality of instruction was more directly linked with positive developmental outcome and skills acquisition than proximity to typical peers, concluding that only strong, high-quality educational settings should be chosen as integration options. Wolery (1994) suggests a continuum of classroomwide and individual interventions, ranging from child-directed to teacher-directed activities that can support inclusion of children with disabilities into regular education settings. Buysse and Bailey (1993) reviewed 22 studies of the behavioral and developmental outcomes of young children in integrated and segregated settings, and identified the following variables related to program quality: (1) ratio of children to staff, (2) ratio of children with disabilities to typically developing children, (3) types of disabilities included within the classroom, (4) severity of disabilities included, (5) chronological age of typically developing children, (6) match between the developmental levels of the typically developing children and the children with disabilities, (7) preparation of the typically developing children for inclusion of children with disabilities, (8) developmental model of program, (9) physical arrangement of the classroom and toy selection, (10) level of teacher preparedness and training, (11) quality of classroom interventions, (12) interpersonal skills of teachers and staff, and (13) presence of resource specialists.

Bruder (1993) described a statewide inclusion demonstration project utilizing community early childhood programs as placements for 30 children with disabilities, highlighting factors facilitating program success. These included (1) an inclusive program philosophy, (2) a consistent and ongoing system for family involvement, (3) multidisciplinary team involvement using a transdisciplinary model, (4) collaboration with community agencies; (5) presence of a well-constructed Individualized Education Program or Individualized Family Services Plan, (6) related service delivery integrated within educational settings, (7) ongoing inservice training for staff, and (8) a system for evaluating the efficacy of service delivery.

The Effects of Integration on Children without Disabilities

Integration and inclusion should meet the educational and social needs of all children. A question that comes to mind for many parents and educators is the potential effects of integration for children without disabilities. As mentioned earlier, many program variables are likely to affect the outcomes for children who participate in integrated or inclusive programs, making it difficult to generalize across early intervention programs.

Wolery et al. (1993) surveyed university faculty and early childhood classroom teachers regarding the benefits of inclusion of children with disabilities into regular education settings. Respondents cited increased acceptance of individual differences by children with and without disabilities in addition to aforementioned benefits. Buysse, Wesley, Keyes, and Bailey (1996) used structured interviews and rating scales with educational professionals in inclusive settings. These individuals concurred that inclusive settings gave typical children an opportunity to learn about individual differences.

McLean and Hanline (1990) reviewed 10 years of research findings and found no reported negative effects for typically developing children. Esposito (1987) found that eight of nine studies reviewed did not find any deleterious effects of integration, while one study suggested that nonintegrated settings may be more positively related to social development for typically developing peers. Odom, Hoyson, Jamieson, and Strain (1985) reported beneficial outcomes for typical peers participating in an integrated special education program.

Interventions to Increase Social Interactions in Inclusive Settings

As mentioned earlier, across research studies, improvement in social interactions and play skills has been the consistently positive outcome for children with disabilities educated with typically developing peers. An impressive number of research studies have addressed successful methods for facilitating social interaction between typically developing peers and children with disabilities in integrated or inclusive settings.

We have discussed social behaviors in several places. Earlier, we introduced the roles of various change agents and basic social behavior intervention methods (Chapter 7). Here we discuss a range of interventions and outcomes for social behaviors as keystones for inclusion. Our discussion continues in the next chapter when we look further at research on play and change efforts related to social behaviors. Several studies have examined the role of teacher prompting, praise, peer initiations, and structured play activities in increasing social, communicative, and play behaviors (Cole, Meyer, Vandercook, & McQuarter, 1986; Hundert & Hopkins, 1992; Lowenthal, 1996; Odom & Strain, 1986; Stafford & Green, 1996). Strain and Odom (1986) found that an intervention package consisting of teacher prompting and verbal reinforcement of peer play initiations, along with teacher-arranged play activities incorporating specific child roles, increased positive social responses and occasional positive initiations from children with disabilities and increased the length of social exchanges between typically developing children and children with disabilities. Jenkins et al. (1989) used teacher proximity, teacher prompting of peers, modeling, and structured play activities with typical children to increase social initiations by children with disabilities and to increase the length of their social exchanges. Shearer, Kohler, Buchan, and McCullough (1996) used prompts, monitoring, and reinforcement to increase social engagement of 3 preschool children with autism. Intervention was equally effective when delivered by teachers or by peers.

The structure of teacher-planned classroom activities also impacted social interaction and engagement. Burstein (1986) found that large-group structured activities decreased social interactions for all children, and informal settings led to inappropriate or isolated behavior on the part of children with disabilities. Small-group activities, on the other hand, were more likely to facilitate peer interactions (McCormick et al., 1998).

Hundert and Houghton (1992) examined the effectiveness of a classwide social skills program in promoting social interactions of children with disabilities in integrated preschools. During training, children with disabilities were (1) given instruction in specific social skills, (2) prompted to exhibit these skills during training play sessions, and (3) praised and reinforced for using them successfully. During training, children with disabilities increased their rates of positive social interactions to levels of typical children, but these rates did not generalize to nontraining play sessions, highlighting the need for ongoing teacher support. Kohler and Strain (1993) taught a range of specific interaction skills (e.g., offering play suggestions) to children in inclusive settings. They found increased positive social interactions for children with diverse disabilities.

Several studies found that initial teacher instruction and intervention was helpful, while later teacher proximity and intervention was intrusive, interrupting social interactions between children with and without disabilities (Cole et al., 1986; File, 1994; McGee et al., 1992). Focusing teacher attention on groups that include children with disabilities was more successful in increasing peer interaction than individual-teacher focus on the child with a disability (Hundert, Mahoney, & Hopkins, 1993).

In a very different direction, affection activities have been used as easy and natural interventions to promote social interaction between children with and without disabilities in inclusive settings. McEvoy, Twardosz, and Bishop (1990) describe affection activities as typical preschool games and songs modified to include affectionate responses during large- and small-group activities. The teacher incorporates individual or group greetings, patting backs or shoulders, or hugging into preschool songs or fingerplays. The teacher then reinforces expressions of affection or friendship during affection activities and free play. In a similar vein, Bergan (1993) encourages classroom teachers to rethink their roles in facilitating close friendships. She advocates (1) establishing a classroom climate that encourages peer interaction between diverse children; (2) pairing competent children with children with disabilities in play partnerships within classroom activities; (3) staying alert to potential friendships between children with and without disabilities, and mentioning common interests to parents for possible interactions outside the classroom; and (4) implementing formal social skills training.

Peer-initiation strategies have been found to be highly effective in developing and sustaining interactions with children with disabilities. Strain and Kohler (1995) taught peers strategies for sharing, organizing play, assisting peers with disabilities, and reinforcing their play initiations. These authors found that peer persistence in responding to and initiating social interaction was effective in increasing social interaction with 3 preschool children with autism.

Goldstein (1993) found that an intervention package incorporating peer-initiation strategies and sociodramatic play scripts instructing children in role-related behaviors was a cost-effective and powerful way to expand communicative interactions between children with and without disabilities. McGee et al. (1992) instructed 3 typically developing children in peer-incidental teaching to increase reciprocal social interactions among 3 boys with autism and classroom children without disabilities. Increased social interactions were maintained after fading of the peer-incidental teaching intervention, possibly because children had learned effective techniques to elicit and sustain responses from their peers with disabilities.

Environmental arrangement and classroom materials were also important in facilitating social interactions. Strain and Odom (1986) used dolls, house materials, blocks, wagons, and dramatic play activities to facilitate social interactions. Lowenthal (1996) found that use of smaller activity areas, increasing proximity with peers, was effective in lengthening social interactions of children with disabilities during dramatic play. Russell-Fox (1997) stressed the importance of tailoring activities and materials to the specific disability of the child to be included, and designing cooperative play situations to facilitate inclusion.

Need for Ongoing Teacher Support and Training

In order to facilitate successful inclusion of children with disabilities into early childhood settings, researchers and practitioners agree that teachers need ongoing support that is responsive to their individual needs and ongoing staff development and training (Buysse et al., 1996; Fleming et al., 1991; Gemmell-Crosby & Hanzlik, 1994; McLean & Hanline, 1990; Wolery et al., 1993, 1995). Rose and Smith (1993) surveyed administrators and parents, and found that lack of teacher training, resources, and support may be major barriers to inclusion. Bruder (1998) advocates a training for inclusion model that incorporates adult learning techniques, is easily accessible to early childhood professionals, advocates recommended practices, and is focused around building collaborative relationships.

Eiserman et al. (1995) surveyed preschool providers' attitudes toward readiness for preschool inclusion. They found generally positive attitudes, depending on the type of disability of the child to be included. Preschool providers identified needs for materials, equipment, resources, access to consultation with a specialist, in-service training, and in-classroom aides to successfully facilitate inclusion.

TRANSITIONS BETWEEN SETTINGS

Planning for transitions between settings requires consideration of many factors (Rous, Hemmeter, & Schuster, 1994). Strategies that have been introduced earlier include planning for "entry into natural communities of reinforcement" (Baer & Wolf, 1970) and template matching. Meetings between sending and receiving schools or agencies are helpful in order to clarify expectations and skills that tend to enhance or impede transitions. Brown, Horn, Heiser, and Odom (1996) describe the use of transition follow-up activities (telephone conversations, home and school visits). In this section, we give major emphasis to organizational strategies and to the parental role.

Organizational Strategies

One major organizational strategy to help with transitions is to identify functional skills that are related to adequate performance in the receiving setting. One of the greatest problems is deciding the likelihood of successful transitions to kindergarten. While a broad array of factors typically are considered, such as global developmental level or IQ, a functional and ecobehavioral approach may prove to be more effective in making predictions and planning transitions.

Teacher ratings of "transition" behaviors may be very useful. These include the degree that a child (1) stays on task without undue teacher attention; (2) sits appropriately; (3) focuses attention on the speaker and shifts focus appropriately; (4) follows directions in large groups; (5) responds appropriately in groups; (6) participates appropriately by waiting for a turn, or waiting to be recognized; (7) works and plays without bothering peers; (8) waits appropriately; and (9) modifies behavior upon receiving a verbal directive (Sainato & Lyon, 1989; Strain, 1988). Other likely transition behaviors include the ability to complete directions with two or three steps, to stay task-engaged while the teacher is absent, and to follow routines at the end of work periods (Sainato & Lyon, 1989).

An obvious advantage of an ecobehavioral and functional approach is that attention is focused on factors that will enable children to benefit from instruction without requiring excessive teacher monitoring and effort. Alternatively, potential problems are that individual instructional needs are not necessarily addressed solely through improving group adaptation. A promising technique to assess skills related to kindergarten success has been developed by Atwater, Carta, and Schwartz (1989).

Sainato, Strain, Lefebvre, and Rapp (1990) developed a self-evaluation treatment package to help integrate preschoolers with disabilities into regular kindergartens based on self-assessments of appropriate academic behavior. An important feature of the intervention was an "independent seatwork rating scale" comprising nine behaviors (such as "listening to the teacher's directions"). The rating scale was used to assess the match between teacher's ratings and children's self-ratings. Children were photographed modeling appropriate behaviors and "happy faces" (or "yes" for appropriate work behavior), and "sad faces" (or "no" for inappropriate work behavior), were placed next to the photographs. At the end of "table time," children were instructed to rate session behaviors. They then met with the teacher to compare ratings. Praise was given for appropriate behavior and accurate assessment. A reinforcement component also was included, where children were able to select small toys for accurate self-assessments (seven out of nine behaviors). Later intervention phases enabled comparisons with components of the package removed. The final phase included only children's self-assessments.

We summarize some of their results. Agreement in the initial phase between teacher and child ratings ranged from 60% to 95%. In later phases, the ranges were from 91% to 100%. The treatment package overall had positive effects on children's behavior and also reduced the need for excessive prompting of appropriate behavior. The results were maintained over systematic reductions in the complexity of the treatment package.

While emphasizing the importance of preparing the new environment and involving parents, Daniel (1995) stresses the importance of a new beginning, suggesting that sharing a child's difficult behavioral history with the receiving teacher may result in stereotyping and decreased expectations. The pros and cons of sharing intervention scripts across settings needs to be weighed carefully by parents.

Parental Strategies

Parents can help with transitions in a number of ways. First, they assist others with understanding their child's educational and developmental needs. Second, they can become aware of program alternatives and strategies to help make choices. It is important that the parents visit alternative sites to make informed decisions.

Preschool programs are often the first setting where complex educational service-delivery strategies are presented to parents. Some parents will have many years ahead of them in making difficult decisions and in unraveling the complexities of service delivery. They can be given assistance in learning to identify and resolve problems as a part of the transition process. Once the child is enrolled in a new school program, for many children and parents, new issues are likely to arise. Identifying effective problem-solving strategies for parents to deal with program modifications and changes may be a significant part of the process. Special attention also should be given to their understanding of legal rights.

For example, parents can be provided with questioning strategies, with the goal of obtaining information while minimizing defensiveness. They can ask for the teacher's perceptions of problems and focus on behaviors and problems to be solved, while not seeking sources to "blame," and can demonstrate concern and willingness to share responsibility. Parents may find ways to facilitate home–school communications.

SUMMARY AND CONCLUSIONS

The range of early education philosophies and practices is enormous. In this chapter, we focused on organizational and systems issues, and possible roles of teachers and peers in intervention design. Major emphasis is given to the class as an ecosystem. The first step in many referral situations is to consult with teachers concerning the overall functioning of the group throughout the day.

With regard to learning and behavior problems, an important point of teacher consultation is the child's progress through a coherent and functional curriculum that includes a wide range of personal, social, and preacademic objectives, and corresponding teaching and classroom-management strategies. Inclusion of children with special needs was discussed as a part of an overall early intervention philosophy and practice that includes preparation for the next environment.

CHAPTER 11

◆◆◆

Classroom Social and Safety-Related Interventions

◆

Regardless of theoretical differences, well-functioning classrooms hold the potential for a broad range of learning opportunities. However, children referred for behavioral or learning difficulties may require specific plans founded on the intervention design components discussed in earlier chapters, and creative and practical intervention strategies based on an analysis of settings and behavior, problem solving, and research.

SOCIAL SKILLS AND PLAY

One of the most important developmental accomplishments is successful play with peers, and the literature is voluminous (Goldstein, 1994; Saracho & Spodek, 1998). Social competence is a foundation of integration and early intervention efforts. Successful peer play is dependent on a range of social skills that frequently is the target of intervention efforts. Building on earlier discussions (Chapters 7 and 10), we review additional social behavior research for a wide range of referral questions. We describe examples of studies from the research explosion in social behavior that have investigated entry into play groups and the maintenance of play behaviors. Age, gender, cultural differences, factors associated with poverty, and severity and type of disabling conditions all have been shown to have differential effects on play behaviors.

Greenwood, Walker, Todd, and Hops (1981) analyzed social interactions of preschool children in free play to provide descriptions and norms for play behaviors extending classic work by Parten (1932). The behaviors measured included the frequency of interactions, initiations (the social responses beginning an interaction), continuing responses (interactive behavior exchanges following the original initiation and the response), and termination (cessation of communication for longer than 5 seconds).

The results are briefly summarized. Significant differences existed across classrooms (the means for interaction rates varied from 0.48 to 0.96; overall, there were 0.63 interactions per minute). Thus, as might be expected, variables such as location, class size, space, program structure, toys, and child–teacher ratio were significant. These figures are not likely to be comparable to other play areas such as outdoor play. Males had more interactions than females for all age levels, but the differences in interaction rate were not numerically very great (0.68 vs. 0.58). The analysis showed similarities in interaction rates for ages 4, 5, and 6. However, significant differences were found between ages 3 and 5 and older. Children termed "low interactors" had low initiation rates and lower probabilities of responding to peer initiations (for females), and received more initiations from peers than they made to members of the peer group.

The intervention implications of the study are at least twofold. First, it is necessary to "establish reciprocity in social responding" (Greenwood et al., 1981, p. 364). The intervention methods include teaching or modifying children's skills to increase reciprocal interactions. Second, it is necessary to "transfer stimulus control" associated with reciprocity "to the social bids occurring in the peer group" (p. 364). An example is initiating an appropriate response after receiving attention from another child. These strategies are examined in detail in the studies that are discussed next.

In contrast to normative social interactions, Hendrickson, et al. (1982) studied social interactions of children described as having behavioral handicaps. They reported studies that examined the potential utility of play behaviors exhibited by typically developing children (from Hendrickson et al., 1982, p. 325; Tremblay, Strain, Hendrickson, & Shores, 1981):

1. *Play organizers* (such as "Let's play school," "Let's play ball").
2. *Shares* (basic exchange of ball, blocks, cars).
3. *Assists* (such as help child onto a play object).

In two phases, a peer confederate was trained in the three social initiation behaviors. The first phase, an extensive preintervention component, introduced the child to the "helper role," taught different ways to initiate the target behaviors, and gave practice in initiating the behaviors and using play materials. The second component was described as follows (adapted from Hendrickson et al., 1982, p. 331).

1. The experimenter began by telling the confederate she was to try and get (*name of child*) to play with her for the next 5 minutes.

2. The experimenter reminded the confederate to use "asking," "sharing," and "helping" to get the other child to play.

3. The experimenter then questioned the confederate about what she was going to try to get [name of child] to play. If the child did not know (or answer), the experimenter made suggestions.

4. The experimenter also asked the confederate what she should do if [name of child] did not respond. . . . The experimenter would prompt the confederate to initiate if she did not begin a new initiation within 15 seconds of the last initiation or interaction.

5. A reward system (session, daily, and weekly) was also used for the confederate.

The three types of initiations by the confederate were highly effective in promoting responses from the socially withdrawn child. The results were replicated across two other socially withdrawn children. A second study replicated the effects with a confederate described as having a handicapping condition. However, the children were older (ages 6 and 7) and the confederate training took longer to accomplish.

Despite the changes in interactive play during the intervention, there was an immediate return to baseline when the intervention was withdrawn. Through confederate prompts and praise, but not spontaneously, interactions generalized to another play area. For future research, the authors suggested that generalization and maintenance may be improved by (1) using multiple peer confederates for individual target children, (2) teaching *approach* behaviors to target children, and (3) examining more intensive training efforts by expanding interventions to other parts of the school day. Other factors that may impact upon such efforts include the relative numbers of socially unresponsive children in various settings, established friendship networks, and prior histories of negative social contacts between target children and peers. In other words, such efforts may require extensive ecobehavioral analysis and modification.

Hecimovic et al. (1985) built on the intervention by Hendrickson and others. They examined the differential effects of returning the socially withdrawn children on alternating days to either developmentally segregated or developmentally integrated free-play settings where the peer confederates also were located. The results are complicated and suggest again the need for considerable analysis. Among the results, the training procedures increased the target children's initiations and interactions with confederates. However, the behaviors were not maintained by 2 of 3 children when the intervention was briefly withdrawn. While the integrated classroom provided the target children with more "social opportunities in the form of initiations from other children" (p. 385), these bids mostly came from children not involved in the research. The segregated setting produced more adult-target children interactions than the integrated setting. Adult–child interactions may interfere with subsequent play interactions between children. Overall, there was a lack of generalization to both integrated and segregated settings.

Kohler and Fowler (1985) studied the effects of a social skills training package for 3 young girls (ages 5–7). Two of the target children were described as domineering, the other was described as passive. As in the earlier studies, the behaviors of interest were play invitations. These included (1) verbally and physically offering to share play materials, (2) offering assistance ("Can I help you?"), (3) inviting another child to join a play activity, and (4) requesting permission to join an ongoing play activity ("Can I play?") (p. 189). They also studied the use of amenities for two children ("Please," "Thank you," "I'm sorry"). The authors found training for play invitations resulted in reciprocated play behaviors for 2 children. Outcomes associated with amenities were less clear but, overall, appeared somewhat promising. For one child, the use of amenities appeared to increase as a result of training in play invitations. For a second child, reciprocal peer responses were delayed until after the training phase. In both cases, peer responses to the use of amenities were variable.

For a third child, the intervention was unsuccessful. However, a change in group contingencies to increase invitations from peers resulted in an increased rate of reciprocated invitations. This phase consisted of appointing 3 volunteer children to offer an invitation to the target child in free play, and to have a fourth child prompt the peers to make social invitations. Different children were used each day. The target child was instructed to offer between three and six invitations, and not to emit negative behaviors. The target child and peer confederates received stickers on days that the specified criterion for invitations was met. The whole class received a reward for meeting the criterion on 3 successive days. A subsequent phase included only training for the target child's peers. The target child spontaneously increased her use of social amenities to peers during the group contingency phase. After the group contingencies were withdrawn, the acceptance ratio for play invitations was maintained but at a lower level. Follow-up observations suggested modest improvements over baseline in overall rates of reciprocated play invitations.

The results show that it may be important to train target children in behaviors likely to be reciprocated by peers, but that this may be insufficient for some children. It also may be important to train peers in reciprocating the targeted behavior to help with the problem of limited generalization of social behaviors. Kohler and Fowler (1985) pointed out that the following conditions may be necessary for the reciprocation of play invitations: "(a) a decrease in (or absence of) behaviors that compete with invitations . . . ; (b) an appropriate rate of invitations, distributed across members of the peer group; and (c) the availability of a peer, not already engaged in an activity who can respond" (p. 197).

A report by Lefebvre and Strain (1989) focused on group-oriented contingencies to further interactions between children with autism and typically developing preschoolers, while also examining the teacher's role in prompting integrated social activities. All children, including those described as having disabilities, participated in the peer-training activities, and all peers acted as change agents. The study was conducted during daily 7-minute sociodramatic play activities (such as grocery store or camping). Each child with disabilities was paired with 2 peer confederates. To improve maintenance and generalizability, the confederates were rotated every 3 days.

In the training phase of the intervention, the "morning circle time" lasting 10–15 minutes per session was used to demonstrate strategies for engaging peers in play. The strategies were role-played by the teacher and a second caregiver. Each child was given the opportunity to role play, and the strategies were reviewed 1 minute before the play activity began. The strategies included (p. 332):

"Say your friend's name."
"Face him or her."
"Keep trying."
"Ask for a toy and hold out your hand."
"Listen and help."
"Give a toy to your friend by placing it in his or her hand."
"Ask a friend to wait (after a request by the peer) and remember to give (the toy requested)."

The training phase was continued until the peers without disabilities met an 80% criterion level; this took 9 days. A token reinforcement system was then implemented during the "morning circle time"; children were given an opportunity to earn tokens by engaging in appropriate strategies. During the intervention, tokens were exchanged for the "reinforcer of the day." Each morning, when the children arrived, they would place their names in one of four boxes, indicating the reinforcer of their choice. Reinforcers included a "popcorn party, popsicle . . . , photographs with friends, listening to records" (p. 333). The group reinforcer was determined by the box that contained the most names. Response categories used to determine the effectiveness of the intervention included appropriate and inappropriate initiations and responses, play organizers, teacher prompts and consequences, and children's responses to teacher prompts.

Three different conditions were compared to assess the most effective way to implement the treatment package. First, the teacher was trained to limit the use of verbal models and prompts. The teacher continued rein-forcing appropriate interactions, strategies, and correction procedures, in-cluding prompting the targeted child to engage in peer interactions, ex-panding the targeted child's verbalizations, and modeling articulation. Prompts were allowed only after 1 minute of no interactions between tar-get children and peers.

The second intervention condition was implemented after peer train-ing and the group contingency were presented. It was built on a poster dis-playing the reinforcer of the day, with empty circles surrounding the rein-forcer. The circles contained the number of appropriate interactions needed by each of the three groups to obtain reinforcement. Every time the teacher observed the targeted child and peer confederate engaged in appropriate interaction, a token was placed in the circle, and the peer or target child was praised. If all three groups met the established criterion, reinforcement was awarded. During this phase, the teacher was again in-structed to refrain from prompts. Thus, all children were able to monitor group progress.

The third, and most effective, condition continued the limited use of prompts, but a change was made in the type of group contingency. Each group could obtain reinforcement noncontingent on the other groups' success. In other words, on any day, one, two, or all three groups could ob-tain backup reinforcement. Overall, teacher prompts were significantly re-duced for all three groups. The most effective teacher strategy for target children was that of verbal expansion, which not only increased the tar-geted child's utterances but also provided models for the peer confeder-ates. *Verbal expansion* was defined as adding to the length of a target child's verbal response or providing a verbal response for a target child's nonver-bal response. Generalization of strategies occurred for 1 of 3 targeted children and a specific peer confederate during other activities, and 1 peer confederate used the strategies with a child with disabilities not targeted in the study.

Sharing and Prosocial Behaviors

A prosocial behavior that is worthy of facilitation is sharing. This behavior is often regarded as a major component of interactive play. Many preschool children may have difficulties with interpersonal relationships because of problems with sharing behaviors. In addition, sharing and oth-er prosocial behaviors are alternative responses for disruptive behaviors. The potential social benefits are great. In other sections of this chapter and earlier, we have addressed applications of sharing with socially with-drawn children as well as children described as disabled. This section specifically reviews sharing interventions.

In a comprehensive study, Barton (1981) compared several different techniques used to teach sharing. The interventions consisted of instructions, modeling, modeling plus praise, behavioral rehearsal, in-session prompts, and in-session praise. Only the last three interventions demonstrated substantial changes in sharing behaviors; in-session praise showed the greatest effects. However, the experimental design could not tease out the potential additive effects of the prior instruction and modeling conditions. Barton concluded that children must be given (1) opportunities to practice sharing, (2) feedback concerning the adequacy of their performance, and (3) praise for practicing sharing. Research has found that the intervention effects may generalize to untrained peers (Barton & Bevirt, 1981). Barton and Osborne (1978) documented the effectiveness of teacher-administered positive practice for increasing classroom sharing with preschoolers with hearing impairments.

Barton and Ascione (1979) concluded that teaching sharing should include both physical and verbal strategies. Physical sharing was defined as "(a) handing a material to another child, (b) allowing another child to take his/her material, (c) using a particular material that another had used during the same observation interval, or (d) simultaneously using a material with another to work on a common project" (p. 420). Verbal sharing included "(a) requests to share another's materials, (b) compliance with a request to share materials, (c) invitations to share one's own materials, or (d) acceptance of invitations to share" (p. 420).

Bryant and Budd (1984) implemented a multicomponent intervention aimed at improving sharing that replicated and extended the study by Barton and Ascione. The intervention was mainly conducted by a teacher with 6 young children. Behaviors measured were (1) offers to share, (2) requests to share, (3) responses to offers or requests to share, (4) refusals to share, (5) taking without asking, (6) "opposing" play, and (7) aggression. The intervention occurred in the classroom, using toys and materials from a specified area. Two children at a time received instruction in sharing by the teacher during the first 10 minutes of freeplay for 4 days. At the end of each session, sharing was briefly reviewed, and the children were instructed to share with other children in the dramatic play or building area ("Sharing . . . is using the same things together" p. 50). On the first day, a rationale for sharing and examples were given: "We can share by giving other children things when they ask nicely for them . . . by asking for toys that other children have. It is not sharing to hit or push . . . , take toys they are playing with, or tell them they cannot play" (p. 50). The teacher modeled the behavior and verbalized appropriate sharing. The second day, the teacher reviewed sharing behaviors, and a second child practiced with the teacher. Two children then played together and received praise and examples of sharing and prompts (if needed). On the third and fourth days, sharing was practiced by the children. After the training sessions, children were reminded to share with all of the children in the classroom and the teacher praised and prompted sharing. Contingent observation was used for severe aggressive behavior. Overall, 5 out of 6 children increased their rate of sharing and decreased negative behaviors.

Correspondence training was used by Rogers-Warren and Baer (1976) to increase sharing behaviors. This type of intervention is important because of its potential for improving generalization, and for possible cost benefits. However, as Barton (1986) noted, direct training may be important. Rogers-Warren and Baer also included modeling in their intervention. Barton stressed that correspondence training may be more effective for maintenance once sharing behavior is well established.

Cooperation is another social skill that may be taught through play involving cooperative games (board games and modified games such as musical chairs). Cooperation, as defined in children's play, may include sharing, assisting, helping, instructing, supporting, or executing a task with another child (Bay-Hinitz, Peterson, & Quilitch, 1994, p. 438). These researchers also included affectionate behaviors in their definition.

In summary, multicomponent training of prosocial behaviors appears effective. Barton (1986) further discussed many related aspects of intervention design, such as the potential effects of different activities and materials, number of children, adult presence, different change agents, and other considerations. Both the target behaviors and training methods must fit the individual needs of children and settings. Cooperative, in contrast to competitive, games also may help to reduce aggressive behaviors and increase positive social behaviors (Bay-Hinitz et al., 1994).

Improving Social Interactions by Modifying Activities or Contingencies

Many interventions to help increase social interactions of withdrawn children have been described in the literature. Previously described interventions involving play behaviors and other social skills have been applied. In this section, additional interventions are reviewed that may help with withdrawn or isolated behaviors, but they are not based directly on play behaviors.

Sainato et al. (1986) described a "classroom manager" intervention whereby socially withdrawn children were placed into leadership positions: "They were required to direct their peers in activities that had previously been designated as being highly preferred by the class" (p. 188). The rationale was described as follows: "By placing withdrawn children in 'status' positions and making them the dispensers of preferred activities, their positive peer interactions would be increased and new friendships would be formed" (p. 188).

Three target children described as socially withdrawn were selected to participate, based on a variety of measures: direct observation, teacher rankings, and peer sociometrics. The setting was a regular kindergarten classroom with 16 children.

Four behavioral measures were used: (1) positive vocal–verbal (verbalizations directed to another child, except for shouting, crying, whining); (2) positive motor–gestural (such as hugging or sharing toys); (3) negative vocal–verbal (such as crying or whining); and (4) negative motor–gestural (hitting or punching). The behaviors were coded as either "initiated" or "responded" events. The measures were obtained during 20-minute free-play periods. Sociometric measures were also obtained to help evaluate the intervention.

The classroom manager intervention was initiated with the teacher announcing to the class that she had selected a new helper. The child was called to the front of the class and given a large "manager" button to wear for a 2-week period. The manager's job was leading and/or directing preferred activities such as feeding a class pet, collecting lunch money, and so on. Each day, the manager's duties were reviewed and a picture board displaying the activities was used to prompt the child. Following a 10-day period, the teacher complimented the children on a "great job" and the class was encouraged to clap for the helper. Each child in the study assumed the role of classroom manager for a 10-day period. The procedure was discontinued after the third child had participated, and follow-up measures were used to assess maintenance effects 4 weeks later.

The results were analyzed for the number of interactions, the positive-versus-negative quality of interactions, and initiations by peers or target children. Baseline conditions revealed that social interactions were relatively rare. The intervention demonstrated effectiveness, indicated by significant level changes for positive behaviors of both target children and peers. Level changes dropped slightly following the end of the classroom manager role, but the change was still higher than the baseline condition. The sociometric ratings similarly reflected positive changes.

The results demonstrate the effectiveness of the technique and the possibility of durable changes. While interactions diminished somewhat following the withdrawal of the intervention when the classroom manager role changed to another child, the results also can be considered reasonable. The experimenters discussed other potential benefits of the intervention: (1) little teacher time was required; (2) children were not removed from ongoing activities; and (3) changes to the usual classroom routines were minimal. Furthermore, similar practices may exist in many preschool classrooms that may be "systematically 'tapped' to derive social benefits for infrequent interactors" (p. 193).

Tarpley and Saudargas (1981) described a teacher-mediated intervention that resulted in rapid increases in peer interactions and expressions of positive affect (laughing or smiling) and decreases in crying for a 4-year-old boy. The intervention consisted of the following five teacher behaviors (pp. 410–411).

1. The teacher would "conspicuously" participate with the child's peers as much as possible.
2. After group activities, the class discussed positive aspects and "feelings" associated with group activities and play.
3. Brief comments were made during group play about satisfying aspects of interactions.
4. Private social reinforcement or praise was given to the withdrawn child contingent on joining a peer group.
5. Ignoring was used when the child was not participating or was distanced from other children. Importantly, the child's withdrawal served as a cue for the teacher to increase the first three steps.

Social reinforcement by teachers has been used to increase the social interactions of an isolated preschool child (Allen, Hart, Buell, Harris, & Wolf, 1964). The intervention consisted of attention to the isolated child contingent on play with another peer, and minimum attention contingent on isolate behavior or interaction with an adult.

Reluctant Speech and Selective Mutism

Children having some but minimal verbal behavior in social situations outside the home may be described as having *reluctant speech*. Morin, Ladouceur, and Cloutier (1982) used a contingency management procedure with a 6-year-old boy described as having "reluctant speech" within a kindergarten classroom. The child received "school money" for verbal responses to questions by the teacher. The tokens were exchanged for tangible reinforcers selected by the child, such as arts and crafts materials. During the intervention, nonverbal communication by the child was ignored. Verbal responses also received teacher attention. Calhoun and Koenig (1973) also investigated the use of classroom interventions for children who talked only infrequently. Classroom rewards, agreed upon by the teachers, were contingent on verbal interaction by the targeted student. Results indicated that the children significantly increased their rate of verbalization and that gains were maintained at 1-year follow-up.

Selective mutism is a similar but more serious condition that describes a child who can comprehend and speak (perhaps with family members), but refuses to do so in certain social situations such as school (American Psychiatric Association, 1994). In environments where the children do not use language, they typically interact using nonverbal means such as gestures and facial expressions. The syndrome typically becomes manifest when the child begins preschool or day care; parents of young, selectively mute children may report no speech difficulties in the home. The literature related to other aspects of personal, social, and family functioning for selectively mute children is mixed. Some children seem to be without other major difficulties, while many other concomitant problems also have been reported for children described as selectively mute (Cunningham, Cataldo, Mallion, & Keyes, 1983; Wilkins, 1985).

Behavioral interventions generally have been found to be successful in eliminating the problem. Social and tangible reinforcement have been the most common methods used for encouraging selectively mute children to speak in the school setting (Labbe & Williamson, 1984); relatedly, shaping and fading techniques also have been implemented (Kratochwill, 1981). Contingency management procedures are likely to be the most effective for children with reluctant speech; additional procedures (such as stimulus fading and response cost) may be needed for selectively mute children (Cunningham et al., 1983; Labbe & Williamson, 1984).

We now mention several representative interventions. Lipton (1980) combined stimulus fading with contingency management in the treatment of an electively mute kindergartner. Activities were used to elicit speech: "structured game playing requiring verbal interaction, working on an exercise book using verbal instructions, and doing picture completion tasks orally" (pp. 147–148), along with shaping and reinforcement. Williamson, Sanders, Sewell, Haney, and White (1977) used a variety of behavioral interventions to treat two children with selective mutism including reinforcement, shaping, modeling, and fading. Cunningham, Cataldo, Mallion, and Keyes (1983) also reported the successful treatment of selective mutism. Schill, Kratochwill, and Gardner (1996) evaluated functional-analytic methods for selective mutism based on parental participation.

In summary, children with selective mutism traditionally have been viewed as difficult to treat; interventions must be carefully developed. However, there are many reported successes based on behavioral interventions.

DISRUPTIVE BEHAVIORS

Disruptive behaviors are often linked to social skills, and many previously discussed interventions are likely to reduce the overall impact of these behaviors. The consultant's initial considerations should include qualities of instructional and social environments, basic rules, routines, and classroom-management procedures. In this section, we summarize tactics and further describe classroom interventions for disruptive and aggressive behaviors.

Examples of Basic Interventions for Disruptive Behaviors

As first steps, we recommend making certain that the child can perform the social and preacademic tasks that create the context for the problem behaviors. Differential reinforcement alone and combined with other intervention components, have been used extensively and effectively to reduce disruptive behaviors. These are likely interventions for many lively preschool situations.

Allen, Turner, and Everett (1970) and Pinkston, Reese, LeBlanc, and Baer (1973) described differential attention and extinction procedures to eliminate aggressive behaviors. In both reports, teachers were instructed to ignore the disruptive behavior of children and attend only to the victims. Teachers also were instructed to attend to the children described as disruptive when they were engaged in appropriate social interaction with their peers. The results of these studies support the use of differential attention and extinction to reduce aggressive behavior and increase positive peer social interaction.

Contingent observation, a mild form of time out that includes teaching about behavior, has been used to decrease disruptive behaviors. Tyroler and Lahey (1980) compared the effectiveness of contingent observation and redirection procedures with a 2-year-old girl. Disruptive behaviors included aggression, crying, fussing, destruction of toys, and creating dangerous situations (throwing objects, standing on a counter).

During the redirection phase, when the child engaged in disruptive behavior, she was told of the inappropriateness of her behavior and was redirected to a more appropriate activity ("Look at the book"). Contingent observation was implemented, following procedures described in Chapter 7. Results demonstrated that contingent observation was more effective in decreasing disruptive behaviors than redirection procedures.

Another natural intervention is choice making. As an example, two conditions were compared with a 5-year-old child referred for extremely aggressive, disruptive, and noncompliant behaviors (Dunlap et al., 1994): (1) teacher-selected books for 15-minute reading sessions or (2) child-selected books (including changing books within a session). Other features of the intervention included specific praise and affection for appropriate listening and participating, ignoring mild transgressions, occasional prompts ("I really like it when children listen and pay attention"; p. 511), and graduated physical guidance to redirect a child contingent on the child leaving the area. The choice-making condition showed positive results for both engagement and disruptive behaviors.

The "Good Behavior Clock"

An early study is instructive in providing creative examples of measuring engagement and methods for self-monitoring, combined with group contingencies. Kubany, Weiss, and Sloggett (1971) described the "good behavior clock" procedure for reducing disruptive classroom behavior in a 6-year-old boy. This intervention incorporated reinforcement for 2-minute intervals of appropriate classroom behavior (i.e., engagement). Reinforcement consisted of receiving "treats" which were placed in a sharing jar, for distribution to classmates at the end of the day. Many of our Head Start teachers have found a "sharing jar" acceptable.

Comprehensive Classroom Packages

We have had consultations when the disruptions in the classroom were extensive and involved several or, at times, many of the children. Even though some individual children have higher rates of disruptive behaviors than others, it may still be helpful to plan for class-wide interventions. These referrals typically include social behaviors as targets, although children may have a variety of developmental or other concerns that may need to be addressed. Comprehensive classroom programming may be helpful for inclusionary practices, especially when social behaviors or adaptation to routines are significant concerns across children. Some relatively inexperienced or new teachers also have requested consultation about classroom management techniques. In situations when classrooms are the focus, ecobehavioral classroom variables are sound initial targets of consultation. Individual children not responding to successful class-wide interventions can then be referred for further consultation, with decisions made about additional individual intervention based on the improvements shown by the class-wide intervention. Successful but demanding class-wide interventions may help demonstrate the need for more extensive resources and support for children and teachers.

As an example, we have had teachers make referrals because of more than one child throwing objects, being aggressive toward other children (aggressive theme play, wrestling, hitting, kicking, spitting) and using loud voices or inappropriate language (yelling, cursing), as well as exhibiting disruptive actions not directly related to social behavior (climbing, running from the class, high rates of activity changes). The teachers reported that children did not listen to them, and that they had difficulty controlling the classroom once these behaviors began. Beyond disrupting classroom routines, the safety of children (and teachers) was of concern.

We have used the problem-solving process to develop ways to reduce these classroom disruptions. Because of stress, other unpleasant emotions, and threats to self-efficacy related to the potentially devastating effects of disruptive behaviors on teachers, it may be helpful during problem analysis to examine a teacher's routine use of effective positive teaching and managing practices. These practices include: setting clear expectations; using effective scheduling and time management, especially during transitions; using positive attention; using physical proximity and clear requests to children; providing natural consequences for appropriate and inappropriate behavior; redirecting behavior as necessary; modeling of appropriate behavior; and applying calming techniques or rest for children if needed. While these proactive management strategies help set the stage for classwide interventions, they may not be sufficient. Plans developed from the problem-solving process typically had many if not all of the following steps, strategies, and components.

1. Consider the full classroom schedule, and make the structure and sequence of planned activities, routines, and events more salient and predictable, from greeting children in the morning to transitioning children to the bus. Based on a functional assessment (waking day interview for classrooms and observations), develop a "whole day" plan, or plans specific to high-risk activities. Activities or time periods can be identified that are most likely related to disruptive behaviors (e.g., "down time" between snacks and the bus at the end of the day, sitting too long at lunch, free play), and these can be buttressed by adding high interest activities (novel, stimulating) and management routines. Greeting children and brief communication with parents may give staff clues about setting events (or what happens before school that may increase the probability of disruptive behavior) and the need for an individualized entry (or neutralizing) routine for that day.

2. Build, as necessary, communication and cooperation between teachers and assistants, other staff, and parents. Disruptive classroom events may cause disharmony among staff members. Intervention design requires cooperation in monitoring interventions and behaviors. After a plan is agreed upon, clarify specific responsibilities. Unobtrusive "signal" systems or prompts between teachers may be helpful for carrying out various features of the intervention plans. Scheduling meeting times for teaming, reviewing procedures, and evaluating effectiveness based on data, will be critical.

3. Clarify, teach, review, and implement rules and limits for social behaviors. Model, practice, guide, and prompt clear classroom, transition,

lunch, gym, and transportation *routines* ("what to do" in a situation in a developmentally appropriate way for an individual child; how to ask another child to play; how to play with each other). As necessary, identify and teach individual skills needed to perform expected social and other tasks. Skills may be briefly introduced, prompted, and practiced incidentally throughout the day. We have used picture prompts—prominently displayed photographs of children engaged appropriately in activities or routines.

4. Introduce new activity centers and effectively manage them (e.g., choice making, limit setting) to reduce classroom disruptions. Lotteries may be used to gain access to centers (Peters, 1995; Stollar, Dye-Collins, & Barnett, 1996). Activities can be rotated (e.g., every week) thereby maintaining interest. High interest activity centers can be used to help provide effective consequences (see #8 of this list).

5. Plan transitions between activities. As with activity centers, teachers can develop alternative transition activities. As an example, a transition between activities may include giving a 5-minute "alert" or using game board themes such as "getting on the train" or "plane" showing the progression of daily events to children ("If I move the marker here, what is it time for?" "Group" "Lunch" "Free play!"). In this classroom routine, a classroom helper could move the marker for transitions (or give a signal such as ringing a bell or flashing the lights).

6. Increase positive scanning, responsiveness, and positive interactions between teachers and children. Teachers may develop a script to include the prompts: "Move slowly and steadily around the room in an unpredictable way. Pause to provide specific positive attention to individual children. Scan the room in a series of spot checks to note quickly whether students are engaging in appropriate behaviors."

7. Improve commands and requests made to children, and, at the same time, reduce "power struggles." Ways to accomplish this include clarifying rules and limits, using choice making, and providing effective consequences (next).

8. Use routine sequences to respond to disruptive behaviors, including positive rules, guides, or scripts for social behaviors, positive reminders, a consequence hierarchy that includes giving the child choices (redirection, offering a choice), warnings, contingent observation, and brief and mild consequences for behaviors. Setting limits and choice making may lead to powerful consequences for disruptive behaviors. Instead of time outs, children can *briefly* lose time or a turn in high interest areas by selecting another activity in the classroom (a mild response cost component; make certain that child responses are not avoidance or escape from the activity). Examples discussed in earlier chapters include neutralizing routines (those that would reduce reinforcement of inappropriate behaviors), rear-

ranging existing contingencies of reinforcement, using high probability request sequences, and adding noncontingent reinforcers.

We recommend procedures for collaborative script development and implementation assistance for classwide interventions. Scripts can be written for key features of the plans. These may include adhering to the classroom schedule (including entering, transitions, and activity periods); making effective requests or commands (to groups or individuals); ways to scan and spot check behavior; and reviewing limits and rules.

Relatively simple observation systems may be used to track changes in classwide disruptions through the use of strategic sampling and scan checking for disruptive behaviors. In addition, with parent permission, we have tracked the behavior of 1 to 5 children, by using interval recording (see micronorm procedures), who had greater probability of disruptive behaviors in order to evaluate the effects of the classwide intervention on individual behavior. Spot checking for intervention script use, the need for assistance in carrying out the scripts, and review, also are helpful in building fluency in using the procedures and for maintenance.

When we have carried out these procedures, classwide intervention measures have shown substantial decreases in disruptive behaviors and significant increases in the use of positive attention, as well as teacher satisfaction. Many classrooms will not need a comprehensive intervention, but the effectiveness of individual components of interventions can be checked and revised if necessary.

SAFETY- AND HEALTH-RELATED INTERVENTIONS

Accidental injuries are the leading cause of children's deaths, and health and safety programs have a broad base of research support. We describe several interventions that may be adapted for children with risk behaviors or in risk situations.

Pedestrian Safety Skills

Yeaton and Bailey (1978) evaluated an instructional package for street crossing. They noted that although many schools may contain curricular materials for safety, the skills may not transfer to real-life situations. The study was conducted at actual intersections where an adult crossing guard was present, and also at streets with a crossing guard nearby, to assess generalization. The ages of the children ranged from 5 to 9.

The training procedure involved four phases, with eight steps in each phase: (1) Wait at the curb; (2) look all ways; (3) watch vehicle distance; (4)

walk (do not stop in street); (5) continue to look; (6) use crosswalk; (7) walk on sidewalk; and (8) cross on corner. In the first phase (Tell Them), the trainer described correct behaviors for all steps. In the second phase (Show Them), the trainer demonstrated the street-crossing sequence by verbalizing and modeling the steps. In the third phase (Ask Them), the trainer questioned the children about the steps and praised correct responses. In the fourth phase (Let Them), children practiced the steps with the crossing guard, who gave feedback for correct and incorrect responses. After the instructional package was presented, the children practiced the safety steps. At one school, the crossing guard signaled each child from the center of the street. At the other, children were allowed safely to initiate the steps with a crossing guard in close proximity but behind the children. After formal instruction, the guard administered a prompt each day to use all the safety steps.

The results showed very positive changes in pedestrian skills, and the level of performance was maintained by the prompts. A 1-year follow-up demonstrated the maintenance of skills at "high levels" or skills that "could be quickly recovered from intermediate levels with only a minimum of remedial training" (Yeaton & Bailey, 1978, p. 327).

The procedure was successful and easy to implement. The training time was reported to average from 10 to 25 minutes for 11 sessions. The procedure potentially can be administered by a range of personnel including crossing guards or other adults. However, the authors noted that generalization was more of a problem and that research is necessary to improve generalization.

In a later study, Yeaton and Bailey (1983) evaluated two training packages. Critical training components include the opportunity to practice newly learned skills and to receive feedback and praise from the adults implementing the training. Still, street crossing supervision is necessary.

Bus Behavior

Disruptive behavior by children while riding in a bus can have extreme negative consequences for all involved.

Allen et al. (1970) used praise and consumable reinforcers to improve the bus behavior of a 4-year-old boy with multiple problem behaviors. We could find little other research on young children's bus behavior. Because of many referrals, the following procedures have been developed at the Northern Kentucky Head Start building on child transportation development plans that cover basic safety issues and responsibilities for staff and parents. For individual children with disruptive bus behavior, we suggest consultation with parents, bus personnel, and teachers to develop bus interventions and to link them to other possible home, community, or classroom interventions as necessary. Interventions may include classwide instruction. In addition, ways to reduce route length, such as changes in child-care arrangements, may be examined. Also, peer-seating arrangements and proximity to the bus monitor may be considered. Other environmental interventions such as bringing small toys, playing group games, and contingent music (McCarty, McElfresh, Rice, & Wilson, 1978) or singing, have helped reduce disruptive behaviors, but without modification (e.g., whisper singing; safe toys and contingencies for appropriate play), they have not been acceptable to drivers and monitors. It also may be important to develop skills in scanning bus behavior, and to implement observing and recording methods appropriate to the situation (e.g., frequency count of disruptive behaviors included in rule development; scan or zone sampling).

In consultation with parents, bus drivers, monitors, and teachers, we recommend developing bus *waiting, entering, riding* (e.g., sitting, using inside voices, hands to self), and *exiting* rules, and written scripts for parents and bus personnel, that can be reviewed daily with children by parents and others. Scripts describe child-appropriate parent and teacher ways to remind children about bus behavior prior to boarding (e.g., give a positive example to help a child follow a specific rule) and redirecting children as necessary. Referred children also have been given bus responsibilities (e.g., helping to line up). Compliance training may be helpful. Classwide, small group, and individualized instruction *and* practice may be used for bus behavior while *not* en route (e.g., classroom chairs are set up like the bus and rules are reviewed; large cardboard box is made into a bus). The bus driver also may review the rules in class.

Many young children will understand the safety reasons. Children can "tell" and/or "show" the driver, monitor or teacher a bus rule. Other steps may include making certain that all children are following the rules before the bus leaves, and providing recognition for children who are following the rules.

For more intensive bus interventions, consider breaking the bus ride into "checkpoints" (smaller individualized units using the odometer, natural landmarks, or time intervals) for reinforcements. These smaller units may be structured as DROs. Furthermore, they can be combined with home–school or school–home notes by including drivers and monitors' observations on a bus behavior checklist.

It is important to evaluate the dangerousness of the situation for the child exhibiting disruptive behaviors, other children, and the driver. Based on the crisis nature of a situation, we recommend consulting with parents about alternative transportation while plans are developed (e.g., having them pick the child up from the center) or other ways to get help for the driver. We also recommend contracts with parents to underscore mutual responsibilities associated with a behavioral plan (Chapters 5 and 9). In extreme situations, parents and staff have agreed to adapting the use of a safety belt/harness by combining it with choice making and the use of contingencies (the harness may also serve as a negative reinforcer) in the following way. First, specific permissions are required outlining the pros and cons associated with aversives, and consideration of alternatives (Chapter 5). The use of a harness should be combined with teaching steps and the introduction of positives (above). Use a script for explaining the expectations ("If you do not follow the bus rules, you will be given one warning. If you break the rules one more time after that warning, you will have to wear the harness for the rest of the bus ride"). Sit in close proximity to the child and monitor any child in a belt/harness. Encouragement (e.g., "Let's try harder today") and the contingencies are reviewed before the next bus ride. Good quality data for intervention outcomes are essential. In our experience, by using sequenced or hierarchical interventions as described, the use of a safety harness has not been needed or its use has been minimal and has been quickly faded.

Seat-Belt Usage

Each year, many young children suffer fatalities or are injured in vehicle collisions. Many states have implemented mandatory seat-belt and child-restraint laws, although parental compliance is questionable (Roberts & Layfield, 1987).

In a study by Sowers-Hoag, Thyer, and Bailey (1987), 16 children ranging in age from 4 to 7, who were never observed to be restrained while riding in a car, were trained to initiate seat-belt usage and ask for assistance when needed. The children were educated about the importance of seat-belt usage, and famous persons who used seat belts were discussed (airline and jet fighter pilots, race car drivers, and television stars). Role playing of scenarios was used to teach children to assert themselves to gain assistance in fastening seat belts before the car was in motion. Behavioral rehearsal was then used, and the children practiced putting on and taking off seat belts. Three cars with different types of seat belts were used for practice, until children were able to buckle and unbuckle the seat belts in less than 10 seconds. Training lasted 10 minutes or less.

Children who were observed to have their seat belts on when arriving at school were then eligible to participate in a lottery. Of the eligible children, half were selected each day to receive stickers, small toys, or "safety award certificates." Results indicated that seat-belt usage significantly increased during intervention as compared to baseline. and gains were maintained at follow-up 2–3 months later. Relatedly, Roberts and Layfield

(1987) found that rewarding children for use of seat belts was more effective than providing information to parents.

Responding to Emergencies

Jones and Kazdin (1980) evaluated the effectiveness of a program designed to teach young children skills necessary in making emergency phone calls. Such skills may be especially important for children who are not well supervised in the home.

The study was implemented based on the interest of the preschool staff. The ages ranged from 3 to 6 years. However, some children were excluded due to absences, change of programs, or a lack of skills, as determined by a pretest. The training was carried out by the preschool teachers in the classroom. Three conditions were compared: a behavioral program, a "teacher-devised method," and a control group of children without training experiences. The behavioral program included instructions, modeling, prompting, remediation, feedback, review, and reinforcement. Each teacher was supplied with a telephone training device that allowed children to simulate calls with an operator. A checklist of emergency dialing skills included using the phone, reporting the emergency, and stating one's full name and address. Each task was first taught independently and then in a combined sequence. During the lessons, the children and the teacher role-played being a parent and giving instructions to the child to contact an emergency agency (fire, police, ambulance). Emergency situations included warning "Fire" and pretending to be injured in an accident. As the children completed the component steps and the sequences, reinforcement was provided. Children were taught in a group format but practiced individually. The behavioral training program resulted in a significant difference in comparison to the other method and the group without training.

In a second study, Jones and Kazdin (1980) extended the research to the children's skills necessary to discriminate situations requiring emergency calls. They used a total of 30 pictures to represent three different conditions: "*fire scenes* (e.g., kitchen stove or couch on fire)"; "*injuries* that warranted emergency assistance" (such as cuts or falling down stairs); and "*neutral situations* (child reading a book or lying in bed)" (adapted from p. 515). The pictures were shown daily in random order, and the children were asked whom they should call.

> The training included the direct teaching of responses: "When we see fires like this, we call the fire truck. The fire truck brings water and puts the fire out. Now here are some pictures with fires in them." The child was then shown each fire scene individually and asked, "Can you tell me what's on fire?" (p. 516)

Following direct teaching, the children were prompted by being shown the different scenes. "What should you do when you see this?" (p. 516). A correct answer was praised and reinforced. Incorrect responses "were followed by . . . 'no,' an explanation . . . , and modeling of the desired response" (p. 516). Modifications were made for 2 children who experienced difficulty. The results indicated that improvements occurred as a function of training.

It is likely that telephone training occurs in many preschools and is also conducted by parents in the home. A carefully constructed behavioral training program may have more benefits than other methods. Children's ability to discriminate situations requiring emergency phone calls improved as a result of a straightforward procedure. Jones and Kazdin (1980) gave several suggestions that would be helpful for practice: using more realistic and naturalistic stimuli (such as videotapes); responding to different operators who ask questions in different ways; and including factors such as busy signals. The procedures may be carried out in about 30 days of 15- to 20-minute sessions.

With similar goals but different methods, Rosenbaum, Creedon, and Drabman (1981) evaluated a treatment package to teach preschool children to discriminate emergency situations, to dial 911, and to respond appropriately to questions relating to the emergency. Six emergency and six nonemergency scenes were presented by videotape. Children's responses included the discrimination task, phone-dialing skills, and providing information that included the child's name, address, a description of the emergency, the number of injured people, and whether an ambulance was needed. Experience with push-button phones also was necessary.

Self-Protection Training

Poche, Brouwer, and Swearingen (1981; see also Bevill & Gast, 1998; Gast, Collins, Wolery, & Jones, 1993) presented a program to teach young children (ages 3–5) safe responses to attempted abductions such as kidnapping or molestation. They cited research that suggests that force is less likely to be used than enticement. Thus, training children to resist enticement may be important in reducing such threats. Three preschool children were included in the study. To aid in generalization, life-like schoolground settings were used. "Suspects" or adult confederates were used in training to resemble possible molesters. Each molester used a ploy, such as a simple request to accompany the molester, a request that the child's parents (or other authority figure) had approved of the child's leaving, or a request to leave with the promise of an incentive. In consultation with the children's parents, definitions of appropriate responses to the lures were developed. In general, the parents wanted the children to make a brief verbal statement to the adult confederate, so as not to offend a kind person, but not so long that the child might be abducted, and to then move quickly from the area. Two adults served as trainers, with one playing the suspect role, while the other modeled appropriate child responses. Behavioral rehearsal and reinforcement were used to train the children using three "lures" per day. The research has been extended to incorporate videotape training (Poche, Yoder, & Miltenberger, 1988; see also Miltenberger & Olsen, 1996).

In a study by Harvey, Forehand, Brown, and Holmes (1988), kindergarten children were provided with a sexual abuse prevention program. Twenty children participated in the program; 20 others served as controls. At preintervention, postintervention, and follow-up, each child was asked to view a series of pictures and to identify whether a picture was depicting good (five pictures) or bad touches (five pictures). Each child also was asked five questions (p. 431): "(1) Is it ok to ever break a promise? (2) Do you think that children should always obey grown-ups? (3) If a person forces or tricks you into a bad touch, should you tell? (4) Do you think that sometimes grown-ups trick children into a bad touch? (5) Do you think that children should decide with whom they want to share their bodies?"

A direct test and generalization tests also were administered to children. Each test contained two stories of sexual abuse: one involved an adult; the other involved a teenager. The child was then asked six questions about whether the abuse was wrong and what he or she should do. Stories presented in the direct test were discussed in the treatment program, while the generalization scenarios were not discussed.

The program consisted of three half-hour sessions over 3 consecutive days, in which sexual abuse was defined, the differences between good, bad, and sexually abusive touches were explained, safety rules to prevent abuse were provided, and the identities of persons who could possibly abuse (strangers, familiar adults, or teenagers) were discussed. The teaching procedures consisted of instruction, modeling, and rehearsal. Stories and a film about sexual abuse also were presented to the children. Results of the study indicated that the children participating in the program demonstrated increased knowledge about abuse, including safety, rules about sexual abuse, and how to handle potential abusive situations, as compared to the control group. The results were maintained at a 7-week follow-up. (See also Chapter 9.)

Comprehensive Programs

Mori and Peterson (1986) extended Peterson's earlier efforts (Peterson, 1984a, 1984b) to demonstrate the successful training of safety skills for preschool children based on the "Safe at Home" game, using preschool teachers as trainers. The game is intended to provide preventive services to children who may be at greater risk for injury or trauma from molestation because of more unsupervised time in the home.

The "Safe at Home" game includes three domains, with two modules within each domain: *emergencies* (cut hand and fire), *encountering strangers* (door and phone), and *food selection and preparation* (nutrition and safe preparation). The game consists of four "safety response rules" for each module; the rules are illustrated and mounted on cards. Several games were used to teach correct responses. Thus, safety rules were presented verbally and visually. Teacher praise was also used, along with social and tangible reinforcement.

The cards were faded gradually, and children were then required to act out and explain the rules without the cards. Rehearsal was used on a repeated basis, and the children also were required to give the rationale for their response. Criteria for discontinuing training were met when "the majority of subjects could act out in proper sequence all four safety responses for each module, while simultaneously reporting its underlying rationale" (p. 110).

Mori and Peterson (1986) warn that the program should be considered only a beginning phase of injury prevention. Furthermore, how well preschool children will actually apply the skills under stress remains untested. Christophersen (1989) also reviewed research-based health interventions for low-income minority groups.

Biting

Biting is an important cause of injury to children and to adults in day care centers (Solomons & Elardo, 1989). In one study of 1,324 accidents in a university day care center composed mostly of children (median age of 38 months) from white, middle-class, two-parent families, 171 accident reports were related to bites received by another child, and 44 were self-induced. Overall, nearly half of the day care children received human bites, the most common circumstance being aggressive acts. However, only four bites actually broke the skin.

Among the recommendations by Solomons and Elardo (1989) are considerations of play materials, anticipation of conflicts and redirecting children, and vigilance in monitoring play behaviors. Factors such as child–adult ratios and in-service training on the management of aggression also are appropriate considerations.

Another potential variable related to biting is functional language. As an example, a 3-year-old girl was referred to Bell for consultation regarding aggressive behaviors, including biting. Direct observation and teacher interviews revealed that she was experiencing significant difficulties in the area of expressive language. She had only a few intelligible words and phrases, and these were not effective in social interactions with her peers. She was taught to use the word "No!" in a forceful voice to signal the teachers, who then intervened and facilitated situational interactions with peers (e.g., negotiated sharing materials, turntaking, sharing space). Aggressive incidents, including biting, decreased to zero levels. For further discussion of functional language use, see Chapter 7.

SUMMARY AND CONCLUSIONS

We reviewed interventions for social competence, disruptive behavior, and other problem behaviors, building on earlier chapters. It is important to establish a range of intervention alternatives for problem behaviors to help fit naturalistic styles of teaching, to promote acceptability, and to help guard against intervention biases. A final section outlined interventions related to safety and health-related issues. Systematic instruction for safety, emergencies, and abduction by a stranger may be a significant part of the preschool curriculum and may help children having special needs.

References

♦

Abraham, M. R., Morris, L. M., & Wald, P. J. (1993). *Inclusive early childhood education: A model classroom.* Tucson, AZ: Communication Skill Builders.

Alessi, G. J. (1988). Direct observation methods for emotional/behavior problems. In E. S. Shapiro & T. R. Kratochwill (Eds.), *Behavioral assessment in schools: Conceptual foundations and practical applications* (pp. 14–75). New York: Guilford Press.

Alessi, G. J., & Kaye, J. H. (1983). *Behavioral assessment for school psychologists.* Washington, DC: National Association of School Psychologists.

Alig-Cybriwsky, C. A., Wolery, M., & Gast, D. L. (1990). Use of constant time delay procedure in teaching preschoolers in a group format. *Journal of Early Intervention, 14,* 99–116.

Allen, K. E., Hart, B., Buell, J. S., Harris, F. R., & Wolf, M. M. (1964). Effects of social reinforcement on isolate behavior of a nursery school child. *Child Development, 35,* 511–518.

Allen, K. E., Turner, K. D., & Everett, P. M. (1970). A behavior modification classroom for Head Start children with behavior problems. *Exceptional Children, 37,* 119–127.

Alpert, C. L., & Rogers-Warren, A. K. (1985). Communication in autistic persons: Characteristics and intervention. In S. F. Warren & A. K. Rogers-Warren (Eds.), *Teaching functional language: Generalization and maintenance of language skills* (pp. 123–155). Austin, TX: Pro-Ed.

Altepeter, T. S., & Walker, C. E. (1992). Prevention of physical abuse of children through parent training. In D. J. Willis, E. W. Holden, & M. Rosenberg (Eds.), *Prevention of child maltreatment: Developmental and ecological perspectives* (pp. 226–248). New York: Wiley.

American Psychiatric Association. (1994). *Diagnostic and statistical manual of mental disorders* (4th ed.). Washington, DC: Author.

American Psychological Association. (1992). *Ethical principles of psychologists and code of conduct.* Washington, DC: Author.

Anastopoulos, A., & Barkley, R. A. (1990). Counseling and training parents. In R.

A. Barkley (Ed.), *Attention-deficit hyperactivity disorder: A handbook for diagnosis and treatment* (pp. 397–431). New York: Guilford Press.

Anderson-Inman, L. (1981). Transenvironmental programming: Promoting success in the regular class by maximizing the effect of resource room assistance. *Journal of Special Education Technology, 4,* 3–12.

Arndorfer, R. E., Miltenberger, R. G., Woster, S. H., Rortvedt, A. K., & Gaffaney, T. (1994). Home-based descriptive and experimental analysis of problem behaviors in children. *Topics in Early Childhood Special Education, 14,* 64–87.

Association for Advancement of Behavior Therapy. (1977). Ethical issues for human services. *Behavior Therapy, 8,* v–vi.

Atkeson, B. M., & Forehand, R. (1979). Home-based reinforcement programs designed to modify classroom behavior: A review and methodological evaluation. *Psychological Bulletin, 86,* 1298–1308.

Atwater, J. B., Carta, J. J., & Schwartz, I. S. (1989). *Assessment code/checklist for the evaluation of survival skills: ACCESS.* Kansas City: Juniper Garden Children's Project, Bureau of Child Research, University of Kansas.

Atwater, J. B., & Morris, E. K. (1988). Teachers' instructions and children's compliance in preschool classrooms: A descriptive analysis. *Journal of Applied Behavior Analysis, 21,* 157–167.

Axelrod, S. (1990). Myths that (mis)guide our profession. In A. C. Repp & N. N. Singh (Eds.), *Perspectives on the use of nonaversive and aversive interventions for persons with developmental disabilities* (pp. 59–72). Sycamore, IL: Sycamore Publishing.

Axelrod, S. (1998). *How to use group contingencies.* Austin, TX: Pro-Ed.

Ayllon, T., & Azrin, N. (1968). *The token economy: A motivational system for therapy and rehabilitation.* New York: Appleton–Century–Crofts.

Azrin, N. H., & Besalel, V. A. (1979). *A parent's guide to bedwetting control: A step-by-step method.* New York: Simon & Schuster.

Azrin, N. H., & Foxx, R. M. (1974). *Toilet training in less than a day.* New York: Simon & Schuster.

Azrin, N. H., Nunn, R. G., & Frantz-Renshaw, S. (1980). Habit reversal treatment of thumbsucking. *Behavior Research and Therapy, 18,* 395–399.

Baer, D. M., & Fowler, S. A. (1984). How should we measure the potential of self-control procedures for generalized educational outcomes. In W. L. Heward, T. E. Heron, D. S. Hill, & J. Trap-Porter (Eds.), *Focus on behavior analysis in education* (pp. 145–161). Columbus, OH: Merrill.

Baer, D. M., & Wolf, M. M. (1970). The entry into natural communities of reinforcement. In R. Ulrich, T. Stachnik, & J. Mabry (Eds.), *Control of human behavior: Vol 11. From cure to prevention* (pp. 319–324). Glenview, IL: Scott, Foresman.

Baer, D. M., Wolf, M. M., & Risley, T. R. (1968). Some current dimensions of applied behavior analysis. *Journal of Applied Behavior Analysis, 1,* 91–97.

Baer, R. A., Detrich, R., & Weninger, J. M. (1988). On the functional role of the verbalization in correspondence training procedures. *Journal of Applied Behavior Analysis, 21,* 345–356.

Baer, R. A., Osnes, P. G., & Stokes, T. F. (1983). Training generalized correspondence between verbal behavior at school and nonverbal behavior at home. *Education and Treatment of Children, 6,* 379–388.

Baer, R. A., Williams, J. A., Osnes, P. G., & Stokes, T. F. (1985). Generalized verbal control and correspondence training. *Behavior Modification, 9,* 477–489.

Bagnato, S. J., & Neisworth, J. T. (1990). *Developmental SPECS (System to Plan Early Childhood Services).* Circle Pines, MN: American Guidance Service.

Bailey, D. B., Jr. (1989). Assessing environments. In D. B. Bailey, Jr., & M. Wolery (Eds.), *Assessing infants and preschoolers with handicaps* (pp. 97–118). New York: Merrill.

Bailey, D. B., Jr., & Wolery, M. (1992). *Teaching infants and preschoolers with disabilities* (2nd ed.). Columbus, OH: Merrill.

Bailey, D. B., Jr., & Wolery, M. (1989). *Assessing infants and preschoolers with handicaps.* Columbus, OH: Merrill.

Bakeman, R., & Gottman, J. M. (1986). *Observing interaction: An introduction to sequential analysis.* New York: Cambridge University Press.

Bandura, A. (1978). The self-system in reciprocal determinism. *American Psychologist, 33,* 344–358.

Bandura, A. (1985). Model of causality in human learning. In M. J. Mahoney & A. Freeman (Eds.), *Cognition and psychotherapy* (pp. 81–99). New York: Plenum Press.

Bandura, A. (1986). *The social foundations of thought and action: A social cognitive theory.* Englewood Cliffs, NJ: Prentice-Hall.

Barkley, R. A. (1987). *Defiant children: A clinician's manual for parent training.* New York: Guilford Press.

Barkley, R. A. (1996). Attention deficit/hyperactivity disorder. In E. J. Mash & L. G. Terdal (Eds.), *Child psychopathology* (pp. 63–112). New York: Guilford Press.

Barkley, R. A. (1997). *Defiant children: A clinician's manual for assessment and parent training* (2nd ed.). New York: Guilford Press.

Barlow, D. H., Hayes, S. C., & Nelson, R. O. (1984). *The scientist-practitioner: Research and accountability in clinical and educational settings.* New York: Pergamon Press.

Barnard, J. D., Christophersen, E. R., & Wolf, M. M. (1977). Teaching children appropriate shopping behavior through parent training in the supermarket setting. *Journal of Applied Behavior Analysis, 10,* 49–59.

Barnett, D. W., Air, A. E., Bell, S. H., Gilkey, C. M., Smith, J. J., Stone, C. M., Nelson, K. I., Maples, K. A., Helenbrook, K., & Hannum, L. E. (in press). Evaluating early intervention: Accountability methods for service delivery innovations. *Journal of Special Education.*

Barnett, D. W., Bauer, A. M., Ehrhardt, K. E., Lentz, F. E., & Stollar, S. A. (1996). Keystone targets for change: Planning for widespread positive consequences. *School Psychology Quarterly, 11,* 95–117.

Barnett, D. W., Bell, S. H., Bauer, A., Lentz, Jr., F. E., Petrelli, S., Air, A., Hannum, L., Ehrhardt, K. E., Peters, C. A., Barnhouse, L., Reifin, L. H., & Stollar, S. (1997). The Early Childhood Intervention Project: Building capacity for service delivery. *School Psychology Quarterly, 12,* 293–315.

Barnett, D. W., Bell, S. H., Gilkey, C. M., Lentz, F. E., Jr., Graden, J. L., Stone, C. M., Smith, J. J., & Macmann, G. M. (in press). The promise of meaningful eligibility determination: Intervention-based multifactored preschool evaluation. *Journal of Special Education.*

Barnett, D. W., & Carey, K. T. (1992). *Designing interventions for preschool learning and behavior problems.* San Francisco: Jossey-Bass.

Barnett, D. W., Collins, R., Coulter, C., Curtis, M. J., Ehrhardt, K., Glaser, A., Reyes, C., Stollar, S., & Winston, M. (1995). Ethnic validity and school psychology: Concepts and practices associated with cross-cultural professional competence. *Journal of School Psychology, 33,* 219–234.

Barnett, D. W., Ehrhardt, K. E., Stollar, S. A., & Bauer, A. M. (1994). PASSKey: A model for naturalistic assessment and intervention design. *Topics in Early Childhood Special Education, 14,* 350–374.

Barnett, D. W., Lentz, F. E., Bauer, A. M., Macmann, G., Stollar, S., & Ehrhardt, K. E. (1997). Ecological foundations of early intervention: Planned activities and strategic sampling. *Journal of Special Education, 30,* 471–490.

Barnett, D. W., & Macmann, G. M. (1992). Decision reliability and validity: Contributions and limitations of alternative assessment strategies. *Journal of Special Education, 25,* 431–452.

Barnett, D. W., Silverstein, B., & Miller, R. (1988). *In vivo language intervention: A case study replication.* Unpublished manuscript, University of Cincinnati.

Barnett, D. W., & Zucker, K. B. (1990). *The personal and social assessment of children: An analysis of current status and professional practice issues.* Boston: Allyn & Bacon.

Barnett, W. S., & Escobar, C. M. (1988). The economics of early intervention for handicapped children: What do we really know? *Journal of the Division for Early Childhood, 12,* 169–181.

Barnett, W. S., & Escobar, C. M. (1990). Economic costs and benefits of early intervention. In S. J. Meisels & J. P. Shonkoff (Eds.), *Handbook of early childhood intervention* (pp. 560–582). New York: Cambridge University Press.

Barone, V. J., Greene, B. F., & Lutzker, J. R. (1986). Home safety with families being treated for child abuse and neglect. *Behavior Modification, 10,* 93–114.

Barrios, B., & Hartmann, D. P. (1986). The contributions of traditional assessment: Concepts, issues, and methodologies. In R. O. Nelson & S. C. Hayes (Eds.), *Conceptual foundations of behavioral assessment* (pp. 81–110). New York: Guilford Press.

Barton, E. J. (1981). Developing sharing: An analysis of modeling and other behavioral techniques. *Behavior Modification, 5,* 386–398.

Barton, E. J. (1986). Modification of children's prosocial behavior. In P. S. Strain, M. J. Guralnick, & H. M. Walker (Eds.), *Children's social behavior: Development, assessment and modification* (pp. 331–372). Orlando, FL: Academic Press.

Barton, E. J., & Ascione, F. R. (1979). Sharing in preschool children: Facilitation, stimulus generalization, response generalization, and maintenance. *Journal of Applied Behavior Analysis, 12,* 417–430.

Barton, E. J., & Bevirt, J. (1981). Generalization of sharing across groups: Assessment of group composition with preschool children. *Behavior Modification, 5,* 503–522.

Barton, E. J., & Osborne, J. G. (1978). The development of classroom sharing by a teacher using positive practice. *Behavior Modification, 2,* 231–250.

Barton, L. E., Brulle, A. R., & Repp, A. C. (1986). Maintenance of therapeutic change by momentary DRO. *Journal of Applied Behavior Analysis, 19*, 277–282.

Bauman, K. E., Reiss, M. L., Rogers, R. W., & Bailey, J. S. (1983). Dining out with children: Effectiveness of a parent advice package on pre-meal inappropriate behavior. *Journal of Applied Behavior Analysis, 16*, 55–68.

Bay-Hinitz, A. K., Peterson, R. F., & Quilitch, H. R. (1994). Cooperative games: A way to modify aggressive and cooperative behaviors in young children. *Journal of Applied Behavior Analysis, 27*, 435–446.

Bell, S. (1997). *Parent preferences for involvement in assessment and intervention design.* Unpublished doctoral dissertation, University of Cincinnati.

Bell, S. H., & Barnett, D. W. (in press). Peer micronorms in the assessment of young children: Methodological review and examples. *Topics in Early Childhood Special Education.*

Belsky, J. (1993). Etiology of child maltreatment: A developmental–ecological analysis. *Psychological Bulletin, 114*, 413–434.

Bem, D. J. (1982). Assessing situations by assessing persons. In D. Magnussen (Ed.), *Toward a psychology of situations: An interactional perspective* (pp. 245–257). Hillsdale, NJ: Erlbaum.

Bennett, C. W. (1973). A four-and-a-half year old as a teacher of her hearing-impaired sister: A case study. *Journal of Communication Disorders, 6*, 67–75.

Bennett, T., Lee, H., & Lueke, B. (1998). Expectations and concerns: What mothers and fathers say about inclusion. *Education and Training in Mental Retardation and Developmental Disabilities, 33*(2), 108–122.

Bereiter, C., & Englemann, S. (1966). *Teaching the disadvantaged child in the preschool.* Englewood Cliffs, NJ: Prentice-Hall.

Bergan, D. (1993). Facilitating friendship development in inclusion classrooms. *Childhood Education, 69*(4), 234–236.

Bergan, J. R., & Tombari, M. L. (1976). Consultant skill and efficiency and the implementation and outcomes of consultation. *Journal of School Psychology, 14*, 3–14.

Berreuta-Clement, J., Schweinhart, L., Barnett, W., Epstein, A., & Weikart, D. (1984). *Changed lives.* Ypsilanti, MI: High/Scope Press.

Bevill, A. R., & Gast, D. L. (1998). Social safety for young children: A review of the literature on safety skills instruction. *Topics in Early Childhood Special Education, 18*, 222–234.

Bijou, S. J. (1995). *Behavior analysis of child development.* Reno, NV: Context Press.

Bijou, S. W. (1975). Development in the preschool years: A functional analysis. *American Psychologist, 30*, 829–837.

Bijou, S. W., & Baer, D. M. (1961). *Child development I: A systematic and empirical theory.* Englewood Cliffs, NJ: Prentice-Hall.

Bijou, S. W., Peterson, R. F., & Ault, M. H. (1968). A method to integrate descriptive and experimental field studies at the level of data and empirical concepts. *Journal of Applied Behavior Analysis, 1*, 175–191.

Bijou, S. W., Peterson, R. F., Harris, F. R., Allen, K. E., & Johnston, M. S. (1969). Methodology for experimental studies of young children in natural settings. *Psychological Record, 19*, 177–210.

Billings, D. C., & Wasik, B. H. (1985). Self-instructional training with preschoolers: An attempt to replicate. *Journal of Applied Behavior Analysis, 18,* 61–67.

Binder, C. (1996). Behavioral fluency: Evolution of a new paradigm. *Behavior Analyst, 19,* 163–197.

Bloom, M., & Fischer, J. (1982). *Evaluating practice: Guidelines for the accountable professional.* Englewood Cliffs, NJ: Prentice-Hall.

Boon, F. F. L., & Singh, N. N. (1991). A model for the treatment of encopresis. *Behavior Modification, 15,* 355–371.

Bornstein, P. H. (1985). Self-instructional training: A commentary and state-of-the-art. *Journal of Applied Behavior Analysis, 18,* 69–72.

Bowers, K. S., & Meichenbaum, D. (Eds.). (1984). *The unconscious reconsidered.* New York: Wiley.

Bracken, B. A., & Myers, D. K. (1986). *Bracken concept development program.* San Antonio, TX: Psychological Corporation.

Bradley-Johnson, S., Sunderman, P., & Johnson, C. M. (1983). Comparison of delayed prompting and fading for teaching preschoolers easily confused letters and numbers. *Journal of School Psychology, 21,* 327–335.

Bramlett, R. K. (1990). *The development of a preschool observation code: Preliminary technical characteristics.* Unpublished doctoral dissertation, University of Cincinnati.

Brassard, M. R., & Gelardo, M. S. (1987). Psychological maltreatment: The unifying construct in child abuse and neglect. *School Psychology Review, 2,* 127–136.

Brassard, M. R., & Hart, S. N. (1987). (Mini-series Eds.). Psychological maltreatment of children. *School Psychology Review, 2.*

Bredekamp, S. (1993). The relationship between early childhood education and early childhood special education: Healthy marriage or family feud? *Topics in Early Childhood Special Education, 13,* 258–273.

Bredekamp, S., & Copple, C. (Eds.). (1997). *Developmentally appropriate practice in early childhood programs* (rev. ed.). Washington, DC: National Association for the Education of Young Children.

Bredekamp, S., & Rosegrant, T. (1995). *Reaching potentials: Transforming early childhood curriculum and assessment* (Vol. 2). Washington, DC: NAEYC.

Bredekamp, S., & Rosegrant, T. (1992). *Reaching potentials: Appropriate curriculum and assessment for young children* (Vol. 1). Washington, DC: NAEYC.

Breiner, J., & Beck, S. (1984). Parents as change agents in the management of their developmentally delayed children's noncompliant behaviors: A critical review. *Applied Research in Mental Retardation, 5,* 259–278.

Bricker, D. D. (1986). *Early education of at-risk and handicapped infants, toddlers, and preschool children.* Glenview, IL: Little, Brown.

Bricker, D., Pretti-Frontczak, K., & McComas, N. (1998). *An activity-based approach to early intervention* (2nd ed.). Baltimore: Paul H. Brookes.

Bricker, D. (1995). The challenge of inclusion. *Journal of Early Intervention, 19*(3), 179–194.

Bricker, D., & Woods Cripe, J. J. (1992). *An activity-based approach to early intervention.* Baltimore: Paul H. Brookes.

Brim, O. G., Jr., & Kagan, J. (Eds.). (1980). *Constancy and change in human development.* Cambridge, MA: Harvard University Press.

Brinckerhoff, J. L., & Vincent, L. J. (1986). Increasing parental decision-making at the individualized educational program meeting. *Journal of the Division for Early Childhood, 11*, 46–58.

Brinker, R. P. (1985). Interactions between severely mentally retarded students and other students in integrated and segregated public school settings. *American Journal of Mental Deficiency, 89*, 587–594.

Brophy, J. E. (1981). Teacher praise: A functional analysis. *Review of Educational Research, 51*(1), 5–32.

Brotherson, M. J., & Goldstein, B. L. (1992). Time as a resource and constraint for parents of young children with disabilities: Implications for early intervention services. *Topics in Early Childhood Special Education, 12*, 508–527.

Brown, J. H., Cunningham, G., & Birkimer, J. C. (1983). A telephone home survey to identify parent–child problems and maintaining conditions. *Child and Family Behavior Therapy, 5*, 85–92.

Brown, L., Nietupski, J., & Hamre-Nietupski, S. (1976). The criterion of ultimate functioning and public school services for severely handicapped students. In M. A. Thomas (Ed.), *Hey, don't forget about me: New directions for serving the severely handicapped* (pp. 2–25). Reston, VA: The Council for Exceptional Children.

Brown, W. H., Horn, E. M., Heiser, J. G., & Odom, S. L. (1996). Project BLEND: An inclusive model of early intervention services. *Journal of Early Intervention, 20*(4), 364–375.

Brown, W. H., McEvoy, M. A., & Bishop, N. (1991, Fall). Incidental teaching of social behavior. *Teaching Exceptional Children*, 35–38.

Bruder, M. (1998). A collaborative model to increase the capacity of child care providers to include young children with disabilities. *Journal of Early Intervention, 21*(2), 177–186.

Bruder, M. B. (1993). The provision of early intervention and early childhood special education within community programs: Characteristics of effective service delivery. *Topics in Early Childhood Special Education, 13*, 19–37.

Bruner, J. (1978). On prelinguistic prerequisites of speech. In N. Campbell, & P. T. Smith (Eds.), *Recent advances in the psychology of language: Language development and mother–child interactions* (Volume III, pp. 199–214). New York: Plenum Press.

Bryant, D. M., & Ramey, C. T. (1987). An analysis of the effectiveness of early intervention programs for environmentally at-risk children. In M. J. Guralnick & F. C. Bennett (Eds.), *The effectiveness of early intervention for at-risk and handicapped children* (pp. 33–78). Orlando, FL: Academic Press.

Bryant, L. E., & Budd, K. S. (1982). Self-instructional training to increase independent work performance in preschoolers. *Journal of Applied Behavior Analysis, 15*, 259–271.

Bryant, L. E., & Budd, K. S. (1984). Teaching behaviorally handicapped preschool children to share. *Journal of Applied Behavior Analysis, 17*, 45–56.

Budd, K. S., Green, D. R., & Baer, D. M. (1976). An analysis of multiple misplaced parental social contingencies. *Journal of Applied Behavior Analysis, 9*, 459–470.

Budd, K. S., Leibowitz, J. M., Riner, L. S., Mindell, C., & Goldfarb, A. L. (1981). Home-based treatment of severe disruptive behaviors: A reinforcement package for preschool and kindergarten children. *Behavior Modification, 5*, 273–298.

Burstein, N. D. (1986). The effects of classroom organization on mainstreamed preschool children. *Exceptional Children, 52,* 425–434.

Buysse, V., & Bailey, D. B., Jr. (1993). Behavioral and developmental outcomes in young children with disabilities in integrated and segregated settings: A review of comparative studies. *Journal of Special Education, 26,* 434–461.

Buysse, V., Wesley, P., Keyes, L., & Bailey, D. B., Jr. (1996). Assessing the comfort zone of child care teachers in serving young children with disabilities. *Journal of Early Intervention, 20,* 189–203.

Cairns, R. B., & Green, J. A. (1979). How to assess personality and social patterns: Observations or ratings? In R. B. Cairns (Ed.), *The analysis of social interactions: Methods, issues, and illustrations* (pp. 209–266). Hillsdale, NJ: Erlbaum.

Caldwell, B. E., & Bradley, R. H. (1979). *Home observation for measurement of the environment.* Little Rock: University of Arkansas.

Calhoun, J., & Koenig, K. P. (1973). Classroom modification of elective mutism. *Behavior Therapy, 4,* 700–702.

Camarata, S. (1993). The application of naturalistic conversation training to speech production in children with disabilities. *Journal of Applied Behavior Analysis, 26,* 173–182.

Campbell, F. A., & Taylor, K. (1996). Early childhood programs that work for children from economically disadvantaged families. *Young Children, 51*(4), 74–80.

Carden Smith, L. K., & Fowler, S. A. (1984). Positive peer pressure: The effects of peer monitoring on children's disruptive behavior. *Journal of Applied Behavior Analysis, 17,* 213–227.

Carey, K. T. (1989). *The treatment utility potential of two methods of assessing stressful relationships in families: A study of practitioner utility.* Unpublished doctoral dissertation, University of Cincinnati.

Carr, E. G., & Durand, V. M. (1985). Reducing behavior problems through functional communication training. *Journal of Applied Behavior Analysis, 18,* 111–126.

Carr, E. G., Levin, L., McConnachie, G., Carlson, J., Kemp, D., & Smith, C. (1994). *Communication-based intervention for problem-behavior: A user's guide for producing positive change.* Baltimore: Paul H. Brookes.

Carr, E. G., Robinson, S., & Palumbo, L. W. (1990). The wrong issues: Aversive vs. nonaversive treatment. The right issue: Functional vs. nonfunctional treatment. In A. C. Repp & N. N. Singh (Eds.), *Perspectives on the use of nonaversive and aversive interventions for persons with developmental disabilities* (pp. 361–379). Sycamore, IL: Sycamore.

Carr, E. G., Taylor, J. C., & Robinson, S. (1991). The effects of severe behavior problems in children on the teaching behavior of adults. *Journal of Applied Behavior Analysis, 24,* 523–535.

Carstens, C. (1982). Application of a work penalty threat in the treatment of a case of juvenile firesetting. *Journal of Behavior Therapy and Experimental Psychiatry, 13,* 159–161.

Carta, J. (1995). Developmentally appropriate practice: A critical analysis as applied to young children with disabilities. *Focus on Exceptional Children, 27*(8), 1–14.

Carta, J. J. (Project Director) (n.d.). *Early childhood classroom survival skills project.* Kansas City: University of Kansas, Juniper Gardens Children's Project.

Carta, J. J., Atwater, J. B., Schwartz, I. S., & McConnell, S. R. (1993). Developmentally appropriate practices and early childhood special education: A reaction to Johnson and McChesney. *Topics in Early Childhood Special Education, 13*, 243–254.

Carta, J. J., Greenwood, C. R., & Atwater, J. B. (1985). *Ecobehavioral system for the complex assessment of preschool environments: ESCAPE.* Kansas City: Juniper Gardens Children's Project, Bureau of Child Research, University of Kansas. *ERIC* (ED 288 268) (EC 200 587).

Carta, J. J., Sainato, D. M., & Greenwood, C. R. (1988). Advances in the ecological assessment of classroom instruction for young children with handicaps. In S. L. Odom & M. B. Karnes (Eds.), *Early intervention for infants and children with handicaps* (pp. 217–239). Baltimore: Paul H. Brookes.

Carta, J. J., Schwartz, I. S., Atwater, J. B., & McConnell, S. R. (1991). Developmentally appropriate practice: Appraising its usefulness for young children with disabilities. *Topics in Early Childhood Special Education, 11*, 1–20.

Cash, W. M., & Evans, I. M. (1975). Training preschool children to modify their retarded siblings' behavior. *Journal of Behavioral Therapy and Experimental Psychiatry, 6*, 13–16.

Chamberlain, P., & Reid, J. B. (1987). Parent observation and report of child symptoms. *Behavioral Assessment, 9*, 97–109.

Chandler, L. K., Lubeck, R. C., & Fowler, S. A. (1992). Generalization and maintenance of preschool children's social skills: A critical review and analysis. *Journal of Applied Behavior Analysis, 25*, 415–428.

Christensen, A. P., & Sanders, M. R. (1987). Habit reversal and differential reinforcement of other behaviour in the treatment of thumb-sucking: An analysis of generalization and side-effects. *Journal of Child Psychology and Psychiatry, 28*, 281–295.

Christophersen, E. R. (1989). Health intervention research. *Education and Treatment of Children, 12*, 391–404.

Christophersen, E. R., Arnold, C. M., Hill, D. W., & Quilitch, H. R. (1972). The home point system: Token reinforcement procedures for application by parents of children with behavior problems. *Journal of Applied Behavior Analysis, 5*, 485–497.

Clark, H. B., Greene, B. F., Macrae, J. W., McNees, M. P., Davis, J. L., & Risley, T. R. (1977). A parent advice package for family shopping trips: Development and evaluation. *Journal of Applied Behavior Analysis, 10*, 605–624.

Clark, H. B., McManmon, L., Smith-Tuten, J. K., & Smith, J. (1985). *The Family Mealtime Game: Advice for parents* (No. 102). Tampa, FL: FMHI Publication Series. (Available from FMHI Publications, Florida Mental Health Institute, University of South Florida, Tampa, FL 33612.)

Clark, L. (1996). *SOS! Help for parents.* Bowling Green, KY: Parents Press.

Cole, D. A., Meyer, L. H., Vandercook, T., & McQuarter, R. J. (1986). Interactions between peers with and without severe handicaps: Dynamics of teacher intervention. *American Journal of Mental Deficiency, 91*(2), 160–169.

Colletti, G., & Harris, S. L. (1977). Behavior modification in the home: Siblings as behavior modifiers, parents as observers. *Journal of Abnormal Child Psychology*, *5*, 21–30.

Cone, J. D. (1978). The behavioral assessment grid (BAG): A conceptual framework and taxonomy. *Behavior Therapy*, *9*, 882–888.

Cone, J. D., & Hoier, T. S. (1986). Assessing children: The radical behavior perspective. In R. Prinz (Ed.), *Advances in behavioral assessment of children and families* (Vol. 2, pp. 1–27). Greenwich, CT: JAI Press.

Conger, R. D., & Lahey, B. B. (1982). Behavioral intervention for child abuse. *Behavior Therapist*, *5*, 49–53.

Consortium for Longitudinal Studies. (1983). *As the twig is bent . . . : Lasting effects of preschool programs*. Hillsdale, NJ: Erlbaum.

Cooper, J. O., Heron, T. E., & Heward, W. L. (1987). *Applied behavior analysis*. Columbus, OH: Merrill.

Corrao, J., & Melton, G. B. (1988). Legal issues in school-based behavior therapy. In J. C. Witt, S. N. Elliott, & F. M. Gresham (Eds.), *Handbook of behavior therapy in education* (pp. 377–399). New York: Plenum Press.

Crowley, C. P., & Armstrong, P. M. (1977). Positive practice, overcorrection and behavioral rehearsal in the treatment of three cases of encopresis. *Journal of Behavior Therapy and Experimental Psychiatry*, *8*, 411–416.

Cunningham, C. E. (1990). A family systems approach to family training. In R. A. Barkley (Ed.), *Attention-deficit hyperactivity disorder: A handbook for diagnosis and treatment* (pp. 432–461). New York: Guilford Press.

Cunningham, C. E., Cataldo, M. F., Mallion, C., & Keyes, J. B. (1983). A review and controlled single case evaluation of behavioral approaches to the management of elective mutism. *Child and Family Behavior Therapy*, *5*, 25–49.

Curtis, M. J., & Watson, K. (1980). Changes in consultee problem clarification skills following consultation. *Journal of School Psychology*, *18*, 210–221.

Dale, P. S., Crain-Thoreson, C., Notari-Syverson, A., & Cole, K. (1986). Parent–child book reading as an intervention technique for young children with language delays. *Topics in Early Childhood Special Education*, *16*, 213–235.

Daniel, J. (1995). New beginnings in transitions for difficult children. *Young Children*, *50*(3), 17–23.

Daro, D., & McCurdy, K. (1994). Preventing child abuse and neglect: Programmatic interventions. *Child Welfare*, *73*, 405–430.

Davis, C. A., & Reichle, J. (1996). Variant and invariant high-probability requests: Increasing appropriate behaviors in children with emotional–behavioral disorders. *Journal of Applied Behavior Analysis*, *29*, 471–482.

Deacon, J. R., & Konarski, E. A., Jr. (1987). Correspondence training: An example of rule-governed behavior? *Journal of Applied Behavior Analysis*, *20*, 391–400.

De Haas-Warner, S. (1992). The utility of self-monitoring for preschool on-task behavior. *Topics in Early Childhood Special Education*, *12*, 478–495.

Deitz, D. E. D., & Repp, A. C. (1983). Reducing behavior through reinforcement. *Exceptional Education Quarterly*, *3*, 34–46.

Deitz, S. M. (1977). An analysis of programming DRL schedules in educational settings. *Behavior Research and Therapy*, *15*, 103–111.

Dishion, T., Gardner, K., Patterson, G., Reid, J., Spyrou, S., & Thibodeaux, S.

(1984). *The Family Process Code: A multidimensional system for observing family interaction*. Eugene: Oregon Social Learning Center.

Division for Early Childhood (DEC) of the Council for Exceptional Children (1993). *Position on inclusion*. Washington, DC: Author.

Division for Early Childhood of the Council for Exceptional Children. (1994). Position on inclusion. *Young Children, 49*(5), 78.

Doleys, D. M. (1979). Assessment and treatment of childhood enuresis. In A. J. Finch & P. C. Kendall (Eds.), *Clinical treatment and research in childhood psychopathology* (pp. 207–233). New York: Spectrum.

Donnellan, A. M., & LaVigna, G. W. (1990). Myths about punishment. In A. C. Repp & N. N. Singh (Eds.), *Perspectives on the use of nonaversive and aversive interventions for persons with developmental disabilities* (pp. 33–57). Sycamore, IL: Sycamore.

Drotar, D., & Crawford, P. (1987). Using home observation in the clinical assessment of children. *Journal of Clinical Child Psychology, 16*, 342–349.

Ducharme, J. M. (1996). Errorless compliance training: Optimizing clinical efficiency. *Behavior Modification, 20*, 259–280.

Dunlap, G., dePerczel, M., Clarke, S., Wilson, S., Wright, S., White, R., & Gomez, A. (1994). Choice making to promote adaptive behavior for students with emotional and behavioral challenges. *Journal of Applied Behavior Analysis, 27*, 505–518.

Dunlap, G., & Kern, L. (1996). Modifying instructional activities to promote desirable behavior: A conceptual and practical framework. *School Psychology Quarterly, 11*, 297–312.

Dunst, C. J., McWilliam, R. A., & Holbert, K. (1986). Assessment of preschool classroom environments. *Diagnostique, 11*, 212–232.

Dunst, C. J., Snyder, S. W., & Mankinen, M. (1990). Efficacy of early intervention. In M.C. Wang, M. C. Reynolds, & H. J. Walberg (Eds.), *Handbook of special education: Research and practice: Volume 3. Low incidence conditions* (pp. 259–294). Elmsford, NY: Pergamon Press.

Dunst, C. J., & Trivette, C. M. (1987). Enabling and empowering families: Conceptual and intervention issues. *School Psychology Review, 16*, 443–456.

Dunst, C. J., Trivette, C. M., & Deal, A. (1988). *Enabling and empowering families: Principles and guidelines for practice*. Cambridge, MA: Brookline.

Durand, V. M. (1990). *Severe behavior problems: A functional communication training approach*. New York: Guilford Press.

Durand, V. M. (1998). *Sleep better: A guide to improving sleep for children with special needs*. Baltimore: Paul H. Brookes.

Durand, V. M., Berotti, D., & Weiner, J. (1993). Functional communication training. In J. Reichle & D. P. Wacker (Eds.), *Communication alternatives to challenging behavior* (Vol. 3, pp. 317–340). Baltimore: Paul H. Brookes.

Durand, V. M., & Mindell, J. A. (1990). Behavioral treatment of multiple childhood sleep disorders: Effects on child and family. *Behavior Modification, 14*, 37–49.

Ehrhardt, K. E., Barnett, D. W., Lentz, F. E., Stollar, S. E., & Reifen, L. (1996). Innovative methodology in ecological consultation: Use of scripts to promote treatment acceptability and integrity. *School Psychology Quarterly, 11*, 149–168.

Eisenberger, R., & Cameron, J. (1996). Detrimental effects of reward: Reality or myth? *American Psychologist, 51,* 1153–1166.

Eiserman, W. D., Shisler, L., & Healey, S. (1995). A community assessment of preschool providers' attitudes toward inclusion. *Journal of Early Intervention, 19*(2), 149–167.

English, K., Goldstein, H., Shafer, K., & Kaczmarek, L. (1997). Promoting interactions among preschoolers with and without disabilities: Effects of a buddy skills-training program. *Exceptional Children, 63,* 229–243.

Esposito, B. G. (1987). The effects of preschool integration on the development of nonhandicapped children. *Journal of the Division of Early Childhood, 12,* 31–46.

Etzel, B. C., LeBlanc, J. M., Schilmoeller, K. J., & Stella, M. E. (1981). Stimulus control procedures in the education of young children. In S. W. Bijou & R. Ruiz (Eds.), *Behavior modification: Contribution to education* (pp. 3–37). Hillsdale, NJ: Erlbaum.

Evans, I. M., & Meyer, L. H. (1985). *An educative approach to behavior problems: A practical decision model for interventions with severely handicapped learners.* Baltimore: Paul H. Brookes.

Evans, I. M., & Meyer, L. H. (1987). Moving to educational validity: A reply to Test, Spooner, and Cooke. *Journal of the Association for Persons with Severe Handicaps, 12,* 103–106.

Fagot, B., & Hagan, R. (1988). Is what we see what we get? Comparisons of taped and live observations. *Behavioral Assessment, 10,* 367–374.

Fantuzzo, J. W., Stevenson, H.C., Weiss, A. D., Hampton, V. R., & Noone, M. J. (1997). A partnership-directed school-based intervention for child physical abuse and neglect: Beyond mandatory reporting. *School Psychology Review, 26*(2), 298–313.

Fantuzzo, J., Weiss, A., & Coolahan, K. C. (1998). Community-based partnership-directed research: Actualizing community strengths to treat child victims of physical abuse and neglect. In J. R. Lutzker (Ed.), *Handbook of child abuse research and treatment* (pp. 31–52). New York: Plenum Press.

Farran, D. C. (1990). Effects of intervention with disadvantaged and disabled children: A decade review. In S. J. Meisels & J. P. Shonkoff (Eds.), *Handbook of early childhood intervention* (pp. 501–539). New York: Cambridge University Press.

Fawcett, S. B., Mathews, R. M., & Fletcher, R. K. (1980). Some promising dimensions for behavioral community technology. *Journal of Applied Behavior Analysis, 13,* 505–518.

Federal Emergency Management Agency (1994). *The National Juvenile Firesetter/Arson Control and Prevention Program.* Washington, DC: U.S. Fire Administration, U.S. Government Printing Office.

Ferber, R. (1985). *Solve your child's sleep problems.* New York: Simon & Schuster.

Fewell, R. R., & Oelwein, P. L. (1990). The relationship between time in integrated environments and developmental gains in young children with special needs. *Topics in Early Childhood Special Education, 10*(2), 104–116.

Field, T. (1984). Play behaviors of handicapped children who have friends. In T. Field, J. L. Roopnarine, & M. Segal (Eds.), *Friendships in normal and handicapped children* (pp. 153–162). Norwood, NJ: Ablex.

File, N. (1994). Children's play, teacher–child interactions, and teacher beliefs in integrated early childhood programs. *Early Childhood Research Quarterly, 9*, 223–240.

File, N., & Kontos, S. (1993). The relationship of program quality to children's play in integrated early intervention settings. *Topics in Early Childhood Special Education, 13*, 1–18.

Firestone, P. (1976). The effects and side effects of timeout on an aggressive nursery school child. *Journal of Behavior Therapy and Experimental Psychiatry, 6*, 79–81.

Flanagan, S., Adams, H. E., & Forehand, R. (1979). A comparison of four instructional techniques for teaching parents to use time-out. *Behavior Therapy, 10*, 94–102.

Fleming, L. A., Wolery, M., Weinzierl, C., Venn, M. L., & Schroeder, C. (1991). Model for assessing and adapting teachers' roles in mainstreamed preschool settings. *Topics in Early Childhood Special Education, 11*(1), 85–98.

Forehand, R., & McMahon, R. J. (1981). *Helping the noncompliant child: A clinician's guide to parent training.* New York: Guilford Press.

Forsythe, W. I., & Redmond, A. (1974). Enuresis and spontaneous cure rate: Study of 1,129 enuretics. *Archives of Disease in Childhood, 49*, 259–263.

Foster, S. L., & Cone, J. D. (1986). Design and use of direct observation. In A. R. Ciminero, K. S. Calhoun, & H. E. Adams (Eds.), *Handbook of behavioral assessment* (2nd ed., pp. 253–324). New York: Wiley.

Fowler, S. A. (1986). Peer-monitoring and self-monitoring: Alternatives to traditional teacher management. *Exceptional Children, 52*, 573–581.

Fowler, S. A., & Baer, D. M. (1981). "Do I have to be good all day?" The timing of delayed reinforcement as a factor in generalization. *Journal of Applied Behavior Analysis, 14*, 13–24.

Fox, J., & McEvoy, M. A. (1993). Assessing and enhancing generalization and social validity of social skills interventions with children and adolescents. *Behavior Modification, 17*, 336–339.

Fox, J., Shores, R., Lindeman, D., & Strain, P. (1986). Maintaining social initiations of withdrawn handicapped and nonhandicapped preschoolers through a response-dependent fading tactic. *Journal of Abnormal Child Psychology, 14*, 387–396.

Fox, L., Dunlap, G., & Philbrick, L. A. (1997). Providing individual supports to young children with autism and their families. *Journal of Early Intervention, 21*, 1–14.

Fox, L., Hanline, M. F., Vail, C. O., & Galant, K. R. (1994). Developmentally appropriate practice: Applications for young children with disabilities. *Journal of Early Intervention, 18*, 243–257.

Foxx, R.M. (1996). Twenty years of applied behavior analysis in treating the most severe problem behavior: Lessons learned. *Behavior Analyst, 19*, 225–235.

Foxx, R. M., & Azrin, N. H. (1973). *Toilet training the retarded: A rapid program for day and nighttime independent toileting.* Champaign, IL: Research Press.

Frankel, F., & Weiner, H. (1990). The Child Conflict Index: Factor analysis, reliability, and validity for clinic-referred and non-referred children. *Journal of Clinical Child Psychology, 19*, 239–248.

Friedlander, S., Weiss, D. S., & Traylor, J. (1986). Assessing the influence of maternal depression on the validity of the child behavior checklist. *Journal of Abnormal Child Psychology, 14*, 123–133.

Friman, P. C., & Jones, K. M. (1998). Elimination disorders in children. In T. W. Watson & F. M. Gresham (Eds.), *Handbook of child behavior therapy* (pp. 239–260). New York: Plenum Press.

Fuchs, L. S., & Fuchs, D. (1986). Linking assessment to instructional interventions: An overview. *School Psychology Review, 15*, 318–323.

Furlong, M. J., & Wampold, B. E. (1982). Intervention effects and relative variation as dimensions in experts' use of visual inference. *Journal of Applied Behavior Analysis, 15*, 415–421.

Garbarino, J. (1982). *Children and families in the social environment.* New York: Aldine.

Garbarino, J., & Stott, F. M. (1989). *What children can tell us.* San Francisco: Jossey-Bass.

Garmezy, N. (1985). Stress-resistant children: The search for protective factors. In J. E. Stevenson (Ed.), *Recent research in developmental psychopathology* (pp. 213–233). New York: Pergamon Press.

Gast, D. L., Collins, B. C., Wolery, M., & Jones, R. (1993). Teaching preschool children with disabilities to respond to the lures of strangers. *Exceptional Children, 59*, 301–311.

Gelfand, D. M., & Hartmann, D. P. (1984). *Child behavior analysis and therapy* (2nd ed.). New York: Pergamon Press.

Gelfand, D. M., Jenson, W. R., & Drew, C. J. (1982). *Understanding child behavior disorders.* New York: Holt, Rinehart & Winston.

Gemmel-Crosby, S., & Hanzlik, J. R. (1994). Preschool teachers' perceptions of including children with disabilities. *Education and Training in Mental Retardation and Developmental Disabilities, 29*(4), 279–290.

Gibbs, J. T., & Huang, L. N. (1989). *Children of color: Psychological interventions with minority youth.* San Francisco: Jossey-Bass.

Goldstein H. (1993.) Use of peers as communication intervention agents. *Teaching Exceptional Children, 25*(2), 37–42.

Goldstein, H., & Cisar, C. L. (1992). Promoting interaction during sociodramatic play: Teaching scripts to typical preschoolers and classmates with disabilities. *Journal of Applied Behavior Analysis, 25*, 265–280.

Goldstein, J. H. (Ed.). (1994). *Toys, play, and child development.* New York: Cambridge University Press.

Gottman, J. M. (1986). Merging social cognition and social behavior. *Monographs of the Society for Research in Child Development, 51*(22, Serial No. 213, 81–85).

Green, G. (1990). Least restrictive use of reductive procedures: Guidelines and competencies. In A. C. Repp & N. N. Singh (Eds.), *Perspectives on the use of nonaversive and aversive interventions for persons with developmental disabilities* (pp. 479–493). Sycamore, IL: Sycamore.

Green, R. B., Hardison, W. L., & Greene, B. F. (1984). Turning the table on advice programs for parents: Using placemats to enhance family interaction at restaurants. *Journal of Applied Behavior Analysis, 17*, 497–508.

Greene, B. F., Clark, H. B., & Risley, T. R. (1977). *Shopping with children: Advice for parents.* San Rafael, CA: Academic Therapy Publications. (Available from

FMHI Publications, Florida Mental Health Institute, University of South Florida, Tampa, FL 33612.)

Greene, B. F., & Kilili, S. (1998). How good does a parent have to be? Issues and examples associated with empirical assessments of parenting adequacy in cases of child abuse and neglect. In J. R. Lutzker (Ed.), *Handbook of child abuse research and treatment* (pp. 53–72). New York: Plenum Press.

Greenwood, C. R., Delquadri, J. C., & Hall, V. R. (1984). Opportunities to respond and student academic performance. In W. L. Heward, T. E. Heron, D. S. Hill, & J. Trap-Porter (Eds.), *Focus on behavior analysis in education* (pp. 58–88). Columbus, OH: Merrill.

Greenwood, C. R., Hops, H., Todd, N. M., & Walker, H. M. (1982). Behavior change targets in the assessment and treatment of socially withdrawn preschool children. *Behavioral Assessment, 4,* 273–297.

Greenwood, C. R., Walker, H. M., Todd, N. M., & Hops, H. (1981). Normative and descriptive analysis of preschool free play social interaction rates. *Journal of Pediatric Psychology, 6,* 343–367.

Greenwood, K. M., & Matyas, T. A. (1990). Problems with the application of interrupted time series analysis for brief single subject data. *Behavioral Assessment, 12,* 355–370.

Gresham, F. M. (1991). Conceptualizing behavior disorders in terms of resistance to intervention. *School Psychology Review, 20,* 23–36.

Gresham, F. M. (1989). Assessment of treatment integrity in school consultation/prereferral intervention. *School Psychology Review, 18,* 37–50.

Gresham, F. M., & Gensle, K. A. (1992). Misguided assumptions of DSM-III-R: Implications for school psychological practice. *School Psychological Quarterly, 7,* 79–95.

Gresham, F. M., & Gresham, G. N. (1982). Interdependent, dependent, and independent group contingencies for controlling disruptive behavior. *Journal of Special Education, 16,* 101–110.

Griest, D. L., Forehand, R., Rogers, T., Breiner, J., Furey, W., & Williams, C. A. (1982). Effects of parent enhancement therapy on the treatment outcome and generalization of a parent training program. *Behaviour Research and Therapy, 20,* 429–436.

Griffith, R. G. (1983) The administrative issues: An ethical and legal perspective. In S. Axelrod & J. Apsche (Eds.), *The effects of punishment on human behavior* (pp. 317–338). New York: Academic Press.

Grigg, N. C., Snell, M. E., & Loyd, B. (1989). Visual analysis of student data: A qualitative analysis of teacher decision making. *Journal of the Association for Persons with Severe Handicaps, 14,* 23–32.

Guevremont, D. C., Osnes, P. G., & Stokes, T. F. (1988). Preschoolers' goal setting with contracting to facilitate maintenance. *Behavior Modification, 12,* 404–423.

Guralnick, M. J. (Ed.). (1997). *The effectiveness of early intervention.* Baltimore: Paul H. Brookes.

Guralnick, M. J. (1987). The peer relationships of young handicapped and non-handicapped children. In P. S. Strain, M. J. Guralnick, & H. M. Walker (Eds.), *Children's social behavior: Development, assessment, and modification* (pp. 93–140). Orlando, FL: Academic Press.

Gutkin, T. B. (1996). Patterns of consultant and consultee verbalizations: Examining communication leadership during initial consultation interviews. *Journal of School Psychology, 34,* 199–219.

Gutkin, T. B., & Curtis, M. J. (1982). School-based consultation: Theory and techniques. In C. R. Reynolds & T. B. Gutkin (Eds.), *Handbook of school psychology* (pp. 796–828). New York: Wiley.

Gutkin, T. B., & Curtis, M. J. (1990). School-based consultation: Theory, techniques, and research. In C. R. Reynolds & T. B. Gutkin (Eds.), *Handbook of school psychology* (2nd ed., pp. 577–611). New York: Wiley.

Hall, R. V., & Hall, M. C. (1998a). *How to use systematic attention and approval* (2nd ed.). Austin, TX: Pro-Ed.

Hall, R. V., & Hall, M. C. (1998b). *How to use planned ignoring* (extinction) (2nd ed.). Austin, TX: Pro-Ed.

Hall, R. V., & Hall, M. C. (1998c). *How to select reinforcers* (2nd ed.). Austin, TX: Pro-Ed.

Hall, R. V., & Van Houten, R. (1983). *Managing behavior: Part 1. Behavior modification: The measurement of behavior.* Austin, TX: Pro-Ed.

Halle, J. W., Baer, D. M., & Spradlin, J. E. (1981). Teachers' generalized use of delay as a stimulus control procedure to increase language use in handicapped children. *Journal of Applied Behavior Analysis, 14,* 389–409.

Halle, J. W., Alpert, C. L., & Anderson, S. R. (1984). Natural environment language assessment and intervention with severely impaired preschoolers. *Topics in Early Childhood Special Education, 4,* 36–56.

Hampel, N. T. (1991). *A teacher interview as a screening tool for a preschool population.* Unpublished doctoral dissertation, University of Cincinnati.

Hancock, T. B., & Kaiser, A. P. (1996). Siblings' use of milieu teaching at home. *Topics in Early Childhood Special Education, 16,* 168–190.

Hanline, M. F. (1993). Inclusion of preschoolers with profound disabilities: An analysis of children's interactions. *Journal of the Association of Persons with Severe Handicaps (JASH), 18,* 28–35.

Hanson, M. J., & Hanline, M. F. (1990). Parenting a child with a disability: A longitudinal study of parent stress and adaptation. *Journal of Early Intervention, 14,* 234–248.

Hansen, D. J., Warner-Rogers, J. E., & Hecht, D. B. (1998). Implementing and evaluating an individualized behavioral intervention program for maltreatng families: Clinical and research issues. In J. R. Lutzker (Ed.), *Handbook of child abuse research and treatment* (pp. 133–158). New York: Plenum Press.

Harding, J., Wacker, D. P., Cooper, L. J., Millard, T., & Jensen-Kovalan, P. (1994). Brief hierarchical assessment of potential treatment components with children in an outpatient clinic. *Journal of Applied Behavior Analysis, 27,* 291–300.

Hardman, M. L., McDonnell, J., & Welch, M. (1997). Perspectives on the future of IDEA. *Journal of the Association for Persons with Severe Handicaps, 22,* 61–77.

Haring, N. G. (Ed.). (1988). *Generalizations for students with severe handicaps: Strategies and solutions.* Seattle: University of Washington Press.

Haring, N. G., Liberty, K. A., & White, O. R. (1980). Rules for data-based strategy decisions in instructional programs. In W. Sailor, B. Wilcox, & L. Brown

(Eds.), *Methods of instruction for severely handicapped students* (pp. 159–192). Baltimore: Paul H. Brookes.

Harms, T., Clifford, R. C., & Cryer, D. (1998). *Early childhood environment rating scale* (rev. ed.). New York: Teachers College Press.

Harris, K. R. (1985). Definitional, parametric, and procedural considerations in timeout interventions and research. *Exceptional Children, 51,* 279–288.

Harris, T. A., Peterson, S. L., Filliben, T. L., & Glassberg, M. (1998). Evaluating a more cost-effective alternative to providing in-home feedback to parents: The use of spousal feedback. *Journal of Applied Behavior Analysis, 31,* 131–134.

Harrop, A., & Daniels, M. (1993). Further appraisal of momentary time sampling and partial interval recording. *Journal of Applied Behavior Analysis, 26,* 277–278.

Hart, B. (1985). Naturalistic language training techniques. In S. F. Warren, & A. Rogers-Warren (Eds.), *Teaching functional language* (pp. 63–85). Austin, TX: Pro-Ed.

Hart, B., & Risley, T. R. (1975). Incidental teaching of language in the preschool. *Journal of Applied Behavior Analysis, 8,* 411–420.

Hart, B., & Risley, T. R. (1980). *In vivo* language intervention: Unanticipated general effects. *Journal of Applied Behavior Analysis, 12,* 407–432.

Hart, B., & Risley, T. R. (1982). *How to use incidental teaching for elaborating language.* Austin, TX: Pro-Ed.

Hart, B., & Risley, T. R. (1995). *Meaningful differences.* Baltimore: Paul H. Brookes.

Hart, S. N. (1991). From property to person status: Historical perspectives on children's rights. *American Psychologist, 46,* 53–59.

Hart, S. N., & Brassard, M. R. (1987). A major threat to children's mental health: Psychological maltreatment. *American Psychologist, 42,* 160–165.

Hartmann, D. P. (1984). Assessment strategies. In D. H. Barlow & M. Hersen (Eds.), *Single case experimental designs: Strategies for studying behavior change* (2nd ed., pp. 107–139). New York: Pergamon Press.

Harvey, P., Forehand, R., Brown, C., & Holmes, T. (1988). The prevention of sexual abuse: Examination of the effectiveness of a program with kindergarten-aged children. *Behavior Therapy, 19,* 429–435.

Haskins, R. (1989). The efficacy of early childhood intervention. *American Psychologist, 44,* 242–282.

Havey, J. M. (1998). Inclusion, the law, and placement decisions: Implications for school psychologists. *Psychology in the Schools, 35*(2), 145–152.

Hawkins, R. P. (1986). Selection of target behaviors. In R. O. Nelson & S. C. Hayes (Eds.), *Conceptual foundations of behavioral assessment* (pp. 331–385). New York: Guilford Press.

Hay, L. R., Nelson, R. O., & Hay, W. M. (1980). Methodological problems in the use of participant observers. *Journal of Applied Behavior Analysis, 13,* 501–504.

Hayes, L. A. (1976). The use of group contingencies for behavioral control: A review. *Psychological Bulletin, 83,* 628–648.

Hayes, S. C. (1981). Single case experimental designs and empirical clinical practice. *Journal of Consulting and Clinical Psychology, 49,* 193–211.

Hayes, S. C., Follette, V. M., Dawes, R. M., & Grady, K. E. (Eds.). (1995). *Scientific standards of psychological practice: Issues and recommendations.* Reno, NV: Context Press.

Hayes, S. C., & Nelson, R. O. (1986). Assessing the effects of therapeutic interventions. In R. O. Nelson & S. C. Hayes (Eds.), *Conceptual foundations of behavioral assessment* (pp. 430–460). New York: Guilford Press.

Hayes, S. C., Nelson, R. O., & Jarrett, R. B. (1986). Evaluating the quality of behavioral assessment. In R. O. Nelson & S. C. Hayes (Eds.), *Conceptual foundations of behavioral assessment* (pp. 461–503). New York: Guilford Press.

Hayes, S. C., Rosenfarb, I., Wulfert, E., Munt, E. D., Korn, Z., & Zettle, R. D. (1985). Self-reinforcement effects: An artifact of social standard setting? *Journal of Applied Behavior Analysis, 18,* 201–214.

Haymes, L. K., Fowler, S. A., & Cooper, A. Y. (1994). Assessing the transition and adjustment of preschoolers with special needs to an integrated program. *Journal of Early Intervention, 18*(2) 184–198.

Haynes, S. N. (1986). The design of intervention programs. In R. O. Nelson & S. C. Hayes (Eds.), *Conceptual foundations of behavioral assessment* (pp. 386–429). New York: Guilford Press.

Hecimovic, A., Fox, J. J., Shores, R. E., & Strain, P. S. (1985). An analysis of developmentally integrated and segregated free play settings and the generalization of newly acquired social behaviors of socially withdrawn preschoolers. *Behavioral Assessment, 7,* 367–388.

Hendrickson, J. M., Strain, P. S., Tremblay, A., & Shores, R. E. (1982). Interactions of behaviorally handicapped children: Functional effects of peer social initiations. *Behavior Modification, 6,* 323–353.

Hepting, N. H., & Goldstein, H. (1996). What's natural about naturalistic language intervention? *Journal of Early Intervention, 20,* 249–265.

Herrnstein, R. J. (1970). On the law of effect. *Journal of the Experimental Analysis of Behavior, 13,* 243–266.

Hitz, R., & Driscoll, A. (1988). Praise or encouragement? New insights into praise: Implications for early childhood teachers. *Young Children, 43*(5), 6–13.

Hobbs, N. (1966). Helping disturbed children: Psychological and ecological strategies. *American Psychologist, 21,* 1105–1115.

Hoier, T. S., McConnell, S., & Pallay, A. G. (1987). Observational assessment for planning and evaluating educational transitions: An initial analysis of template matching. *Behavioral Assessment, 9,* 5–19.

Hopkins, B. L., & Herman, J. A. (1976). Evaluating interobserver reliability of interval data. *Journal of Applied Behavior Analysis, 10,* 121–126.

Hops, H., Fleischman, D., Guild, J., Paine, S., Street, A., Walker, H. M., & Greenwood, C. R. (1978). *Procedures for establishing effective relationships skills (peers).* Eugene: Center at Oregon for Research in the Behavioral Education of the Handicapped, University of Oregon.

Horner, R. D., & Baer, D. M. (1978). Multiple probe technique: A variation of the multiple baseline design. *Journal of Applied Behavior Analysis, 11,* 189–196.

Horner, R. H., Day, H. M., & Day, J. R. (1997). Using neutralizing routines to reduce problem behaviors. *Journal of Applied Behavior Analysis, 30,* 601–614.

Houlihan, D., & Brandon, P. K. (1996). Compliant in a moment: A commentary on Nevin. *Journal of Applied Behavior Analysis, 29,* 549–555.

Hulsey, T. L., Kerkman, D. D., & Pinon, M. F. (1997). What it takes for preschoolers to learn sex abuse prevention concepts. *Early Education & Development, 8,* 187–202.

Humphreys, L., Forehand, R., McMahon, R., & Roberts, M. (1978). Parental behavioral training to modify child compliance: Effects on untreated siblings. *Behavior Therapy and Experimental Psychiatry, 9,* 235–238.

Hundert, J., & Hopkins, B. (1992). Training supervisors in a collaborative team approach to promote peer interactions of children with disabilities in integrated preschools. *Journal of Applied Behavior Analysis, 25,* 385–400.

Hundert, J., & Houghton, A. (1992). Promoting social interaction of children with disabilities in integrated preschools: A failure to generalize. *Exceptional Children, 58*(4), 311–320.

Hundert, J., Mahoney, W. J., & Hopkins, B. (1993). The relationship between the peer interaction of children with disabilities in integrated preschools and resource and classroom teacher behaviors. *Topics in Early Childhood Special Education, 13*(3), 328–343.

Huynen, K. B., Lutzker, J. R., Bigelow, K. M., Touchette, P. E., & Campbell, R. V. (1996). Planned activities training for mothers of children with developmental disabilities: Community generalization and follow-up. *Behavior Modification, 20,* 406–427.

Isaacs, C. D. (1982). Treatment of child abuse: A review of the behavioral interventions. *Journal of Applied Behavior Analysis, 15,* 273–294.

Iwata, B. A. (1987). Negative reinforcement in applied behavior analysis: An emerging technology. *Journal of Applied Behavior Analysis, 20,* 361–368.

Iwata, B. A., Vollmer, T. R., & Zarcone, J. R. (1990). The experimental (functional) analysis of behavior disorders: Methodology, applications, and limitations. In A. C. Repp & N. N. Singh (Eds.), *Perspective on the use of nonaversive and aversive interventions for persons with developmental disabilities* (pp. 301–330). Sycamore, IL: Sycamore.

Jacobson, J. M., Bushell, D., Jr., & Risley, T. (1969). Switching requirements in a Head Start classroom. *Journal of Applied Behavior Analysis, 2,* 43–47.

James, S. D., & Egel, A. L. (1986). A direct prompting strategy for increasing reciprocal interactions between handicapped and nonhandicapped siblings. *Journal of Applied Behavior Analysis, 19,* 173–186.

Jenkins, J. R., Odom, S. L., & Speltz, M. L. (1989). Effects of social integration of preschool children with handicaps. *Exceptional Children, 55,* 420–428.

Jersild, A. T., & Holmes, F. B. (1935). Methods of overcoming children's fears. *Journal of Psychology, 1,* 75–104.

Jewett, J., & Clark, H. B. (1979). Teaching preschoolers to use appropriate dinnertime conversation: An analysis of generalization from home to school. *Behavior Therapy, 10,* 589–605.

Johnson-Martin, N. M., Attermeier, S. M., & Hacker, B. (1990). *The Carolina Curriculum for Preschoolers with Special Needs.* Baltimore: Paul H. Brookes.

Johnston, J. M., & Pennypacker, H. S. (1993). *Strategies and tactics of behavioral research* (2nd ed.). Hillsdale, NJ: Erlbaum.

Jones, M. M., & Carlier, L. L. (1995). Creating inclusionary opportunities for learners with multiple disabilities: A team-teaching approach. *Teaching Exceptional Children, 27*(3), 23–27.

Jones, R. T., & Kazdin, A. E. (1980). Teaching children how and when to make emergency telephone calls. *Behavior Therapy, 11,* 509–521.

Kagan, J. (1996). Three pleasing ideas. *American Psychologist, 51,* 901–908.

Kaiser, A. P. (1993). Parent-implemented language intervention: An environmental system perspective. In A. P. Kaiser & D. B. Gray (Eds.), *Enhancing children's communication: Research foundations for intervention* (pp. 63–84). Baltimore: Paul H. Brookes.

Kaiser, A. P., Hemmeter, M. L., Ostrosky, M. M., Fischer, R., Yoder, P., & Keefer, M. (1996). The effects of teaching parents to use responsive interaction strategies. *Topics in Early Childhood Education, 16,* 375–406.

Kaminski, R. A., & Good, R. H., III. (1996). Toward a technology for assessing basic early literacy skills. *School Psychology Review, 25,* 215–227.

Kamps, D. M., Leonard, B. R., Dugan, E. P., Boland, B., & Greenwood, C. R. (1991). The use of ecobehavioral assessment to identify naturally occurring effective procedures in classrooms serving students with autism and other developmental disabilities. *Journal of Behavioral Education, 1,* 369–397.

Kanfer, F. H. (1985). Target selection for clinical change programs. *Behavioral Assessment, 7,* 7–20.

Kanfer, F. H., & Gaelick, L. (1986). Self-management methods. In F. H. Kanfer & A. P. Goldstein (Eds.), *Helping people change: A textbook of methods* (3rd ed., pp. 283–245). New York: Pergamon Press.

Kanfer, F. H., & Grimm, L. G. (1977). Behavior analysis: Selecting target behaviors in the interview. *Behavior Modification, 1,* 7–28.

Kanfer, F. H., & Karoly, P. (1982). The psychology of self-management: Abiding issues and tentative directions. In P. Karoly & F. H. Kanfer (Eds.), *Self-management and behavior change: From theory to practice* (pp. 571–599). New York: Pergamon Press.

Kara, A., & Wahler, R. G. (1977). Organizational features of a young child's behavior. *Journal of Experimental Child Psychology, 24,* 24–39.

Karoly, P., & Kanfer, F. H. (Eds.). (1982). *Self-management and behavior change: From theory to practice.* New York: Pergamon Press.

Katims, D. S., & Pierce, P. L. (1995). Literacy-rich environments and the transition of young children with special needs. *Topics in Early Childhood Special Education, 15,* 219–234.

Kazdin, A. E. (1977a). Assessing the clinical or applied significance of behavior change through social validation. *Behavior Modification, 1,* 427–452.

Kazdin, A. E. (1977b). *The token economy: A review and evaluation.* New York: Plenum Press.

Kazdin, A. E. (1980). Acceptability of alternative treatments for deviant child behavior. *Journal of Applied Behavior Analysis, 13,* 259–273.

Kazdin, A. E. (1982a). The token economy: A decade later. *Journal of Applied Behavior Analysis, 15,* 431–445.

Kazdin, A. E. (1982b). *Single-case research designs.* New York: Oxford University Press.

Kazdin, A. E. (1984). *Behavior modification in applied settings* (3rd ed.). Homewood, IL: Dorsey.

Kazdin, A. E. (1985). Selection of target behaviors: The relationship of treatment focus to clinical dysfunction. *Behavior Assessment, 7*, 33–47.

Kazdin, A. E. (1994). *Behavior modification in applied settings* (5th ed.). Pacific Grove, CA: Brooks/Cole.

Kazdin, A. E., & Mascitelli, S. (1980). The opportunity to earn oneself off a token system as a reinforcer for attentive behavior. *Behavior Therapy, 11*, 68–78.

Kelly, G. A. (1955). *The psychology of personal constructs* (Vols. I & II). New York: Basic Books.

Kelley, M. L. (1990). *School–home notes: Promoting children's classroom success.* New York: Guilford Press.

Kennedy, C. H., & Itkonen, T. (1993). Effects of setting events on the problem behaviors of students with severe disabilities. *Journal of Applied Behavior Analysis, 26*, 321–327.

Kerr, M. M., & Nelson, C. M. (1998). *Strategies for managing behavior problems in the classroom* (3rd ed.). Columbus, OH: Merrill.

Koegel, R. L., & Frea, W. D. (1993). Treatment of social behavior in autism through the modification of pivotal social skills. *Journal of Applied Behavior Analysis, 26*, 369–377.

Koegel, R. L., & Koegel, L. K. (1988). Generalized responsivity and pivotal behaviors. In R. H. Horner, G. Dunlap, & R. L. Koegel (Eds.), *Generalization and maintenance* (pp. 41–66). Baltimore: Paul H. Brookes.

Koegel, L. K., Koegel, R. L., & Dunlap, G. (Eds.). (1996). *Positive behavioral support: Including people with difficult behavior in the community.* Baltimore: Paul H. Brookes.

Kohler, F. W., & Fowler, S. A. (1985). Training prosocial behaviors to young children: An analysis of reciprocity with untrained peers. *Journal of Applied Behavior Analysis, 18*, 187–200.

Kohler, F. W., & Strain, P. S. (1993). The Early Childhood Social Skills program. *Teaching Exceptional Children, 25*(2), 41–42.

Kohler, F. W., Strain, P. S., Hoyson, M., Davis, L., Donina, W. M., & Rapp, N. (1995). Using a group oriented contingency to increase social interactions between children with autism and their peers. *Behavior Modification, 19*, 10–32.

Kolko, D. (1998). Integration of research and treatment. In J. R. Lutzker (Ed.), *Handbook of child abuse research and treatment* (pp. 159–182). New York: Plenum Press.

Kolko, D. J. (1996). Education and counseling for child firesetters: A comparison of skills training programs with standard practice. In E. D. Hibbs & P. S. Jensen (Eds.), *Psychosocial treatments for child and adolescent disorders: Empirically based strategies for clinical practice* (pp. 409–433). Washington, DC: American Psychological Association.

Kolko, D. J. (1983). Multicomponent parental treatment of firesetting in a six year old boy. *Journal of Behavior Therapy and Experimental Psychiatry, 14*, 349–353.

Kolko, D. J. (1996). Clinical monitoring of treatment course in physical child abuse: Psychometric characteristics and treatment comparisons. *Child Abuse & Neglect, 20*, 23–43.

Kolko, D. J., & Kazdin, A. E. (1989a). Assessment of dimensions of childhood firesetting among patients and nonpatients: The firesetting risk interview. *Journal of Abnormal Child Psychology, 17,* 157–176.

Kolko, D. J., & Kazdin, A. E. (1989b). The children's firesetting interview with psychiatrically referred and nonreferred children. *Journal of Abnormal Child Psychology, 17,* 609–624.

Kolko, D. J., Watson, S., & Faust, J. (1991). Fire safety/prevention skills training to reduce involvement with fire in young psychiatric inpatients: Preliminary findings. *Behavior Therapy, 22,* 269–284.

Konarski, E. A., Jr., Johnson, M. R., Crowell, C. R., & Whitman, T. L. (1981). An alternative approach to reinforcement for applied researchers: Response deprivation. *Behavior Therapy, 12,* 653–666.

Koocher, G. P. (1976). *Children's rights and the mental health professions.* New York: Wiley.

Krantz, P. J., & Risley, T. R. (1977). Behavioral ecology in the classroom. In K. D. O'Leary & S. G. O'Leary (Eds.), *Classroom management: The successful use of behavior modification* (pp. 349–366). New York: Pergamon Press.

Kratochwill, T. R. (1978). Foundations of time series research. In T. R. Kratochwill (Ed.), *Single subject research: Strategies for evaluating change* (pp. 1–100). Orlando, FL: Academic Press.

Kratochwill, T. R. (1981). *Selective mutism: Implications for research and treatment.* Hillsdale, NJ: Erlbaum.

Kratochwill, T. R. (Guest Ed.). (1985). Mini-series on target behavior selection. *Behavioral Assessment, 7*(1).

Kratochwill, T. R., & Bergan, J. R. (1990). *Behavioral consultation in applied settings: An individual guide.* New York: Plenum Press.

Kratochwill, T. R., & Morris, R. J. (Eds.). (1991). *The practice of child therapy* (2nd ed.). New York: Pergamon Press.

Kubany, E. S., Weiss, L. E., & Sloggett, B. B. (1971). The good behavior clock: A reinforcement/timeout procedure for reducing disruptive classroom behavior. *Journal of Behavior Therapy and Experimental Psychiatry, 1,* 173–179.

Labbe, E. E., & Williamson, D. A. (1984). Behavioral treatment of elective mutism: A review of the literature. *Clinical Psychology Review, 4,* 273–292.

Lahey, B. B., Gendrich, J. G., Gendrich, S. I., Schnelle, J. F., Gant, D. S., & McNees, M. P. (1977). An evaluation of daily report cards with minimal teacher and parent contacts as an efficient method of classroom intervention. *Behavior Modification, 1,* 381–394.

Laosa, L. M., & Sigel, I. E. (Eds.). (1982). *Families as learning environments for children.* New York: Plenum Press.

Lattal, K. A., & Neef, N. A. (1996). Recent reinforcement-schedule research and applied behavior analysis. *Journal of Applied Behavior Analysis, 29,* 213–230.

LaVigna, G. W., & Donnellan, A. M. (1986). *Alternatives to punishment: Solving behavior problems with non-aversive strategies.* New York: Irvington.

Le Ager, C., & Shapiro, E. S. (1995). Template matching as a strategy for assessment of an intervention for preschool students with disabilities. *Topics in Early Childhood Special Education, 15,* 187–218.

LeBlanc, J. M., Etzel, B. C., & Domash, M. A. (1978). A functional curriculum for early intervention. In K. E. Allen, V. A. Holm, & R. L. Schiefelbusch (Eds.),

Early intervention-A team approach (pp. 331–381). Baltimore: University Park Press.

Lee, S., & Odom, S. L. (1996). The relationship between stereotypic behavior and peer social interaction for children with severe disabilities. *Journal of the Association for Persons with Severe Handicaps, 21*(2), 88–95.

Lefebvre, D., & Strain, P. S. (1989). Effects of a group contingency on the frequency of social interactions among autistic and nonhandicapped preschool children: Making LRE efficacious. *Journal of Early Intervention, 13*, 329–341.

LeLaurin, K., & Risley, T. R. (1972). The organization of day care environments: "Zone" versus "man-to-man" staff assignments. *Journal of Applied Behavior Analysis, 5*, 225–232.

LeLaurin, K., & Wolery, M. (1992). Research standards in early intervention: Defining, describing, and measuring the independent variable. *Journal of Early Intervention, 16*, 275–287.

Lentz, F. E. (1988). Reductive procedures. In J. C. Witt, S. N. Elliott, & F. M. Gresham (Eds.), *Handbook of behavior therapy in education* (pp. 439–468). New York: Plenum Press.

Lentz, F. E., Jr., Allen, S. J., & Ehrhardt, K. E. (1996). The conceptual elements of strong interventions in school settings. *School Psychology Quarterly, 11*, 118–136.

Lerman, D. C., & Iwata, B. A. (1993). Descriptive and experimental analysis of variables maintaining self-injurious behavior. *Journal of Applied Behavior Analysis, 26*, 293–319.

Lerman, D. C., & Iwata, B. A. (1996). Developing a technology for the use of operant extinction in clinical settings: An examination of basic and applied research. *Journal of Applied Behavior Analysis, 29*, 345–382.

Lewis, M. (1997). *Altering fate: Why the past does not predict the future.* New York: Guilford.

Liberty, K. (1988). Characteristics and foundations of decision rules. In N. G. Haring (Ed.), *Generalization for students with severe handicaps: Strategies and solutions* (pp. 53–72). Seattle: University of Washington Press.

Linehan, M. M. (1980). Content validity: Its relevance to behavioral assessment. *Behavioral Assessment, 2*, 147–159.

Lipsey, M. W. (1990). *Design sensitivity.* Newbury Park, CA: Sage.

Lipton, H. (1980). Rapid reinstatement of speech using stimulus fading with a selectively mute child. *Journal of Behavior Therapy and Experimental Psychiatry, 11*, 147–149.

Litow, L., & Pumroy, D. K. (1975). A review of classroom group-oriented contingencies. *Journal of Applied Behavior Analysis, 8*, 341–347.

Loeber, R., & Schmaling, K. B. (1985). Empirical evidence for overt and covert patterns of antisocial conduct problems: A metaanalysis. *Journal of Abnormal Child Psychology, 13*, 337–352.

Lohrmann-O'Rouke, S., & Zirkel, P. (1998). The case law on aversive interventions for students with disabilities. *Exceptional Children, 65*, 101–123.

Lovaas, O. I. (1981). *Teaching developmentally disabled children: The me book.* Austin, TX: Pro-Ed.

Lovaas, O. I., & Favell, J. E. (1987). Protection for clients undergoing aversive/restrictive interventions. *Education and Treatment of Children, 10*, 311–325.

Lowenthal, B. (1996). Teaching social skills to preschoolers with special needs. *Childhood Education, 72,* 137–140.

Lutzker, J. R., Bigelow, K. M., Doctor, R. M., Gershater, R. M., & Greene, B. F. (1998). An ecobehavioral model for the prevention and treatment of child abuse and neglect: History and applications. In J. R. Lutzker (Ed.), *Handbook of child abuse research and treatment* (pp. 239–266). New York: Plenum Press.

Lutzker, J. R., Frame, R. E., & Rice, J. M. (1982). Project 12-ways: An ecobehavioral approach to the treatment and prevention of child abuse and neglect. *Education and Treatment of Children, 5,* 141–155.

MacDonald, J. D. (1985). Language through conversation: A model for intervention with language-delayed persons. In S. F. Warren & A. K. Rogers-Warren (Eds.), *Teaching functional language: Generalization and maintenance of language skills* (pp. 89–122). Austin, TX: Pro-Ed.

Mace, F. C., Hock, M. L., Lalli, J. S., West, B. J., Belfiore, P., Pinter, E., & Brown, D. K. (1988). Behavioral momentum in the treatment of noncompliance. *Journal of Applied Behavior Analysis, 21,* 123–141.

Mace, F. C., & Kratochwill, T. R. (1988). Self-monitoring. In J. C. Witt, S. N. Elliott, & F. M. Gresham (Eds.), *Handbook of behavior therapy in education* (pp. 489–522). New York: Plenum Press.

Mace, F. C., Page, T. J., Ivancic, M. T., & O'Brien, S. (1986). Effectiveness of brief time-out with and without contingent delay: A comparative analysis. *Journal of Applied Behavior Analysis, 19,* 79–86.

Macmann, G. M., & Barnett, D. W. (1999). Diagnostic decision making in school psychology: Understanding and coping with uncertainty. In C. R. Reynolds & T. B. Gutkin (Eds.), *The handbook of school psychology* (3rd ed., pp. 519–548). New York: Wiley.

Macmann, G. M., Barnett, D. W., Allen, S. J., Bramlett, R. K., Hall, J. D., & Ehrhardt, K. E. (1996). Problem solving and intervention design: Guidelines for the evaluation of technical adequacy. *School Psychology Quarterly, 11,* 137–148.

MacMillan, D. L., & Turnbull, A. P. (1983). Parent involvement with special education: Respecting individual differences. *Education and Training of the Mentally Retarded, 18,* 4–9.

MacPhee, D., Ramey, C. T., & Yeates, K. O. (1984). Home environment and early cognitive development: Implications for intervention. In A. W. Gottfried (Ed.), *Home environment and early cognitive development: Longitudinal research* (pp. 343–369). Orlando, FL: Academic Press.

Mahoney, G., O'Sullivan, P., & Robinson, C. (1992). The family environments of children with disabilities: Diverse but not so different. *Topics in Early Childhood Special Education, 12*(3), 386–402.

Mahoney, G., Spiker, D., & Boyce, G. (1996). Clinical assessments of parent–child interactions: Are professionals ready to implement this practice? *Topics in Early Childhood Special Education, 16,* 26–50.

Marcus, B. A., & Vollmer, T. R. (1996). Combining noncontingent reinforcement and differential reinforcement schedules as treatment for aberrant behavior. *Journal of Applied Behavior Analysis, 29,* 43–51.

Martens, B. K., Halperin, S., Rummel, J. E., & Kilpatrick, D. (1990). Matching theory applied to contingent teacher attention. *Behavioral Assessment, 12,* 139–155.

Martens, B. K., & Kelly, S. Q. (1993). A behavioral analysis of effective teaching. *School Psychology Quarterly, 8,* 10–26.

Martens, B. K., Witt, J. C., Daly, E. J., III, & Vollmer, T. R. (1999). Behavior analysis: Theory and practice in educational settings. In C. R. Reynolds & T. B. Gutkin (Eds.), *The handbook of school psychology* (3rd ed., pp. 638–663). New York: Wiley.

Martin, J. A. (1989). Personal and interpersonal components of responsiveness. In M. H. Bornstein (Ed.), *Maternal responsiveness: Characteristics and consequences* (pp. 5–14). San Francisco: Jossey-Bass.

Martin, R. (1975). *Legal challenges to behavior modification: Trends in schools, mental health, and corrections.* Champaign, IL: Research Press.

Mash, E. J., & Barkley, R. A. (1998). *Treatment of childhood disorders* (2nd ed.). New York: Guilford Press.

Mash, E. J., & Barkley, R. A. (Eds.). (1997). *Assessment of childhood disorders* (3rd ed.). New York: Guilford Press.

Mason, S. A., McGee, G. G., Farmer-Dougan, V., & Risley, T. (1989). A practical strategy for ongoing reinforcer assessment. *Journal of Applied Behavior Analysis, 22,* 171–179.

Matson, J. L., & DiLorenzo, T. M. (1984). *Punishment and its alternatives: A new perspective for behavior modification.* New York: Springer.

McCormick, L., Noonan, M. J., & Heck, R. (1998). Variables affecting engagement in inclusive preschool classrooms. *Journal of Early Intervention, 21*(2), 160–176.

McCarty, B. C., McElfresh, C. T., Rice, S. V., & Wilson, S. J. (1978). The effect of contingent background music on inappropriate bus behavior. *Journal of Music Therapy, 15,* 150–156.

McCloskey, C. M. (1996). Taking positive steps toward classroom management in preschool: Loosening up without letting it all fall apart. *Young Children, 51*(3), 14–16.

McDonnell, A., & Hardman, M. (1988). A synthesis of "best practice" guidelines for early childhood services. *Journal of the Division for Early Childhood, 12,* 328–341.

McDowell, J. J. (1982). The importance of Herrnstein's mathematical statement of the law of effect for behavior therapy. *American Psychologist, 37,* 771–779.

McEvoy, M. A. (1990). The organization of caregiving environments: Critical issues and suggestions for future research. *Education and Treatment of Children, 13,* 269–273.

McEvoy, M. A., Twardosz, S., & Bishop, N. (1990). Affection activities: Procedures for encouraging young children with handicaps to interact with their peers. *Education and Treatment of Children, 13,* 159–167.

McGee, G. G., Almeida, C., Sulzer-Azaroff, B., & Feldman, R. S. (1992). Promoting reciprocal interactions via peer incidental teaching. *Journal of Applied Behavior Analysis, 25,* 117–126.

McGee, G. G., Paradis, T., & Feldman, R. S. (1993). Free effects of integration on levels of autistic behavior. *Topics in Early Childhood Special Education, 13*(1), 57–67.

McGillicuddy-Delisi, A. V. (1985). The relationship between parental beliefs and children's cognitive level. In I. E. Sigel (Ed.), *Parental belief systems: The psychological consequences for children* (pp. 7–24). New York: Plenum Press.

McGimsey, J. F., Greene, B. F., & Lutzker, J. R. (1995). Competence in aspects of behavioral treatment and consultation: Implications for service delivery and graduate training. *Journal of Applied Behavior Analysis, 28*, 301–315.

McGinnis, E., & Goldstein, A. P. (1990). *Skillstreaming in early childhood: Teaching prosocial skills to the preschool and kindergarten child.* Champaign, IL: Research Press.

McGrath, P., Marshall, P. G., & Prior, K. (1979). A comprehensive treatment program for a fire setting child. *Journal of Behavior Therapy and Experimental Psychiatry, 10*, 69–72.

McLaughlin, T. F., & Williams, R. L. (1988). The token economy. In J. C. Witt, S. N. Elliott, & F. M. Gresham (Eds.), *Handbook of behavior therapy in education* (pp. 469–487). New York: Plenum Press.

McLean, M., & Hanline, M. F. (1990). Providing early intervention service in integrated environments: Challenges and opportunities for the future, *Topics in Early Childhood Special Education, 10*(2), 62–77.

McLinden, S. E. (1990). Mothers' and fathers' reports of the effects of a young child with special needs on the family. *Journal of Early Intervention, 14*, 249–259.

McMahon, R. J. (1987). Some current issues in the behavioral assessment of conduct disordered children and their families. *Behavioral Assessment, 9*, 235–252.

McManmon, L., Peterson, C. R., Metelenis, L., McWhirter, J., & Clark, H. B. (1982). The development of a parental advice protocol for enhancing family mealtime. *Behavioral Counseling Quarterly, 2*, 156–167.

McMillen, J. C. (1997). A practice model for enhancing effective coping in child welfare families. *Child Welfare, 76*(6), 781–799.

McWilliam, R. A. (1991). Targeting teaching at children's use of time: Perspective on preschooler's engagement. *Teaching Exceptional Children, 23*, 42–43.

McWilliam, R. A., & Bailey, D. B. (1995). Effects of classroom social structure and disability on engagement. *Topics in Early Childhood Special Education, 15*, 123–147.

McWilliam, R. A., Trivette, C. M., & Dunst, C. J. (1985). Behavior engagement as a measure of the efficacy of early intervention. *Analysis and Intervention in Developmental Disabilities, 5*, 33–45.

Meichenbaum, D., & Goodman, J. (1971). Training impulsive children to talk to themselves: A means of developing self-control. *Journal of Abnormal Psychology, 77*, 115–126.

Melton, G. B. (1991). Socialization in the global community: Respect for the dignity of children. *American Psychologist, 46*, 66–71.

Melton, G. B., & Wilcox, B. L. (1989). Changes in family law and family life: Challenges for psychology. *American Psychologist, 44*, 1213–1216.

Messick, S. (1983). The assessment of children. In P. H. Mussen (Ed.), *Handbook of child psychology* (Vol. 1, pp. 477–526). New York: Wiley.

Messick, S. (1989). Validity. In R. L. Linn (Ed.), *Educational measurement* (3rd ed., pp. 13–103). New York: Macmillan.

Messick, S. (1995). Validity of psychological assessment: Validation of inferences from persons' responses and performances as scientific inquiry into score meaning. *American Psychologist, 50,* 741–749.

Meyer, L. H., & Evans, I. M. (1993). Science and practice in behavioral intervention: Meaningful outcomes, research validity, and usable knowledge. *Journal for the Association of Persons with Severe Handicaps, 18,* 224–234.

Michael, J. (1982). Distinguishing between discriminative and motivational functions of stimuli. *Journal of the Experimental Analysis of Behavior, 37,* 149–155.

Miller, L. J., Strain, P. S., Boyd, K., Hunsicker, S., McKinley, J., & Wu, A. (1992). Parental attitudes toward inclusion. *Topics in Early Childhood Special Education, 12*(2), 230–246.

Miller, N. B. (1994). *Nobody's perfect: Living and growing with children who have special needs.* Baltimore: Paul H. Brookes.

Miller, N. B., & Cantwell, D. P. (1976). Siblings as therapists: A behavioral approach. *American Journal of Psychiatry, 133*(4), 447–450.

Miltenberger, R. G., & Olsen, L. A. (1996). Abduction prevention training: A review of findings and issues for future research. *Education and Treatment of Children, 19,* 69–82.

Mischel, W. (1981). A cognitive-social learning approach to assessment. In T. V. Merluzzi, C. R. Glass, & M. Genest (Eds.), *Cognitive assessment* (pp. 479–502). New York: Guilford Press.

Mischel, W. (1984). Convergences and challenges in the search for consistency. *American Psychologist, 39,* 351–364.

Moncher, F. J., & Prinz, R. J. (1991). Treatment fidelity in outcome studies. *Child Psychology Review, 11,* 247–266.

Mori, L., & Peterson, L. (1986). Training preschoolers in safety skills to prevent inadvertent injury. *Journal of Clinical Child Psychology, 15,* 106–114.

Morin, C., Ladouceur, R., & Cloutier, R. (1982). Reinforcement procedure in the treatment of reluctant speech. *Journal of Behavior Therapy and Experimental Psychiatry, 13,* 145–147.

Morris, R. J., Kratochwill, T. R., & Aldridge, K. (1988). Fears and phobias. In J. C. Witt, S. N. Elliott, & F. M. Gresham (Eds), *Handbook of behavior therapy in education* (pp. 679–717). New York: Plenum Press.

Morrow, L. M., & Rand, M. K. (1991). Promoting literacy during play by designing early childhood classroom environments. *The Reading Teacher, 44,* 396–402.

National Association for the Education of Young Children. (September, 1986). Position statement on developmentally appropriate practice in early childhood programs serving children from birth through age 8. *Young Children,* 4–16.

National Association for the Education of Young Children. (1993). *Position on inclusion.* Washington, DC: Author.

National Association for the Education of Young Children. (1996). NAEYC position statement: Technology and young children—Ages three through eight. *Young Children, 51*(6), 11–16.

National Association of School Psychologists. (1984a). *Standards for the provision of school psychological services*. Washington, DC: Author.

National Association of School Psychologists. (1984b). *Principles for professional ethics*. Washington, DC: Author.

National Association of School Psychologists. (1993). *Position statement on inclusive programs for students with disabilities*. Washington, DC: Author.

Nelson, C. M., & Rutherford, R. B. (February, 1983). Timeout revisited: Guidelines for its use in special education. *Exceptional Education Quarterly, 56–67*.

Nelson, R. O., Hay, L. R., Devany, J., & Koslow-Green, L. (1980). The reactivity and accuracy of children's self-monitoring: Three experiments. *Child Behavior Therapy, 2*, 1–24.

Nelson, R. O., & Hayes, S. C. (1986). The nature of behavioral assessment. In R. O. Nelson & S. C. Hayes (Eds.), *Conceptual foundations of behavior assessment* (1–40). New York: Guilford Press.

Nevin, J. A. (1996). The momentum of compliance. *Journal of Applied Behavior Analysis, 29*, 535–547.

Niemeyer, J. A., & Fox, J. (1990). Reducing aggressive behavior during car riding through parent-implemented DRO and fading procedures. *Education and Treatment of Children, 13*, 21–35.

Noell, G. H., & Gresham, F. M. (1993). Functional outcome analysis: Do the benefits of consultation and prereferral intervention justify the cost? *School Psychology Quarterly, 8*, 200–227.

Nordquist, V. M., & Twardosz, S. (1990). Preventing behavior problems in early childhood special education classrooms through environmental organization. *Education and Treatment of Children, 13*, 274–287.

Nordquist, V. M., Twardosz, S., & McEvoy, M. A. (1991). Effects of environmental reorganization in classrooms for children with autism. *Journal of Early Intervention, 15*, 135–152.

Northup, J., George, T., Jones, K., Broussard, C., & Vollmer, T. R. (1996). A comparison of reinforcement assessment methods: The utility of verbal and pictorial choice procedures. *Journal of Applied Behavior Analysis, 29*, 201–212.

Novak, M. A., Olley, J. G., & Kearney, D. S. (1980). Social skills of children with special needs in integrated and separate preschools. In T. M. Field (Ed.), *High risk infant and children: Adult and peer interactions* (pp. 327–345). New York: Academic Press.

Odom, S. L., Bender, M. K., Stein, M. L., Doran, L. P., Houden, P. M., McInnes, M., Gilbert, M. M., Deklyen, M., Speltz, M. L., & Jenkins, J. R. (1988). *The integrated preschool curriculum: Procedures for socially integrating young handicapped and normally developing children*. Seattle: University of Washington Press.

Odom, S. L., Hoyson, M., Jamieson, B., & Strain, P. S. (1985). Increasing handicapped preschoolers' peer social interactions: Cross-setting and component analysis. *Journal of Applied Behavior Analysis, 18*, 3–16.

Odom, S. L., & Strain, P. S. (1984). Peer-mediated approaches to promoting children's social interaction: A review. *American Journal of Orthopsychiatry, 54*, 544–557.

Odom, S. L., & Strain, P. S. (1986). A comparison of peer-initiation and teacher-antecedent interventions for promoting reciprocal social interaction of autistic preschoolers. *Journal of Applied Behavior Analysis, 19*, 59–71.

Ollendick, T. H., & Francis, G. (1988). Behavioral assessment and treatment of childhood phobias. *Behavior Modification, 12*(2), 165–204.

O'Neill, R. E., Horner, R. H., Albin, R. W., Sprague, J. R., Storey, K., & Newton, J. S. (1997). *Functional assessment and program development for problem behavior: A practical handbook* (2nd ed). Pacific Grove, CA: Brooks/Cole.

Osnes, P. G., Guevremont, D. C., & Stokes, T. F. (1986). If I say I'll talk more, then I will: Correspondence training to increase peer-directed talk by socially withdrawn children. *Behavior Modification, 10*, 287–299.

Pace, G. M., Ivancic, M. T., Edwards, G. L., Iwata, B. A., & Page, T. J. (1985). Assessment of stimulus preference and reinforcer value with profoundly retarded individuals. *Journal of Applied Behavior Analysis, 18*, 249–255.

Page, T. J., & Iwata, B. A. (1986). Interobserver agreement: History, theory, and current methods. In A. Poling & R. W. Fuqua (Eds.), *Research methods in applied behavior analysis* (pp. 99–126). New York: Plenum Press.

Paine, S. C., Radicchi, J., Rosellini, L. C., Deutchman, L., & Darch, C. B. (1983). *Structuring your classroom for academic success.* Champaign, IL: Research Press.

Panaccione, V. F., & Wahler, R. G. (1986). Child behavior, maternal depression, and social coercion as factors in the quality of child care. *Journal of Abnormal Child Psychology, 14*, 263–278.

Panyan, M. (1980). *How to use shaping.* Austin, TX: Pro-Ed.

Parker, R., Tindal, G., & Stein, S. (1992). Estimating trend in progress monitoring data: A comparison of simple line-fitting methods. *School Psychology Review, 21*, 300–312.

Parpal, M., & Maccoby, E. E. (1985). Maternal responsiveness and subsequent child compliance. *Child Development, 56*, 1326–1334.

Parsonson, B. S., & Baer, D. M. (1978). The analysis and presentation of graphic data. In T. R. Kratochwill (Ed.), *Single subject research: Strategies for evaluating change* (pp. 101–165). Orlando, FL: Academic Press.

Parsonson, B. S., & Baer, D. M. (1986). The graphic analysis of data. In A. Poling & W. R. Fuqua (Eds.), *Research methods in applied behavior analysis* (pp. 157–186). New York: Plenum Press.

Parten, M. B. (1932). Social participation among preschool children. *Journal of Abnormal and Social Psychology, 27*, 243–269.

Patterson, G. R. (1975a). *Families.* Champaign, IL: Research Press.

Patterson, G. R. (1975b). *Professional guide for families and living with children.* Champaign, IL: Research Press.

Patterson, G. R., & Bank, L. (1986). Bootstrapping your way in the nomological thicket. *Behavioral Assessment, 8*, 49–73.

Patterson, G. R., Reid, J. B., Jones, R. R., & Conger, R. E. (1975). *A social learning approach to family intervention* (Vol. 1). Eugene, OR: Castalia.

Pazulinec, R., Meyerrose, M., & Sajwaj, T. (1983). Punishment via response cost. In S. Axelrod & J. Apsche (Eds.), *The effects of punishment on human behavior* (pp. 71–86). New York: Academic Press.

Peck, S. M., Wacker, D. P., Berg, W. K., Cooper, L. J., Brown, K. A., Richman, D., McComas, J. J., Frischmeyer, P., & Millard, T. (1996). Choice-making treatment of young children's severe behavior problems. *Journal of Applied Behavior Analysis, 29*, 263–290.

Peters, C. (1995). *Preschool activity centers: Effects on opportunities to engage in social interactions.* Unpublished doctoral dissertation, University of Cincinnati.

Peterson, D. R. (1968). *The clinical study of social behavior.* New York: Appleton–Century–Crofts.

Peterson, L. (1984a). The "Safe at Home" game: Training comprehensive prevention skills in latchkey children. *Behavior Modification, 8,* 474–494.

Peterson, L. (1984b). Teaching home safety and survival skills to latch-key children: A comparison of two manuals and methods. *Journal of Applied Behavior Analysis, 17,* 279–293.

Peterson, L. (1988). Preventing the leading killer of children: The role of the school psychologist in injury prevention. *School Psychology Review, 17,* 593–600.

Petrakos, H., & Howe, N. (1996). The influence of the physical design of the dramatic play center on children's play. *Early Childhood Research Quarterly, 11,* 63–77.

Piazza, C. C., & Fisher, W. (1991). A faded bedtime with response cost protocol for treatment of multiple sleep problems in children. *Journal of Applied Behavior Analysis, 24,* 129–140.

Pinkston, E. M., Reese, N. M., LeBlanc, J. M., & Baer, D. M. (1973). Independent control of a preschool child's aggression and peer interaction by contingent teacher attention. *Journal of Applied Behavior Analysis, 6,* 115–124.

Plomin, R. (1987). Behavior genetics and intervention. In J. J. Gallagher & C. T. Ramey (Eds.), *The malleability of children* (pp. 15–24). Baltimore: Paul H. Brookes.

Plomin, R., DeFries, J. C., McClearn, G. E., & Rutter, R. (1997). *Behavioral genetics* (3rd ed.). New York: W. H. Freeman.

Poche, C., Brouwer, R., & Swearingen, M. (1981). Teaching self-protection to young children. *Journal of Applied Behavior Analysis, 14,* 169–176.

Poche, C., Yoder, P., & Miltenberger, R. (1988). Teaching self-protection to children using television techniques. *Journal of Applied Behavior Analysis, 21,* 253–261.

Poling, A., & Ryan, C. (1982). Differential reinforcement-of-other-behavior schedules: Therapeutic applications. *Behavior Modification, 6,* 3–21.

Poole, D. A., & Lindsay, D. S. (1995). Interviewing preschoolers: Effects of non-suggestive techniques, parental coaching, and leading questions on reports of nonexperienced events. *Journal of Experimental Child Psychology, 60,* 129–154.

Porterfield, J. K., Herbert-Jackson, E., & Risley, T. R. (1976). Contingent observation: An effective and acceptable procedure for reducing disruptive behavior of young children in a group setting. *Journal of Applied Behavior Analysis, 9,* 55–64.

Portwood, S. G., Repucci, N. D., & Mitchell, M. S. (1998). Balancing rights and responsibilities: Legal perspectives on child maltreatment. In J. R. Lutzker (Ed.), *Handbook of child abuse research and treatment* (pp. 31–52). New York: Plenum Press.

Positive behavioral support. (1999, Winter). *Research Connections in Special Education, 4,* 1–8.

Poth, R. L., & Barnett, D. W. (1983). Reduction of a behavioral tic with a preschooler using relaxation and self-control techniques across settings. *School Psychology Review, 12,* 472–476.

Powell, T. H., & Ogle, P. A. (1985). *Brothers and sisters—A special part of exceptional families.* Baltimore: Paul H. Brookes.

Power, T. J., & DuPaul, G. J. (1996). Attention-deficit hyperactivity disorder: The reemergence of subtypes. *School Psychology Review, 25,* 284–296.

Premack, D. (1959). Toward empirical behavior laws I. Positive reinforcement. *Psychological Review, 66,* 219–233.

Project Sunrise. (1989). *Preschool assessment of the classroom environment—Revised.* Morganton, NC: Family, Infant, and Preschool Program, Western Carolina Center.

Prutting, C. A. (1982). Pragmatics as social competence. *Journal of Speech and Hearing Disorders, 47,* 123–134.

Ramey, C. T., & Campbell, F. A. (1987). The Carolina Abedecarian project: An educational experiment. In J. J. Gallagher & C. T. Ramey (Eds.), *The malleability of children* (pp. 127–139). Baltimore: Paul H. Brookes.

Ramey, C. T., & Ramey, S. L. (1998). Early intervention and early experience. *American Psychologist, 53,* 109–120.

Redmon, W. K., & Farris, H. E. (1987). Application of basic research to the treatment of children with autistic and severely handicapped repertoires. *Education and Treatment of Children, 10,* 326–337.

Reichle, J., & Wacker, D. P. (Eds.). (1993). *Communication alternatives to challenging behavior* (Vol. 3). Baltimore: Paul H. Brookes.

Reid, J. B. (Ed.). (1978). *A social learning approach to family intervention. Vol. 2: Observation in home settings.* Eugene, OR: Castalia.

Reid, J. B. (1985). Behavioral approaches to intervention and assessment with child abusive families. In P. H. Bornstein & A. E. Kazdin (Eds.), *Handbook of clinical behavior therapy with children* (pp. 772–812). Homewood, IL: Dorsey.

Reimers, T. M. (1996). A biobehavioral approach toward managing encopresis. *Behavior Modification, 20,* 469–479.

Rekers, G. A. (1984). Ethical issues in child behavior assessment. In T. H. Ollendick & M. Hersen (Eds.), *Child behavior assessment: Principles and procedures* (pp. 244–262). New York: Pergamon Press.

Repp, A. C., Nieminen, G. S., Olinger, E., & Brusca, R. (1988). Direct observation: Factors affecting the accuracy of observers. *Exceptional Children, 55,* 29–36.

Repp, A. C., & Singh, N. N. (Eds.). (1990). *Perspectives on the use of nonaversive and aversive interventions for persons with developmental disabilities.* Sycamore, IL: Sycamore.

Rimmerman, A. (1989). Provision of respite care for children with developmental disabilities: Changes in maternal coping and stress over time. *Mental Retardation, 27,* 99–103.

Rimmerman, A., & Duvdevani, I. (1996). Parents of children and adolescents with severe mental retardation: Stress, family resources, normalization, and their application for out-of-home placement. *Research in Developmental Disabilities, 17,* 487–494.

Risley, T. (1972). Spontaneous language and the preschool environment. In J. C. Stanley (Ed.), *Preschool programs for the disadvantaged: Five experimental approaches to early childhood education* (pp. 92–110). Baltimore: Johns Hopkins University Press.

Roberts, M. C., & Layfield, D. A. (1987). Promoting child passenger safety: A comparison of two positive methods. *Journal of Pediatric Psychology, 12,* 257–271.

Roberts, M. W. (1982). The effects of warned versus unwarned time-out procedures on child noncompliance. *Child and Family Behavior Therapy, 4,* 37–53.

Roberts, M. W. (1985). Praising child compliance: Reinforcement or ritual? *Journal of Abnormal Child Psychology, 13,* 611–629.

Roberts, M. W. (1988). Enforcing chair timeouts with room timeouts. *Behavior Modification, 12*(3), 353–370.

Roberts, M. W., & Powers, S. W. (1988). The Compliance Test. *Behavior Assessment, 10,* 375–398.

Roberts, M. W., & Powers, S. W. (1990). Adjusting chair timeout enforcement procedures for oppositional children. *Behavior Therapy, 21,* 257–271.

Robinson, E. A., & Eyberg, S. M. (1981). The dyadic parent–child interaction coding system: Standardization and validation. *Journal of Consulting and Clinical Psychology, 49,* 245–250.

Rogers-Warren, A. K. (1982). Behavior ecology in classrooms for young, handicapped children. *Topics in Early Childhood Special Education, 2,* 21–32.

Rogers-Warren, A., & Baer, D. M. (1976). Correspondence between saying and doing: Teaching children to share and praise. *Journal of Applied Behavior Analysis, 9,* 335–354.

Rogers-Warren, A., & Warren, S. F. (1980). Mands for verbalization: Facilitating the display of newly trained language in children. *Behavior Modification, 4,* 361–382.

Rolider, A., & Van Houten, R. (1984). The effects of DRO alone and DRO plus reprimands on the undesirable behavior of three children in home settings. *Education and Treatment of Children, 7,* 17–31.

Rolider, A., & Van Houten, R. (1990). The role of reinforcement in reducing inappropriate behavior: Some myths and misconceptions. In A. C. Repp & N. N. Singh (Eds.), *Perspectives on the use of nonaversive and aversive interventions for persons with developmental disabilities* (pp. 119–127). Sycamore, IL: Sycamore.

Rose, D. F., & Smith, B. J. (1993). Preschool mainstreaming: Attitude barriers and strategies for addressing them. *Young Children, 48*(4), 59–62.

Rosen, C. E. (1974). The effects of sociodramatic play on problem-solving behavior among culturally disadvantaged preschool children. *Child Development, 45,* 920–927.

Rosenbaum, M. S., Creedon, D. L., & Drabman, R. S. (1981). Training preschool children to identify emergency situations and make emergency phone calls. *Behavior Therapy, 12,* 425–435.

Ross, A. O.(1980). *Psychosocial disorders of children* (2nd edition). New York: McGraw-Hill.

Rous, B., Hemmeter, M. L., & Schuster, J. (1994). Sequenced transition to education in the public schools: A systems approach to transition planning. *Topics in Early Childhood Special Education, 14,* 374–393.

Rowbury, T. G., Baer, A. M., & Baer, D. M. (1976). Interactions between teacher guidance and contingent access to play in developing preacademic skills of deviant preschool children. *Journal of Applied Behavior Analysis, 9*, 85–104.

Russell-Fox, J. (1997). Together is better: Specific tips on how to include children with various types of disabilities. *Young Children, 52*(4), 81–83.

Russo, D. C., & Koegel, R. L. (1977). A method for integrating an autistic child into a normal public-school classroom. *Journal of Applied Behavior Analysis, 10*, 579–590.

Rutter, M. (1981). Stress, coping, and development: Some issues and some questions. *Journal of Child Psychology and Psychiatry, 22*, 323–356.

Rutter, M. (1984). Continuities and discontinuities in socioemotional development: Empirical and conceptual perspectives. In R. M. Emde & J. R. Harmon (Eds.), *Continuities and discontinuities in development* (pp. 41–68). New York: Plenum Press.

Rutter, M. (1987). Psychosocial resilience and protective mechanisms. *American Journal of Orthopsychiatry, 57*, 316–331.

Sackett, G. P. (1978). Measurement in observational research. In G. P. Sackett (Ed.), *Observing behavior: Vol. 2. Data collection and analysis methods* (pp. 25–43). Baltimore: University Park Press.

Safford, P. I. (1989). *Integrated teaching in early childhood.* White Plains, NY: Longman.

Sainato, D. M., & Lyon, S. R. (1989). Promoting successful mainstreaming transitions for handicapped preschool children. *Journal of Early Intervention, 13*, 305–314.

Sainato, D. M., Maheady, L., & Shook, G. L. (1986). The effects of a classroom manager role on the social interaction patterns and social status of withdrawn kindergarten students. *Journal of Applied Behavior Analysis, 19*, 187–195.

Sainato, D. M., Strain, P. S., Lefebvre, D., & Rapp, N. (1987). Facilitating transition times with handicapped preschool children: A comparison between peer-mediated and antecedent prompt procedures. *Journal of Applied Behavior Analysis, 20*, 285–291.

Sainato, D. M., Strain, P. S., Lefebvre, D., & Rapp, N. (1990). Effects of self-evaluation on the independent work skills of preschool children with disabilities. *Exceptional Children, 56*, 540–549.

Sainato, D. M., Strain, P. S., & Lyon, S. R. (1987) Increasing academic responding of handicapped preschool children during group instruction. *Journal of the Division for Early Childhood, 12*, 23–30.

Salisbury, C. L., & Vincent, L. J. (1990). Criterion of the next environment and best practices: Mainstreaming and integration 10 years later. *Topics in Early Childhood Special Education, 10*, 78–89.

Saltz, E., Dixon, D., & Johnson, J. (1977). Training disadvantaged preschoolers on various fantasy activities: Effects on cognitive functioning and impulse control. *Child Development, 48*, 367–380.

Saltz, E., & Johnson, J. (1974). Training for thematic-fantasy play in culturally disadvantaged children: Preliminary results. *Journal of Educational Psychology, 66*, 623–630.

Sanders, M. R., & Christensen, A. P. (1985). A comparison of the effects of child management and planned activities training in five parenting environments. *Journal of Abnormal Child Psychology, 13*, 101–117.

Sanders, M. R., & Dadds, M. R. (1982). The effects of planned activities and child management procedures in parent training: An analysis of setting generality. *Behavior Therapy*, *13*, 452–461.

Sanders, M. R., & Dadds, M. R. (1993). *Behavioral family intervention*. Boston: Allyn & Bacon.

Sanders, M. R., & Glynn, T. (1981). Training parents in behavioral self-management: An analysis of generalization and maintenance. *Journal of Applied Behavior Analysis*, *14*, 223–237.

Sanders, M. R., & Plant, K. (1989). Programming for generalization to high and low risk parenting situations in families with oppositional developmentally disabled preschoolers. *Behavior Modification*, *13*, 283–305.

Sansbury, L. L., & Wahler, R. G. (1992). Pathways to maladaptive parenting with mothers and their conduct disordered children. *Behavior Modification*, *16*, 574–592.

Sapon-Shevin, M. (1982). Ethical issues in parent training programs. *Journal of Special Education*, *16*, 341–357.

Saracho, O. N., & Spodek, B. (Eds.). (1998). *Multiple perspectives on play in early childhood education*. Albany, NY: State University of New York Press.

Saudargas, R. A. (1980). *The State–Event Classroom Observation System*. Knoxville: University of Tennessee.

Saudargas, R. A., & Lentz, F. E., Jr. (1986). Estimating percept of time and rate via direct observation: A suggested observation procedure. *School Psychology Review*, *15*, 36–48.

Schill, M. T., Kratochwill, T. R., & Gardner, W. I. (1996). An assessment protocol for selective mutism: Analogue assessment using parents as facilitators. *Journal of School Psychology*, *34*, 1–21.

Schön, D. A. (1983). *The reflective practitioner: How professionals think in action*. New York: Basic Books.

Schrader, C., & Gaylord-Ross, R. (1990). The eclipse of aversive technology: A triadic approach to assessment and treatment. In A. C. Repp & N. N. Singh (Eds.), *Perspectives on the use of nonaversive and aversive interventions for persons with developmental disabilities* (pp. 403–417). Sycamore, IL: Sycamore.

Schreibman, L., O'Neill, R. E., & Koegel, R. L. (1983). Behavioral training for siblings of autistic children. *Journal of Applied Behavior Analysis*, *16*, 129–138.

Schuster, J. W., & Griffin, A. K. (1990). Using time delay with task analyses. *Teaching Exceptional Children*, *22*, 49–53.

Schwartz, I. S., & Baer, D. M. (1991). Social validity assessment: Is current practice state of the art? *Journal of Applied Behavior Analysis*, *24*, 189–204.

Schwartz, I. S., Carta, J. J., & Grant, S. (1996). Examining the use of recommended language intervention practices in early childhood special education classrooms. *Topics in Early Childhood Special Education*, *16*, 251–272.

Sechrest, L., West, S. G., Phillips, M. A., Redner, R., & Yeaton, W. (1979). Some neglected problems in evaluation research: Strength and integrity of treatments. In L. Sechrest, S. G. West, M. A. Phillips, R. Redner, & R. Yeaton (Eds.), *Evaluation studies annual review* (pp. 15–35). Beverly Hills, CA: Sage.

Seligman, M., & Darling, R. E. (1997). *Ordinary families, special children: A systems approach to childhood disability* (2nd ed.). New York: Guilford Press.

Seymour, F. W. (1987). Parent management of sleep difficulties in young children. *Behaviour Change, 4*, 39–48.

Shapiro, E. S. (1979). Restitution and positive practice overcorrection in reducing aggressive–disruptive behavior: A long-term follow-up. *Journal of Behavior Therapy and Experimental Psychiatry, 10*, 131–134.

Shearer, D. D., Kohler, F. W., Buchan, K. A., & McCollough, K. M. (1996). Promoting independent interactions between preschoolers with autism and their nondisabled peers: An analysis of self-monitoring. *Early Education and Development, 7*(3), 205–220.

Shearer, D. E., & Shearer, M. S. (1976). The Portage Project: A model for early intervention. In T. D. Tjossen (Ed.), *Intervention strategies for high risk infants and young children* (pp. 335–350). Baltimore: University Park Press.

Shearer, M. S., & Shearer, D. E. (1972). The Portage Project: A model for early childhood education. *Exceptional Children, 38*, 210–217.

Sherburne, S., Utley, B., McConnell, S., & Gannon, J. (1988). Decreasing violent or aggressive theme play among preschool children with behavior disorders. *Exceptional Children, 55*, 166–172.

Shriver, M., & Allen, K. D. (1997). Defining child noncompliance: An examination of temporal parameters. *Journal of Applied Behavioral Analysis, 30*, 173–176.

Sigel, I. E., McGillicuddy-DeLisi, A. V., & Goodnow, J. J. (Eds.). (1992). *Parental belief systems: The psychological consequences for children* (2nd ed.). Hillsdale, NJ: Erlbaum.

Skinner, B. F. (1953). *Science and human behavior.* New York: Free Press.

Skinner, B. F. (1957). *Verbal behavior.* Englewood Cliffs, NJ: Prentice-Hall.

Smilansky, S. (1968). *The effects of sociodramatic play on disadvantaged children: Preschool children.* New York: Wiley.

Snell, M. E., Lowman, D. K., & Canady, R. L. (1996). Parallel block scheduling: Accommodating students' diverse needs in elementary schools. *Journal of Early Intervention, 20*(3), 266–278.

Snow, C. E. (1977). Mother's speech research: From input to interaction. In C. E. Snow & C. A. Furgeson (Eds.), *Talking to children: Language input and acquisition.* New York: Cambridge University Press.

Snow, C. E., Burns, M. S., & Griffin, P. (Eds.). (1998). *Preventing reading difficulties in young children.* Washington, DC: National Academy Press.

Solomons, H. C., & Elardo, R. (1989). Bite injuries at a day care center. *Early Childhood Research Quarterly, 4*, 89–96.

Sowers-Hoag, K. M., Thyer, B. A., & Bailey, J. S. (1987). Promoting automobile safety belt use by young children. *Journal of Applied Behavior Analysis, 20*, 133–138.

Spiegler, M. D. (1983). *Contemporary behavioral therapy.* Palo Alto, CA: Mayfield.

Spradley, J. P. (1980). *Participant observation.* New York: Holt, Rinehart & Winston.

Sroufe, L. A. (1979). The coherence of individual development: Early care, attachment, and subsequent developmental issues. *American Psychologist, 34*, 834–841.

Sroufe, L. A., & Rutter, M. (1984). The domain of developmental psychopathology. *Child Development, 55*, 17–29.

Stafford, S. H., & Green, V. P. (1996). Preschool integration: Strategies for teaching. *Childhood Education, 72*(4), 214–218.

Stokes, T. F., & Baer, D. M. (1977). An implicit technology of generalization. *Journal of Applied Behavior Analysis, 19,* 349–367.

Stokes, T. F., Fowler, S. A., & Baer, D. M. (1978). Training preschool children to recruit natural communities of reinforcement. *Journal of Applied Behavior Analysis, 11,* 285–303.

Stokes, T. F., & Osnes, P. G. (1986). Programming the generalization of children's social behavior. In P. S. Strain, M. J. Guralnick, & H. M. Walker (Eds.), *Children's social behavior: Development, assessment, and modification* (pp. 407–443). Orlando, FL: Academic Press.

Stokes, T. F., & Osnes, P. G. (1988). The developing applied technology of generalization and maintenance. In R. H. Horner, G. Dunlap, & R. L. Koegel (Eds.), *Generalization and maintenance: Life-style changes in applied settings* (pp. 5–19). Baltimore, MD: Paul H. Brookes.

Stokes, T. F., & Osnes, P. G. (1989). An operant pursuit of generalization. *Behavior Therapy, 20,* 337–355.

Stollar, S. A., Dye Collins, P. A., & Barnett, D. W. (1994). Structured free-play to reduce disruptive activity changes in a Head Start classroom. *School Psychology Review, 23,* 310–322.

Stolz, S. B., & Associates (1978). *Ethical principles in behavior modification.* San Francisco: Jossey-Bass.

Strain, P. S. (1985). Social and nonsocial determinants of acceptability in handicapped preschool children. *Topics in Early Childhood Special Education, 4,* 47–58.

Strain, P. S. (April 1988). *Early intervention.* Workshop presented at the National Association of School Psychologists, Washington, DC.

Strain, P. S., Hoyson, M., & Jamieson, B. (Spring, 1985). Normally developing preschoolers as intervention agents for autistic-like children: Effects on class deportment and social interaction. *Journal of the Division for Early Childhood,* 105–115.

Strain, P. S., & Kohler, F. W. (1995). Analyzing predictors of daily social skill performance. *Behavioral Disorders, 21*(1), 79–88.

Strain, P. S., Lambert, D. L., Kerr, M. M., Stagg, V., & Lenkner, D. A. (1983). Naturalistic assessment of children's compliance to teachers' requests and consequences for compliance. *Journal of Applied Behavior Analysis, 16,* 243–249.

Strain, P. S., & Odom, S. L. (1986). Peer social initiations: Effective intervention for social skills development of exceptional children. *Exceptional Children, 52,* 543–551.

Strayhorn, J. M., & Strain, P. S. (1986). Social and language skills for preventative mental health: What, how, who, and when. In P. S. Strain, M. J. Guralnick, & H. M. Walker (Eds.), *Children's social behavior: Development, assessment, and modification* (pp. 287– 330). Orlando, FL: Academic Press.

Striefel, S. (1981). *How to teach through modeling and imitation.* Austin, TX: Pro-Ed.

Striefel, S. (1998). *How to teach through modeling and imitation* (2nd ed.). Austin, TX: Pro-Ed.

Strosahl, K. D., & Linehan, M. M. (1986). Basic issues in behavioral assessment. In A. R. Ciminero, K. S. Calhoun, & H. E. Adams (Eds.), *Handbook of behavioral assessment* (2nd ed., pp. 12–46). New York: Wiley.

Suen, H. K., & Ary, D. (1989). *Analyzing quantitative behavioral observation data.* Hillsdale, NJ: Erlbaum.

Sulzer-Azaroff, B., & Mayer, G. R. (1991). *Behavior analysis for lasting change.* Fort Worth: Holt, Rinehart & Winston.

Tarpley, B. S., & Saudargas, R. A. (1981). An intervention for a withdrawn child based on teacher recorded levels of social interaction. *School Psychology Review, 10,* 409–412.

Taverne, A., & Sheridan, A. M. (1995). Parent training in interactive book reading: An investigation of its effects with families at risk. *School Psychology Quarterly, 10,* 41–64.

Taylor, E. (1988). Attention deficit and conduct disorder syndromes. In M. Rutter, A. H. Tuma, & I. S. Lann (Eds.), *Assessment and diagnosis in child psychopathology* (pp. 377–407). New York: Guilford Press.

Tertinger, D. A., Greene, B. F., & Lutzker, J. R. (1984). Home safety: Development and validation of one component of an ecobehavioral treatment program for abused and neglected children. *Journal of Applied Behavior Analysis, 17,* 159–174.

Test, D. W., Spooner, F., & Cooke, N. L. (1987). Educational validity revisited. *Journal of the Association for Persons with Severe Handicaps, 12,* 96–102.

Thibadeaux, S. F. (1998). *How to use response cost.* Austin, TX: Pro-Ed.

Thibodeaux, S., Gardner, K., Forgatch, M., & Reid, J. (1984). *Observer training.* Eugene, OR: Oregon Social Learning Center.

Thompson, R. H., Fisher, W. W., Piazza, C. C., & Kuhn, D. E. (1998). The evaluation and treatment of aggression maintained by attention and automatic reinforcement. *Journal of Applied Behavior Analysis, 31,* 103–116.

Thomson, C., Holmberg, M. & Baer, D. M. (1974). A brief report on a comparison of time-sampling procedures. *Journal of Applied Behavior Analysis, 7,* 623–626.

Thurman, S. K., & Widerstrom, A. H. (1990). *Infants and young children with special needs: A developmental and ecological approach* (2nd ed.). Baltimore: Paul H. Brookes.

Timberlake, W., & Allison, J. (1974). Response deprivation: An empirical approach to instrumental performance. *Psychological Review, 81,* 146–164.

Tirapelle, L., & Cipani, E. (1992). Developing functional requesting: Acquisition, durability, and generalization of effects. *Exceptional Children, 58,* 260–269.

Tremblay, A., Strain, P. S., Hendrickson, J. M., & Shores, R. E. (1981). Social interactions of normal preschool children: Using normative data for subject and target behavior selection. *Behavior Modification, 5,* 237–253.

Trivette, C. M., Dunst, C. J., & Hamby, D. W. (1996). Factors associated with perceived control appraisals in a family-centered early intervention program. *Journal of Early Intervention, 20,* 165–178.

Tryon, W. W. (1983). Further implications of Herrnstein's Law of Effect. *American Psychologist, 38,* 613–614.

Turnbull, A. P., & Turnbull, H. R., III (1986). *Families, professionals, and exceptionality: A special partnership*. Columbus, OH: Merrill.

Tversky, A., & Kahneman, D. (1984). The framing of decisions and the psychology of choice. In G. Wright (Ed.), *Behavioral decision making* (pp. 25–41). New York: Plenum Press.

Tyroler, M. J., & Lahey, B. B. (1980). Effects of contingent observation on the disruptive behavior of a toddler in a group setting. *Child Care Quarterly, 9*, 265–274.

Umbreit, J. (1995). Functional analysis of disruptive behavior in an inclusive classroom. *Journal of Early Intervention, 20*, 18–29.

United Nations Convention on the Rights of the Child. (1991). *American Psychologist, 46*, 50–52.

Van Houten, R. (1980). *How to use reprimands*. Austin, TX: Pro-Ed.

Van Houten, R. (1984). Setting up performance feedback systems in the classroom. In W. L. Heward, T. E. Heron, D. S. Hill, & J. Trapp-Porter (Eds.), *Focus on behavior analysis in education* (pp. 114–125). Columbus, OH: Merrill.

Van Houten, R., Axelrod, S., Bailey, J. S., Favell, J. E., Foxx, R. M., Iwata, B. A., & Lovaas, O. I. (1988). The right to effective behavioral treatment. *Journal of Applied Behavior Analysis, 21*, 381–384.

Vedder-Dubocq, S. A. (1990). *An investigation of the utility of the Parenting Stress Index for intervention decisions*. Unpublished doctoral dissertation, University of Cincinnati.

Vincent, L. J., Salisbury, C., Walter, G., Brown, P., Gruenewald, L. J., & Powers, M. (1980). Program evaluation and curriculum development in early childhood/special education. Criteria of the next environment. In W. Sailor, B. Wilcox, & L. Brown (Eds.), *Methods of instruction for severely handicapped students* (pp. 303–328). Baltimore: Paul H. Brookes.

Voeltz, L. M., & Evans, I. M. (1982). The assessment of behavioral interrelationships in child behavior therapy. *Behavioral Assessment, 4*, 131–165.

Volkmar, F. R. (1993). Autism and the pervasive developmental disorders. In C. H. Zeanah, Jr., (Ed.), *Handbook of infant mental health* (pp. 236–249). New York: Guilford Press.

Vollmer, T. R. (1994). The concept of automatic reinforcement: Implications for behavioral research in developmental disabilities. *Research in Developmental Disabilities, 15*, 187–207.

Vollmer, T. R., & Iwata, B. A. (1991). Establishing operations and reinforcement effects. *Journal of Applied Behavior Analysis, 24*, 279–291.

Vollmer, T. R., Ringdahl, J. E., Roane, H. S., & Marcus, B. A. (1997). Negative side effects of noncontingent reinforcement. *Journal of Applied Behavior Analysis, 30*, 161–164.

Wahler, R. G. (1975). Some structural aspects of deviant child behavior. *Journal of Applied Behavior Analysis, 8*, 27–42.

Wahler, R. G. (1980). The insular mother: Her problems in parent–child treatment. *Journal of Applied Behavior Analysis, 13*, 207–219.

Wahler, R. G., & Afton, A. D. (1980). Attentional processes in insular and noninsular mothers: Some differences in their summary reports about child problem behaviors. *Child Behavior Therapy, 2*, 25–41.

Wahler, R. G., & Cormier, W. H. (1970). The ecological interview: A first step in outpatient child behavior therapy. *Journal of Behavior Therapy and Experimental Psychiatry, 1,* 279–289.

Wahler, R. G., & Dumas, J. E. (1986). "A chip off the old block": Some interpersonal characteristics of coercive children across generations. In P. S. Strain, M. J. Guralnick, & H. M. Walker (Eds.), *Children's social behavior: Development, assessment, and modification* (pp. 49–91). New York: Academic Press.

Wahler, R. G., & Fox, J. J. (1980). Solitary toy play and time out: A family treatment package for children with aggressive and oppositional behavior. *Journal of Applied Behavior Analysis, 13,* 23–39.

Wahler, R. G., & Fox, J. J. (1981). Setting events in applied behavior analysis: Toward a conceptual and methodological expansion. *Journal of Applied Behavior Analysis, 14,* 327–338.

Wahler, R. G., & Hann, D. M. (1984). The communication patterns of troubled mothers: In search of a keystone in the generalization of parenting skills. *Education and Treatment of Children, 7,* 335–350.

Wahler, R. G., House, A. E., & Stambaugh, E. E. (1976). *Ecological assessment of child problem behavior.* New York: Pergamon Press.

Wahler, R. G., & Meginnis, K. L. (1997). Strengthening child compliance through positive parenting practices: What works? *Journal of Clinical Child Psychology, 26,* 433–440.

Wahler, R. G., Winkel, G. H., Peterson, R. F., & Morrison, D. C. (1965). Mothers as behavior therapists for their own children. *Behaviour Research and Therapy, 3,* 113–124.

Walker, C. E., Kenning, M., & Faust-Campanile, J. (1989). Enuresis and encopresis. In E. J. Mash & R. A. Barkley (Eds.), *Treatment of childhood disorders* (pp. 423–448). New York: Guilford Press.

Walker, H. M. (February, 1983). Applications of response cost in school settings: Outcomes, issues and recommendations. *Exceptional Education Quarterly,* 47–55.

Walker, H. M., & Hops, H. (1976). Use of normative peer data as a standard for evaluating classroom treatment effects. *Journal of Applied Behavior Analysis, 9,* 159–168.

Walker, H. M., & Rankin, R. (1983). Assessing the behavioral expectations and demands of less restrictive settings. *School Psychology Review, 12,* 274–284.

Walker, H. M., Reavis, H. K., Rhode, G., & Jenson, W. R. (1985). A conceptual model for the delivery of behavioral services to behavior disordered children in educational settings. In P. H. Bornstein & A. E. Kazdin (Eds.), *Handbook of clinical behavior therapy with children* (pp. 700–741). Homewood, IL: Dorsey.

Walle, D. L., Hobbs, S. A., & Caldwell, H. S. (1984). Sequencing of parent training procedures: Effects on child noncompliance and treatment acceptability. *Behavior Modification, 8,* 540–552.

Warren, S. F. (1992). Facilitating basic vocabulary acquisition with milieu teaching procedures. *Journal of Early Intervention, 16,* 235–251.

Warren, S. F., & Gazdag, G. (1990). Facilitating early language development with milieu intervention procedures. *Journal of Early Intervention, 14,* 62–86.

Warren, S. F., & Kaiser, A. P. (1986). Incidental language teaching: A critical review. *Journal of Speech and Hearing Disorders, 51,* 291–299.

Wasik, B. H. (1998). Implications for child abuse and neglect interventions from early educational interventions. In J. R. Lutzker (Ed.), *Handbook of child abuse research and treatment* (pp. 519–541). New York: Plenum Press.

Watson, D. L., & Tharp, R. G. (1996). *Self-directed behavior: Self-modification for personal adjustment* (7th ed.). Pacific Grove, CA: Brooks/Cole.

Webster-Stratton, C. (1981a). Modification of a mother's behaviors and attitudes through a videotape modeling group discussion program. *Behavior Therapy, 12,* 634–642.

Webster-Stratton, C. (1981b, Summer). Videotape modeling: A method of parent education. *Journal of Clinical Child Psychology,* 93–97.

Webster-Stratton, C. (1982). The long-term effects of a videotape modeling parent-training program: Comparison of immediate and 1-year follow-up results. *Behavior Therapy, 13,* 702–714.

Webster-Stratton, C. (1998a). Parent training with low-income families: Promoting parental engagement through a collaborative approach. In J. R. Lutzker (Ed.), *Handbook of child abuse research and treatment* (pp. 183–210). New York: Plenum Press.

Webster-Stratton, C. (1998b). Preventing conduct problems in Head Start children: Strengthening parenting competencies. *Journal of Consulting and Clinical Psychology, 66*(5), 715–730.

Webster-Stratton, C., & Hammond, M. (1988). Maternal depression and its relationship to life stress, perceptions of child behavior problems, parenting behaviors, and child conduct problems. *Journal of Abnormal Child Psychology, 16,* 299–315.

Webster-Stratton, C., & Herbert, M. (1993). "What really happens in parent training?" *Behavior Modification, 17,* 407–456.

Webster-Stratton, C., Hollingsworth, T., & Kolpacoff, M. (1989). The long-term effectiveness and clinical significance of three cost-effective programs for families with conduct-problem children. *Journal of Consulting and Clinical Psychology, 57,* 550–553.

Weintraub, S., Winters, K. C., & Neale, J. M. (1986). Competence and vulnerability in children with an affectively disordered parent. In M. Rutter, C. E. Izard, & P. B. Read (Eds.), *Depression in young children: Developmental and clinical perspectives* (pp. 205–220). New York: Guilford Press.

Weiss, R. S. (1981). INREAL intervention for language handicapped and bilingual children. *Journal of the Division for Early Childhood, 4,* 40–52.

Weitzman, J. (1985). Engaging the severely dysfunctional family in treatment: Basic considerations. *Family Process, 24,* 473–485.

Weninger, J. J., & Baer, R. A. (1990). Correspondence training with time delay: A comparison of reinforcement compliance. *Education and Treatment of Children, 13,* 36–44.

Werner, E. E. (1986). A longitudinal study of perinatal risk. In D. C. Farran & J. D. McKinney (Eds.), *Risk in intellectual and psychosocial development* (pp. 3–27). Orlando, FL: Academic Press.

Whalen, C. K. (1989). Attention deficit and hyperactivity disorders. In T. H. Ollendick & M. Hersen (Eds.), *Handbook of child psychopathology* (2nd ed., pp. 131–169). New York: Plenum Press.

White, K. R. (1985–1986). Efficacy of early intervention. *Journal of Special Education, 19*, 401–416.

White, O. R., & Haring, N. G. (1980). *Exceptional teaching* (2nd ed.). Columbus, OH: Merrill.

Wilkins, R. (1985). A comparison of elective mutism and emotional disorders in children. *British Journal of Psychiatry, 146*, 198–203.

Willems, E. P. (1977). Steps toward an ecobehavioral technology. In A. Rogers-Warren & S. F. Warren (Eds.), *Ecological perspectives in behavior analysis* (pp. 39–61). Baltimore: University Park Press.

Williamson, D. A., Sanders, S. H., Sewell, W. R., Haney, J. N., & White, D. (1977). The behavioral treatment of elective mutism: Two case studies. *Journal of Behavior Therapy and Experimental Psychiatry, 8*, 143–149.

Wilson, F. E., & Evans, I. M. (1983). The reliability of target-behavior selection in behavioral assessment. *Behavioral Assessment, 5*, 15–32.

Witt, J. C., & Elliott, S. N.(1982). The response cost lottery: A time efficient and effective classroom intervention. *Journal of School Psychology, 20*, 155–161.

Witt, J. C., & Elliott, S. N. (1985). Acceptability of classroom management strategies. In T. R. Kratochwill (Ed.), *Advances in school psychology* (Vol. 4, pp. 251–288). Hillsdale, NJ: Erlbaum.

Witt, J. C., & Martens, B. K. (1988). Problems with problem-solving consultation: A re-analysis of assumptions, methods, and goals. *School Psychology Review, 17*, 211–226.

Wolery, M. (1989). Using direct observation in assessment. In D. B. Bailey, Jr. & M. Wolery (Eds.), *Assessing infants and preschoolers with handicaps* (pp. 64–96). Columbus, OH: Merrill.

Wolery, M. (1994). Implementing instruction for young children with special needs in early childhood classrooms. In M. Wolery & J. S. Wilbers (Eds.), *Including children with special needs in early childhood programs* (pp. 151–166). Washington, DC: National Association for the Education of Young Children.

Wolery, M., Ault, M. J., & Doyle, P. M. (1992). Naturalistic teaching procedures. *Teaching students with moderate to severe disabilities: Use of response prompting strategies* (pp. 169–200). New York: Longman.

Wolery, M., Bailey, D. B., & Sugai, G. M. (1988). *Effective teaching: Principles and procedures of applied behavior analysis with exceptional students.* Boston: Allyn & Bacon.

Wolery, M., & Bredekamp, S. (1994). Developmentally appropriate practices and young children with disabilities: Contextual issues in the discussion. *Journal of Early Intervention, 18*, 331–341.

Wolery, M., & Gast, D. L. (1990). Re-framing the debate: Finding middle ground and defining the role of social validity. In A. C. Repp & N. N. Singh (Eds.), *Perspectives on the use of nonaversive and aversive interventions for persons with developmental disabilities* (pp. 129–143). Sycamore, IL: Sycamore.

Wolery, M., Holcombe, A., Venn, M., Brookfield, J., Huffman, K., Schroeder, C., Martin, C. G., & Fleming, L. A. (1993). Mainstreaming in early childhood programs: Current status and relevant issues. *Young Children, 49*(1), 78–84.

Wolery, M., Strain, P. S., & Bailey, D. B. (1992). Reaching potentials of children with special needs. In S. Bredekamp & T. Rosegrant (Eds.), *Reaching potentials: Appropriate curriculums and assessment for young children* (Vol. 1, pp. 92–111).

Washington, DC: National Association for the Education of Young Children.

Wolery, M., Werts, M. G., Caldwell, N. K., Snyder, E. D., & Lisowski, L. (1995). Experienced teachers' perceptions of resources and supports for inclusion. *Education and Training in Mental Retardation and Developmental Disabilities*, 30(1), 15–26.

Wolery, M., & Wilburs, J. (Eds.). (1994). *Including children with special needs in early childhood programs* (pp. 151–166). Washington, DC: National Association for the Education of Young Children.

Wolf, M. M. (1978). Social validity: The case for subjective measurement or how applied behavior analysis is finding its heart. *Journal of Applied Behavior Analysis, 11*, 203–214.

Wolfe, D. A. (1987). *Child abuse: Implications for child development and psychopathology.* Newbury Park, CA: Sage.

Wolfe, D. A. (1991). *Preventing physical and emotional abuse of children.* New York: Guilford Press.

Wolfe, D. A. (1994). The role of intervention and treatment services in the prevention of child abuse and neglect. In G. B. Melton & F. D. Barry (Eds.), *Protecting children from abuse and neglect: Foundations for a new national strategy* (pp. 224–303). New York: Guilford Press.

Wolfe, D. A., & McEachran, A. (1997). Child physical abuse and neglect. In E. J. Mash & L. G. Terdal (Eds.), *Assessment of childhood disorders* (3rd ed., pp. 523–568). New York: Guilford Press.

Wolfe, V. V., & Birt, J. (1997). Child sexual abuse. In E. J. Mash & L. G. Terdal (Eds.), *Assessment of childhood disorders* (3rd ed., pp. 569–623). New York: Guilford Press.

Wolfensberger, W. (1972). *The principle of normalization in human services.* Toronto: National Institute on Mental Retardation.

Wolfensberger, W. (1983). Social role valorization: A proposed new term for the principle of normalization. *Mental Retardation, 21*, 234–239.

Wolff, R. (1984). Satiation in the treatment of inappropriate firesetting. *Journal of Behavior Therapy and Experimental Psychiatry, 15*, 337–340.

Wright, H. F. (1967). *Recording and analyzing child behavior.* New York: Harper & Row.

Wurtele, S. K., & Drabman, R. S. (1984). "Beat the Buzzer" for classroom dawdling: A one-year trial. *Behavior Therapy, 15*, 403–409.

Yarrow, L. J. (1960). Interviewing children. In P. H. Mussen (Ed.), *Handbook of research methods in child development* (pp. 561–602). New York: Wiley.

Yates, B. T. (1985). Cost-effectiveness analysis and cost–benefit analysis: An introduction. *Behavioral Assessment, 7*, 207–234.

Yeaton, W. H., & Bailey, J. S. (1978). Teaching pedestrian safety skills to young children: An analysis and one-year follow up. *Journal of Applied Behavior Analysis, 11*, 315–329.

Yeaton, W. H., & Sechrest, L. (1981). Critical dimensions in the choice and maintenance of successful treatments: Strength, integrity, and effectiveness. *Journal of Consulting and Clinical Psychology, 49*, 156–167.

Zangwill, W. M. (1984). An evaluation of a parent training program. *Child and Family Behavior Therapy, 5*, 1–16.

Zigler, E., & Valentine, J. (Eds.). (1979). *Project Head Start: A legacy of the war on poverty.* New York: Free Press.

Author Index

◆

Abraham, M. R., 265
Adams, H. E., 185, 241
Afton, A. D., 230
Air, A., 93, 101, 113
Albin, R. W., 49, 83
Aldridge, K., 228
Alessi, G. J., 23, 24, 25, 59, 60
Alig-Cybriwsky, C. A., 267
Allen, K. D., 236
Allen, K. E., 36, 46, 49, 299, 301, 306
Allen, S. J., 107, 265
Allison, J., 165
Almeida, C., 161, 281, 284, 285
Alpert, C. L., 158
Altepeter, T. S., 255
Anastopoulos, A., 245
Anderson, S. R., 158
Anderson-Inman, L., 80
Armstrong, P. M., 224
Arndorfer, R. E., 39
Arnold, C. M., 241
Ary, D., 43, 46, 52, 56
Ascione, F. R., 296
Atkeson, B. M., 213
Attermeier, S. M., 264
Atwater, J. B., 61, 261, 263, 264, 287
Ault, M. H., 36, 49
Ault, M. J., 148, 172
Axelrod, S., 126, 128, 129, 130, 131,
    183, 184, 197
Ayllon, T., 165, 166, 205
Azrin, N. H., 165, 166, 190, 205, 222,
    224, 226

B

Baer, A. M., 271, 272
Baer, D. M., 4, 52, 57, 59, 69, 78, 85, 89,
    96, 97, 98, 106, 117, 118, 121, 160,
    242, 271, 272, 273, 274, 286, 297,
    301
Baer, R. A., 194, 195
Bagnato, S. J., 16
Bailey, D. B., Jr., 57, 75, 98, 99, 100,
    134, 135, 138, 142, 145, 149, 151,
    171, 172, 186, 191, 261, 262, 281,
    282, 283, 286, 305, 306
Bailey, J. S., 126, 128, 129, 131, 218,
    305, 306, 308
Bakeman, R., 62
Bandura, A., 3, 63, 151, 152
Bank, L., 78, 82, 231, 232, 251
Barkley, R. A., 40, 73, 105, 235, 236,
    239, 241, 242, 244, 245, 247
Barlow, D. H., 4, 5, 30, 86, 114, 125
Barnard, J. D., 215, 216
Barnett, D. W., 1, 2, 11, 26, 29, 45, 60,
    67, 73, 74, 78, 80, 90, 93, 101, 107,
    113, 116, 132, 134, 137, 161, 193,
    247, 269, 270, 304
Barnett, W. S., 9
Barnhouse, L., 101, 113
Barone, V. J., 245
Barrios, B., 67
Barton, E. J., 296, 297
Barton, L. E., 180
Bauer, A. M., 26, 45, 78, 101, 113

357

Subject Index

◆